PHYSIOLOGY OF EXERCISE

PHYSIOLOGY OF EXERCISE
RESPONSES AND ADAPTATIONS

David R. Lamb

Purdue University
West Lafayette, Indiana

Macmillan Publishing Co., Inc.
New York

Collier Macmillan Publishers
London

Macmillan Publishing Co., Inc.
866 Third Avenue, New York, New York 10022

Collier Macmillan Canada, Ltd.

Library of Congress Cataloging in Publication Data

Lamb, David R
  Physiology of exercise.

  Includes bibliographies and index.
    1. Exercise—Physiological aspects. I. Title.
QP301.L27   1978   612'.044   77-5791
ISBN 0-02-367200-5

Printing: 2 3 4 5 6 7 8   Year: 8 9 0 1 2 3 4

To Cozette,
Michelle,
and Jason

Preface

This book is designed to serve as a text for a beginning exercise physiology course. Although intended primarily as an undergraduate text, it has also proved beneficial to many graduate students. No previous chemistry background is assumed as a prerequisite to the use of this book.

As the title suggests, the main goal of the book is to describe and explain the functional responses and adaptations that accompany single and repeated bouts of physical exercise. Many examples from physical education, athletics, and medicine are included to illustrate the practical application of the concepts discussed. The mechanisms underlying the physiological responses and adaptations to exercise are emphasized throughout the text.

To enhance the readability of the text for the typical undergraduate student, documentation includes many review articles that will help the student use his library time more efficiently and yet provide citations of original literature for those who have the time and inclination to seek out that literature.

Professors Robert Kertzer, Robert L. Kurucz, and Edward N. Norris provided comprehensive and helpful reviews of the manuscript, and I gratefully acknowledge their excellent contributions. I will also be grateful to those who will be good enough to inform me of the errors of fact and interpretation that I may have made.

D. R. L.

Contents

ix

11 Muscular fatigue and soreness 177

12 The physiology of aerobic endurance 197

19 Aids and impediments to physical performance: fact and fiction

Appendixes

PHYSIOLOGY OF EXERCISE

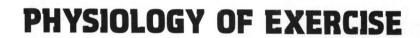

1

The nature of exercise physiology, physical fitness, and athletic conditioning

At the Boston Marathon on April 16th, 1973, the temperature at race time was 79°F, a pleasant temperature for the thousands of onlookers who sat or stood in a shaded spot, cold drink in hand. For most of the runners, however, this 79-degree temperature imposed an enormous burden because at this early date they had not yet become acclimatized to running in a hot environment. Of the 1400 qualifiers supposedly able to complete a marathon in 3½ hours or less, only 600 actually bested that time. Nearly a dozen competitors were hospitalized, and one who collapsed later died from the oppressive heat.

A few years ago at a major Midwestern university a football player died after collapsing during a preseason football practice in 90-degree weather. It was later determined that this young athlete had voluntarily restricted his fluid intake for some days prior to that fateful workout in hopes of losing excess weight and "toughening" himself for the football season. He had not informed either his family doctor or the coaching staff about his self–imposed fluid restriction.

1

These two examples of how the human body was not able to withstand the combined stresses of exercise and heat illustrate the need for an adequate understanding of how the organism reacts, in response to the demands of exercise, so that persons can understand the limits of their bodies and so that they can better prepare their bodies for the rigors of future exercise periods. The remaining chapters in this book are aimed at explaining how the human body responds to a single period of exercise, how its response to exercise changes after several weeks of physical training, and how this knowledge of exercise physiology can be applied for the betterment of physical fitness or for the improvement of athletic conditioning. First, though, let us establish some common ground by developing an understanding of what is meant by three terms that have already been mentioned: *exercise physiology*, *physical fitness*, and *athletic conditioning*.

EXERCISE PHYSIOLOGY

Imagine that you are watching a three-year-old child, Timothy the Terrible, as he plays with a Jack-in-the-Box for the first time. As he sees the colorful box with the top closed, Timothy's first inclination is to see what the thing is good for. After tossing it across the room, banging it on the dining room table, and being scolded for almost launching it into the toilet, Timothy spies a funny little button on the box, presses the button, and squeals with glee as the "Jack" pops out. After repeating his observations about *what* the box does. Timothy begins to wonder, in a childlike way, *how* the box works. How does pushing a button make the little man jump out? Timothy then pries open the box and carefully examines the coil spring and simple catch mechanism. Later, as he carefully observes how his long–suffering father repairs the toy, Timothy comes to understand more thoroughly how it works.

After a few months of repeated openings and closings of the Jack-in-the-box, Timothy notices that the pop-up response of the "Jack" is getting weaker and weaker as the coil spring becomes limp. Thus, Timothy has observed a change in response after repeated trials.

Finally, several years later, Timothy decides to use his knowledge of *what* the box does, *how* it does it, and how it responds to repeated trials to build a "super Jack-in-the-box" for his baby brother. He puts a longer, stronger, more durable spring in the box so that the toy will have an *improved response* to each trail.

This tale of Timothy the Terrible and his toy shows the essential simplicity of this science of exercise physiology. Exercise physiology is the study of *what* happens to the body as it exercises a *single time*, *how* these changes in function are brought about, *what* changes in function occur after *repeated* bouts of exercise and *how* those changes come to pass, and, finally, what can be done to *improve* the body's response to exercise and its adaptation to repeated bouts of exercise. The exercise physiologist's observation, his curiosity and his desire to improve upon what he observes are similar to those described in the story of Timothy. So let there be no mystery about exercise physiology; the only complicated feature of this or any science is the necessity to become familiar with many new terms, and in this book that process will be simplified as much as possible.

A more concise definition of exercise physiology is as follows: *Exercise physiology is the description and explanation of functional changes brought on by single (acute) or repeated bouts of exercise (chronic exercise or training), often with the objective of improving the exercise response.* In this definition the *description of functional changes* refers to *what happens to the body,* and the *explanation* refers to understanding *how the changes occur.* For example, we now know that repeated lifting of heavy weights usually results in greater ability to lift even heavier weights. This functional change brought on by repeated bouts of exercise can be explained partly by an increased growth of muscle tissue, so that more protein threads in the muscle are available to exert contractile force, and partly by an improved ability of the nervous system to cause greater numbers of muscle fibers to contract simultaneously for the greatest possible force of contraction of the entire muscle. This understanding of how weight-lifting ability develops has led to better training programs to improve the lifting response.

Note that in the concise definition of exercise physiology, the objective of improving the exercise response was qualified by the word *often.* This qualification is meant to point out that, scientifically speaking, there is no requirement that the study of exercise responses be designed to improve those responses. The basic knowledge of what happens during exercise and how it happens is important in itself, just as obtaining basic knowledge of any sort has been an important trait of human beings throughout history. It is not possible in the present to foretell what sort of knowledge will have "practical" benefits to mankind in the future, just as it was not understood that research in theoretical physics would lead to the development of transistors that have become part of our everyday lives in radios, television sets and computers. As it happens, a great many scientists who study the responses of the body to exercise do so with the hope of improving the capacity of heart patients to work at their jobs, enabling industrial workers to work more efficiently, or establishing a new world record in the 100 meter freestyle swim.

Mechanisms in Exercise Physiology

When one tries to explain *how* some change in body function comes about as a result of exercise, it can be said that he wants to know the *mechanism* underlying the response, that is, he wants to know as much as possible about the physical and chemical laws presumed to be the basis for the change in function. The desire for understanding the mechanisms underlying exercise responses is governed not only by a natural curiosity, but also by the belief that knowing the details of how a response occurs will make it more likely that the response can be better predicted, better controlled and more efficiently improved.

As an example, let us examine the relationship between regular endurance exercise (jogging, cycling, swimming and so on) and the risk of suffering coronary heart disease at an early age. Most studies that have compared the risk of coronary heart disease in groups of people who exercise regularly with the risk in groups who engage in little physical activity show that exercise seems to be protective and thus reduces the risk of suffering early heart disease. Therefore, a change in body function seems to occur as a result of regular exercise—the heart is more resistant to disease. The question in many people's minds is, "How is this protective effect brought about?" In other words, what is it about jogging three miles daily that enables the heart to better resist coronary artery disease? Some authorities believe that exercise has a direct effect on improving the blood-vessel supply to the heart. Others believe the exercise is beneficial because it reduces blood fat, or because it retards blood clotting in the veins, or because it causes one to lose body weight.

Hopefully, if researchers can determine the mechanism underlying the protective effect of exercise on the heart and the resultant reduction in coronary heart–disease risk, it will be easier to prescribe exactly the right kind and amount of exercise; it will be easier to monitor the effect of the exercise program; and, perhaps, it will be possible to locate the exact chemical malfunction involved, so that steps could be taken to prevent heart disease entirely by appropriate diet, medication, surgery or radiation therapy. Although it is not always true that understanding *how* a response works makes it easier to predict, prevent or treat, medical history books are full of examples of how such understanding has made possible far–reaching improvements in medicine. In a similar fashion, the understanding of exercise responses has made possible important gains in exercise treatment of cardiac patients, in athletic conditioning programs, and in selection of athletes for world–class training.

It is also possible to ask *why* or for what *purpose* a particular physiological response to exercise occurs. For example, one may say that the heart beats faster during exercise because it must pump blood to the working muscles, or because the skin needs more blood to help rid the body of excess heat, or because blood pressure would fall too low if the heart did not speed up, or for any number of other plausible reasons. The study of the *purposes* underlying occurences in nature is called *teleology*. Teleological explanations of exercise responses can sometimes prove useful in helping us remember *what* and *how* things happen, but they can also impede the learning process in exercise physiology if one settles for a teleological explanation and neglects to learn *how* a response occurs. For example, a complete understanding of the heart–rate response to exercise does not stop with the declaration that the heart rate increases to provide more blood to the muscles, just as a complete understanding of an automobile's acceleration does not stop with the observation that stepping on the accelerator increases speed. One who truly understands the heart-rate response to exercise knows where the stimuli that begin the response originate, that is, in the brain, the working muscles and joints, or in the heart itself, and knows the nervous or hormonal steps that lie between the initial stimuli and the final speeding up of the heart. Therefore, it is more useful to think about the *how* questions rather than the *why* questions in exercise physiology.

Another problem with trying to determine why physiological responses to exercise occur is that it is usually impossible to judge objectively whether a purpose decided upon is the correct one. We don't really know, for example, whether the purpose behind a reduced amount of blood sugar after prolonged exercise is to signal the body to rest or to enable the body to use more fats for energy. It is indeed quite possible that the fall in blood sugar has no purpose but simply happens as a consequence of the depletion of sugar stores in the liver as exercise progresses.

PHYSICAL FITNESS

Consider the cases of two individuals—Peter Plowfaster, a fullback for the Baskerville Hounds professional football team, and Marybeth Snowperch, librarian at the Simon Smedley School for Sailors. Do these two persons have different requirements for "physical fitness"? Some authorities might say that both Peter and Mary have the same requirements for physical fitness because these authorities rather narrowly define physical fitness as the functional capacity of the cardiovascular system, and they maintain that each person must maximize his cardiovascular potential to remain healthy and free of cardiovascular disease. Such authorities advocate regular, long-distance running, swimming or cycling as the only means of attaining high levels of physical fitness.

Others claim that physical fitness implies *maximal* functional capacity of all systems of the body and, especially, the cardiovascular and musculoskeletal systems. Such a concept means that Peter, Marybeth and all of us should daily concentrate on building our cardiovascular endurance, strength, flexibility, speed and local muscle endurance to maximal levels.

In this book a more moderate stance is taken. *Physical fitness* is defined herein as *the capacity to meet the present and potential physical challenges of life with success.* With this definition, physical fitness requirements for individuals are related to the different types of physical challenges that different persons must face. Peter Plowfaster, for example, must face the grueling challenges of professional football; therefore, he must regularly work to improve and maintain his muscular strength and endurance, flexibility, speed, and cardiorespiratory endurance. On the other hand, Marybeth Snowperch has no reason to believe that she will ever be required to run fast or produce a large amount of muscular force. Her physical fitness goals should probably be aimed at maintaining enough muscular strength, flexibility and cardiorespiratory endurance to participate successfully in any recreational pursuits that interest her, to insure that she can perform her daily tasks with ease, and to help prevent the onset of low back pain, excessive spinal curvatures and cardiovascular disease. Cardiovascular disease and other disabling diseases can be considered physical challenges because those afflicted by these diseases have definite limits placed upon their movements; a high level of cardiorespiratory fitness may help delay this heart disease challenge. Likewise, poor muscular strength of abdomen, shoulders and back may lead to low back pain and spinal curvatures that place chronic, excessive strain on muscles and, therefore, represent physical challenges. The precise levels of various types of fitness that are required to meet physical challenges are often difficult or impossible to determine. Research has provided some guidelines to help in exercise prescription, and these guidelines will be discussed in subsequent chapters.

Physical Fitness and Exercise Physiology

Physical fitness involves preparing the body for a movement or exercise response whether that movement may be shoveling snow, touching one's toes or running a three-hour marathon. Therefore, because exercise physiology is the study of the body's response to single and repeated bouts of exercise, the knowledge from exercise physiology can be used to improve physical fitness. In other words, the *improvement of physical fitness could be defined as the application of the principles of exercise physiology to the improvement of man's response and adaptation to life's physical challenges.* For example, information gained from studies of strength-training methods can be used to design the most effective program for a person who wants to improve strength, and results of research on diet and exercise can be applied to developing a successful weight-control program for those who are obese.

It is unfortunate that many persons do not see the connection between exercise physiology and physical fitness; for better physical fitness programs could be designed to meet individuals' specific fitness needs if knowledge gained from studies of exercise physiology were more frequently applied to the design of fitness programs.

ATHLETIC CONDITIONING

In this text, *"athletic conditioning" is used to describe the process by which individuals become physically fit for specialized athletic competition.* In other words, athletic conditioning is a special case of becoming physically fit. Athletic conditioning in this sense does *not* include the learning of the motor skills involved in athletic performance such as pole vaulting, punting or field goal shooting; nor does it include the care of injuries and taping of limbs sometimes considered in athletic conditioning courses. Thus, being in good athletic condi-

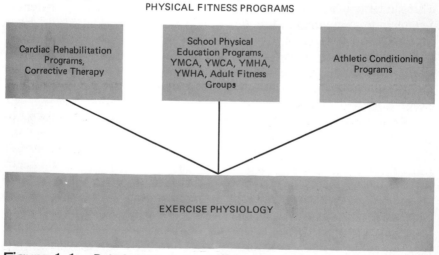

Figure 1.1. Relationship between exercise physiology, physical fitness, and athletic conditioning.

tion in this view is simply the state of being physically fit to meet the unique challenges of athletic competition.

Therefore, the relationship between exercise physiology and athletic conditioning is similar to that between exercise physiology and physical fitness; athletic conditioning is the application of knowledge gained from exercise physiology to improvement of the body's capacity to successfully respond to special physical challenges of athletic competition (Fig. 1.1).

RESPONSES AND ADAPTATIONS: THE EFFECTS OF EXERCISE AND TRAINING

In subsequent chapters, a great deal of time is spent describing the changes in function of the body brought about by single and repeated bouts of exercise. Sometimes a single bout of exercise is called *acute* exercise, whereas repeated bouts of exercise over several days or months may be called *chronic* exercise. Also, *exercise* may be used to indicate a single episode of exercise, and *training* may be used instead of *repeated bouts* or *chronic* exercise. It is important to remember that functional changes that occur with training do not necessarily occur with a single bout of exercise. For example, a single bout of exercise does not affect one's resting heart rate, whereas regular endurance training usually reduces resting heart rate. Two other words—*response* and *adaptation*—are often used interchangeably in exercise physiology texts.

In this book the functional changes that occur when one exercises a single time are called *responses* to exercise. *Responses are the sudden, temporary changes in function caused by exercise. These functional changes disappear shortly after the exercise period is finished.* Examples of responses to exercise are the increase in heart rate, the rise in blood pressure and the increase in breathing that accompanies exercise. Each of these responses is no longer present a few minutes after the exercise is over.

An adaptation is a more or less persistent change in structure or function following training that apparently enables the body to respond more easily to subsequent exercise bouts. Ordinarily, adaptations are not seen until several weeks of training have passed, but some occur after only four or five days of training. One example of an adaptation to training is a reduction in heart rate for a submaximal exercise load that nearly always follows several weeks of training. This reduction in exercise heart rate seems to enable the heart to pump the same amount of blood to the working muscles at a lower energy cost for the heart. Another example of an adaptation is the increased muscle size that accompanies a strenuous weight-lifting program and enables the lifter to exert greater muscular force than before training. Much of this increased strength persists for many months after the training program ends.

Homeostasis and the Negative Feedback Character of Responses and Adaptations to Exercise

Nearly all of the changes in body function brought on by exercise or training tend to reduce the stressfulness of exercise for the entire organism. For instance, contracting muscles are severely stressed as they use up oxygen, but as the heart rate and breathing rate increase, more oxygen is delivered to the working muscles to reduce that stress. As another example of this principle, consider the increase in sweat rate that accompanies repeated exercise bouts in hot environments. The heat of the environment puts a stress on all the tissues of the body, but after training in the heat, this stress is reduced because the increased sweat production helps cool the body by evaporation.

The tendency for living organisms to maintain a stable internal environment for their cells is called *homeostasis*. Thus, the human body carefully regulates the temperature, acidity, oxygen, glucose, sodium, potassium, chloride and other characteristics of its body fluids. The most important method of regulation used by the body to maintain homeostasis is *negative feedback* regulation in which a disruption of homeostasis results in a functional change that causes a return of the cells' environment toward normal. For example, if the use of blood sugar (glucose) by the muscles during exercise begins to reduce glucose levels in the blood, the pancreas monitors this fall in blood glucose and responds by the secretion of glucagon, which in turn speeds up the release of glucose into the blood from the glucose stores in the liver. This release of glucose from the liver into the blood brings the blood sugar stores back toward normal, homeostatic levels. Conversely, after a carbohydrate-rich meal, blood glucose levels rise above normal but are soon lowered by the action of pancreatic insulin. Therefore, it can be seen that negative feedback regulation acts to change the cellular environment toward a condition *opposite (negative)* to that produced by stress; if blood glucose levels are too *high*, negative feedback occurs to *lower* glucose, but if glucose levels are too *low*, negative feedback regulation operates to *raise* those levels.

One should keep the principle of negative feedback in mind when studying how exercise responses and adaptations to training occur, because the application of this principle often helps to sort out meaningful relationships between functional changes and to predict what responses or adaptations should occur. For instance, an increase in body temperature during exercise should be rapidly followed, if negative feedback regulation occurs, by increased sweating and increased blood flow to the skin in order to speed heat loss and return body temperature toward normal. Of course, this is exactly what happens.

General Patterns of Physiological Responses and Adaptations to Exercise and Training

Although there are some physiological responses and adaptations to exercise and training that make little sense to exercise physiologists, most are examples of negative feedback regulation apparently designed to help the body minimize changes in homeostasis during exercise. Also, most responses and adaptations fit into general patterns that often prove useful in gaining a clearer insight into those responses and adaptations.

General Pattern of Exercise Responses. A simplified general pattern of physiologic responses to single exercise bouts is shown in Fig. 1.2. In this scheme exercise is the stimulus that causes a disturbance in homeostasis, that is, a change in the physical or chemical environment of the cells. Exercise may cause body temperature to rise, acidity of the blood to increase, oxygen content of the body fluids to fall, carbon dioxide to rise and many other disturbances in homeostasis.

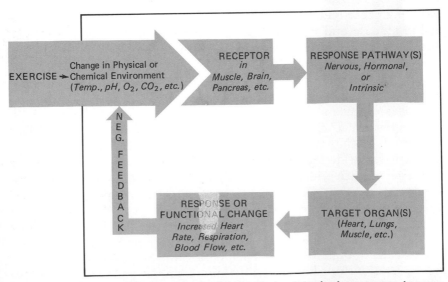

Figure 1.2. Simplified general scheme of physiological responses to exercise.

One or more of these changes in the body's internal environment are sensed in some way by molecules in certain cells of the body that then stimulate a complex response pathway. By means of this pathway a "signal" is transmitted to those organ(s) that will actually change their functions to produce the observed response to exercise. The exercise response in its turn has a negative feedback influence on the homeostatic disturbances caused by the exercise. As a specific example of this general scheme, consider the increase in breathing (ventilation) that accompanies strenuous exercise. The exercise causes a buildup of carbon dioxide, a reduction in oxygen and an increased acidity (reduced pH) in the working muscles, as well as mechanical pressure or stretch on nerve endings in the muscles and working joints. All of these changes (and others) in the chemical and physical environment of the cells have been implicated in the mechanism underlying the increased breathing that occurs during exercise. The receptors that sense the changes in carbon dioxide, oxygen, and acidity are nerve cells of the brain that control respiration and specialized cells of the aorta and carotid arteries. The receptors that sense the changes in pressure or stretch in working muscles and joints are nerve endings in the joints and muscles themselves. The response pathways from receptors to target organs (in this case, the muscles that control breathing) are nerve pathways; that is, the nerve cells of the brain that sense changes in carbon dioxide, oxygen, and acid generate nerve impulses that are sent directly to the respiratory muscles to speed up the rate and depth of breathing. The response pathways from the pressure or stretch receptors of working muscles and joints generate nerve impulses that reach, by way of the spinal cord, the nerve cells that control respiration at the base of the brain. These respiratory nerve cells in turn send impulses to the breathing muscles to increase the rate and depth of breathing. The exercise response or functional change in this example is obviously the increased rate and depth of breathing that acts in a negative feedback manner to decrease body fluid carbon dioxide, increase oxygen and decrease acidity, thereby minimizing some of the homeostatic disruptions caused by exercise.

Other functional responses to exercise use hormonal or intrinsic pathways rather than nervous pathways. An intrinsic pathway is one located within an organ that serves both as receptor and target organ. For example, one of the responses of skeletal muscles to exercise is that these working muscles take up glucose from the blood more rapidly than when they are at rest. This increased glucose uptake is thought to be caused by some factor in the muscle itself. Therefore, it appears that the working muscle serves as the receptor (perhaps sensing changes in tension or changes in oxygen or carbon dioxide), that the response pathway is intrinsic to (located within) the same muscle, and that the muscle also is the target organ. The response of glucose uptake compensates for the fall in muscle glucose that occurs as the muscle uses glucose for energy.

General Patterns of Training Adaptations.   The general pattern of physiological or anatomical adaptations to training (Fig. 1.3) is similar to that described for responses to a single bout of exercise, but includes an *adaptation pathway* and arrows showing the relationships between the adaptation pathway and other elements in the scheme. It should be noted at this stage that no one is yet certain of the entire scheme for any of the adaptations known to occur with regular physical training. Therefore, the following example of a specific adaptation of skeletal muscle is only deemed probable and has not yet been confirmed.

It is known that skeletal muscle adapts to regular cardiorespiratory endurance training (jogging, cycling, and so on) by increasing its capacity for producing energy for contraction. This increased capacity for energy production is brought about by increases in the number of enzymes needed to speed up the chemical reactions that produce

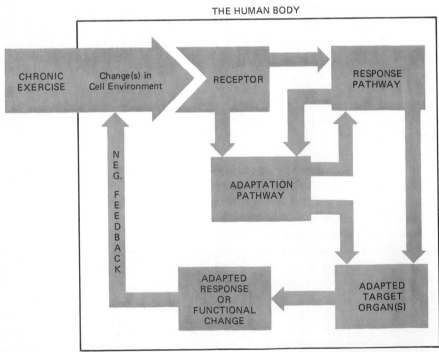

Figure 1.3.   Simplified general scheme of physiological adaptations to training.

energy compounds. Let us now examine each of the elements included in the general adaptation scheme for this specific adaptation. First, the change in the cell environment caused by exercise may be the reduction in certain chemical energy compounds in the working muscles. The receptor is some molecule in the skeletal muscle cell itself, and the response pathway is located within the muscle cell (intrinsic pathway) and involves the *activation of enzyme molecules already present* in the target organ (the same muscle cells), so that reserve energy sources that are stored in the muscle can be released and used to replenish the energy compounds depleted by exercise. This exercise response, of course, tends to compensate (in a negative feedback manner) for the reduction of energy caused by muscle contraction during exercise. Now if this response (releasing more energy as needed) could be made more efficient or faster by some adaptive process, an even greater homeostatic disturbance in energy supplies could be tolerated, and the individual could work at a faster rate, that is, he would become better trained.

The adaptation pathway in the example being discussed may lie entirely within the muscle (intrinsic pathway) and include the stimulation of the synthesis of more enzyme molecules. This stimulation is brought about as a result of a receptor molecule in the muscle cell sensing a change in environment (perhaps chemical energy levels). The arrow in Fig. 1.3 which connects the receptor and the adaptation pathway represents the transfer of information from the receptor molecule to the enzyme-protein synthesis apparatus in the muscle cell (the adaptation pathway). The target organ (muscle cell) would then be better adapted to chronic exercise by virtue of its increased enzyme capacity, and the adapted response or functional change would be the increased number of chemical energy molecules produced during exercise. This increased rate of chemical energy production would tend to act in negative feedback fashion, both to reduce the energy balance disturbance caused by exercise and also to limit the extent of stimulation of the adaptation pathway. As suggested by the arrow connecting the response pathway to the adaptation pathway and vice versa, there are other ways that the adaptation pathway (whether it be intrinsic, hormonal, or nervous) could be stimulated and other influences that the adaptation pathway could have. For example, if some exercise response pathway included hormonal involvement, the change in hormone(s), rather than a signal from the original receptor molecule, could activate the adaptation pathway. Also, the adaptation pathway may have its effect on the target organ indirectly, that is, by somehow altering the exercise response pathway that in turn will affect the target organ.

We can truly understand responses and adaptations to exercise and training, respectively, only when the response schemes and adaptation schemes are fully understood. The serious student of exercise physiology will want to compare his knowledge of a particular response or adaptation with the general schemes shown in Fig. 1.2 and Fig. 1.3. If there are gaps in his knowledge of the elements of a scheme for a specific response or adaptation, the student should seek out the answer. If, as will be true much of the time, this answer is not available, the dedicated student may hypothesize explanations that will fill in the gaps of the scheme and, perhaps, become interested in setting up a research project sometime in the future to determine whether his hypothesis was correct.

These general patterns of responses and adaptations should serve as useful study guides. The more elements of the general schemes that a student is sure he understands for a specific response or adaptation, the more likely it is that the student has mastered that area of exercise physiology.

Review Questions

1. Define the following terms: *exercise, physiology, physical fitness, athletic conditioning*.
2. Explain why it is important to understand the mechanisms underlying physiological responses and adaptations to exercise.
3. What is the relationship between exercise physiology and physical fitness?
4. Distinguish between the terms *response* and *adaptation*.
5. Explain why homeostasis and negative feedback are important concepts in exercise physiology.

References

1. Asmussen, E. Exercise: General statement of unsolved problems. *Circulation Research*, 1967, **20–21** (Supplement I): 12–15.
2. Dill, D. B. (Ed.), *Handbook of Physiology, Section 4: Adaptation to the Environment*. Washington, D.C.: American Physiological Society, 1964.
3. Brooks, C. McC. The nature of adaptive reactions and their initiation. In E. Bajusz (Ed.), *Physiology and Pathology of Adaptation Mechanisms*. New York: Pergamon Press, 1969, pp. 439–451.

2

Skeletal muscle structure and function

An understanding of the structure and function of skeletal muscle is basic to an understanding of how the body responds to a single bout of exercise and adapts to physical training. That skeletal muscle is important for exercise is evident for the following reasons. First, without muscle contraction, of course, there can be no movement. Second, the period of time a movement may continue depends on the relative degree of muscular exertion and the extent of muscular fatigue. Finally, because the skeletal muscles consume most of the oxygen and require most of the body's blood during heavy exercise, the functions of other parts of the body, such as the liver, the kidneys or the stomach, are dependent upon what happens in the skeletal muscle.

The material in this chapter may serve as a brief review for those who have previously studied the anatomy and physiology of skeletal muscles. On the other hand, for those who have only a modest background in physiology the material in this chapter may well be the most difficult of any in the book. There are many complex ideas and what may seem to be an unending stream of strange vocabulary in these pages, but a firm grasp of the contents of this chapter is absolutely essential if the remainder of the text is to be fully comprehended.

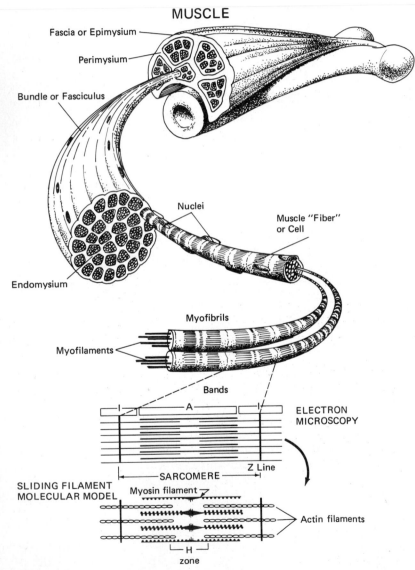

Figure 2.1.   **Skeletal muscle structure.**

THE STRUCTURE OF SKELETAL MUSCLE

If one were to examine a whole skeletal muscle and gradually dissect it into its component parts, he would first discover that the muscle is composed of bundles of fibers. (See Fig. 2.1.) *Endomysium* is the name given to the connective tissue that surrounds individual fibers and binds them together to form bundles of fibers. (See Fig. 2.1.) Each bundle is called a *fasiculus* (plural: fasiculi) and is bound to neighboring fasiculi by white fibrous connective tissue, the *perimysium*. The external connective tissue that binds all the fiber bundles or fasiculi together into a whole muscle is called *epimysium* or *fascia*.

Each fiber is composed of a covering or membrane called the *sarcolemma* and a gelatin-like substance called *sarcoplasm* in which hundreds of contractile *myofibrils* and other important structures such as *mitochondria* and the *sarcoplasmic reticulum* are embedded (Fig. 2.3). Each myofibril in turn contains many fine protein threads (myofilaments). These include the *actin filaments* and thick *myosin filaments* (Fig. 2.4). When thin slices of muscle tissue are stained with the appropriate chemicals and observed under a microscope, they

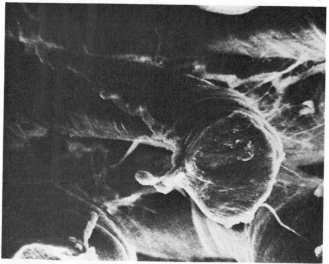

Figure 2.2. Stereo electron micrograph of several muscle fibers that have been teased apart to show web-like connective tissue (endomysium) between fibers. A single capillary is shown along left lower border of the central muscle fiber. (Courtesy of R. E. Carrow, W. W. Heusner and W. D. Van Huss, Michigan State University, E. Lansing, Michigan.)

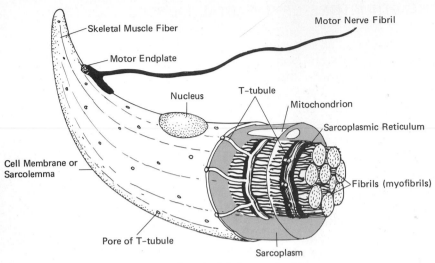

Skeletal Muscle Fiber

Motor Nerve Fibril

Motor Endplate

Nucleus

T-tubule

Mitochondrion

Sarcoplasmic Reticulum

Cell Membrane or Sarcolemma

Fibrils (myofibrils)

Pore of T-tubule

Sarcoplasm

Figure 2.3.   Components of a skeletal muscle fiber.

RELAXED MYOFIBRIL

H Zone

Z Line

A Band   I Band

Sarcomere

Myosin   Actin

H Zone

Z Line or Disc

"Relaxed" Cross Bridges

CONTRACTED MYOFIBRIL

A Band   I Band

Sarcomere

"Activated" Cross Bridges Pull Actin Filaments Toward Each Other

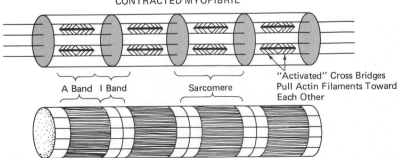

Figure 2.4.   Appearance of relaxed and contracted muscle.

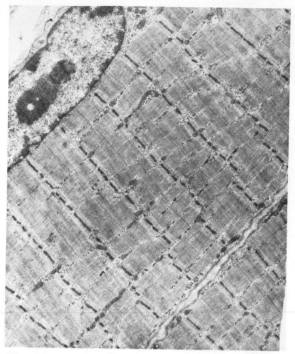

Figure 2.5. Electron micrograph of skeletal muscle (magnification ×7,500). (Courtesy of G. Colin Budd, Physiology Department, Medical College of Ohio, Toledo, Ohio)

take on a banded or *striated* appearance because of the regular arrangement of the myofilaments into dark or *A bands* and light or *I bands* (Fig. 2.1, 2.4). The I bands appear light because they contain mostly the thin actin filaments, whereas the A bands are dark because they have both the thin actin filaments and thicker myosin filaments. (Fig. 2.4). When a muscle is relaxed, the central portion of each A band appears somewhat lighter than the outer portions because the actin filaments do not meet in the center of the A band. This light area of the A band is the *H zone*, and it disappears when the muscle contracts as described in the next paragraph. Each I band is bisected by a *Z line* or disc which seems to anchor the actin filaments. The distance between two Z lines is known as a *sarcomere*. When a muscle fiber contracts, the Z lines move closer together and, thus, the sarcomeres shorten.

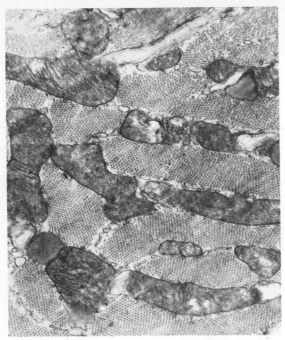

Figure 2.6. Electron micrograph of cross sections of cardiac myofibrils showing thick and thin filaments (magnification ×17,500). Large dark structures are mitochondria. (Courtesy of G. Colin Budd, Physiology Department, Medical College of Ohio, Toledo, Ohio.)

MUSCLE CONTRACTION

With the electron microscope, one can compare the detailed structures of relaxed muscle fibers with those of the contracted fibers. The most common observations are that after contraction the lengths of the A bands have not changed, whereas the I bands are shorter and the H zones of the A bands are obliterated. These observations have led scientists to conclude that muscles contract by the sliding of actin filaments toward each other in the central parts of the A bands. As these actin filaments move toward each other, the Z lines are pulled closer together so that the I bands shorten. Also, the movement of actin filaments toward each other across the myosin filaments causes the H zone of the A band to disappear as it becomes occupied by actin. This notion that the actin filaments slide toward each other during contraction is called the *"sliding filament" theory of muscle contraction* (2, 3, 4).

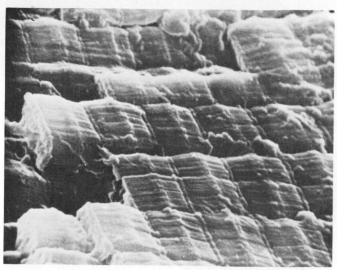

Figure 2.7. Stereo electron micrograph of myofibrils showing striations, z-lines. (Courtesy of R. E. Carrow, W. W. Heusner and W. D. Van Huss, Michigan State University, E. Lansing, Michigan.)

There is still some controversy regarding the specific way in which actin filaments manage to creep past the myosin filaments, but it is thought that the actin is bound to the myosin at the *"cross bridges,"* which are extensions of the myosin molecules that reach out toward the actin filaments. (See Fig. 2.4.) When chemical energy is available, the cross bridges may "bend" toward the center of the A band and carry the actin filaments with them. (See Fig. 2.4.)

The Chemistry of Contraction

Energy is defined as the capacity to do work, and energy must be supplied to myofibrils to cause the movement of actin filaments toward the center of the A bands. This energy is provided when molecules of adenosine triphosphate (ATP) are split into adenosine diphosphate (ADP) and phosphate groups (P) by the action of myosin, which can serve as an enzyme to split ATP. This enzymatic, ATP–splitting property of myosin is called *myosin ATPase activity*, and the essentials of the splitting of ATP for energy are as follows:

$$\text{ATP} \xrightarrow[\substack{\text{Myosin ATPase} \\ \text{activity}}]{} \text{ADP} + \text{P} + \text{energy for contraction}$$

In a resting muscle, myosin does not split ATP because it is inactivated by *troponin*, another protein found in myofibrils. Until the troponin molecules themselves are inactivated, the muscle remains at rest. The chemical which inactivates troponin is calcium, and calcium ions (positively charged calcium atoms, Ca^{++}) are delivered to the troponin molecules when a motor nerve or electric shock stimulates a muscle fiber as described in the following section.

The Contractile Process

When a motor nerve fiber delivers a stimulus or *action potential* to a skeletal muscle fiber at the motor endplate (Fig. 2.3), an action potential subsequently spreads rapidly over the entire sarcolemma. At nearly the same instant, the action potential is transmitted down the *T-tubules* toward the interior of the fiber (Fig. 2.3). These T-tubules lie adjacent to parts of the *sarcoplasmic reticulum*, a system of canals that spreads out over the surfaces of the myofibrils (Fig. 2.3). The transmission of the action potential down the T-tubules causes calcium to be released from the sarcoplasmic reticulum. These calcium ions then diffuse rapidly to the myofilaments and inactivate troponin molecules (1). The inactivated troponin can then no longer interfere with myosin ATPase activity so that myosin ATPase is free to split ATP, probably at the cross bridges, and thus release the energy needed to cause the actin filaments to move toward each other. (Fig. 2.9).

After myosin cross bridges to actin have drawn the actin filaments a minute distance toward the center of the myosin filaments, the cross bridges must disengage and reattach themselves to sites further down on the actin filaments (toward the Z lines) to continue the shortening process. The breaking of the original bridge to actin is accomplished when a fresh ATP molecule is made available to the myosin cross bridge. The myosin-ATP cross bridge is then free to attach itself to a new site on the actin filament (as long as calcium is present to inhibit tropinin). Once the fresh ATP molecule is split by myosin-ATPase activity, the new cross bridge draws the actin filament further toward the center of the myosin filament. This rapid attachment, disengagement, and reattachment of the cross bridges occurs many times per second during a muscle contraction, and stops only when calcium is withdrawn during relaxation of the muscle or when fresh ATP molecules cannot be supplied rapidly enough to recharge the cross bridges.

MUSCLE RELAXATION

When the motor nerve stops firing, so that an action potential no longer spreads across the sarcolemma and down the T-tubules, the

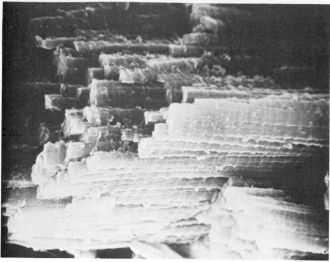

Figure 2.8. Stereo electron micrograph of myofibrils from a single muscle fiber. Note striations for each myofibril. (Courtesy of R. E. Carrow, W. W. Heusner and W. D. Van Huss, Michigan State University, E. Lansing, Michigan.)

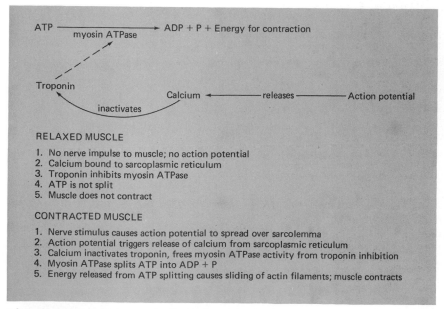

Figure 2.9 Invovement of calcium, troponin and myosin ATPase activity in contraction and relaxation.

sarcoplasmic reticulum withdraws calcium from the myofibrils and, once again, the calcium is bound to the sarcoplasmic reticulum in such a way that calcium cannot inactivate troponin. Since the troponin molecules are then free to inactivate myosin-ATPase, no ATP can be split for energy, and the muscle relaxes. Thus, the sarcoplasmic reticulum is vital not only because of its action in releasing calcium for muscle contraction, but also because of its withdrawal of calcium in the relaxation process (Fig. 2.9).

A knowledge of the chemistry of muscle contraction and relaxation can aid one's appreciation and understanding of possible explanations for various physiological phenomena associated with exercise. For example, changes in the levels of sodium and potassium, which are needed for development of the action potential, could cause disturbances in the excitability of the sarcolemma, and alterations in calcium levels might disrupt the normal release and withdrawal of calcium by the sarcoplasmic reticulum. These factors in turn could play important roles in bringing about muscle weakness, muscle fatigue and muscle cramps.

ENERGY SOURCES FOR MUSCLE CONTRACTION

There is enough ATP stored in skeletal muscle to provide essentially all the chemical energy required for the brief contractions associated with strength-related events such as weightlifting, the shot put and the discus throw. Thus, there is no need for concern about special dietary programs for increasing energy stores for brief, maximal exertions because there is no known way to increase ATP stores by special diets. Adequate dietary protein intake is important for assuring sufficient proteins for muscle growth in those training for strength activities, but protein is *not* used for energy during such activities.

However, stores of adenosine triphosphate are not sufficient to meet the energy demands of more prolonged activities such as a 400 meter run, a distance swim or a basketball game. During these activities the body must call upon its fuel reserves for the energy to produce more ATP as the initial ATP stores are used up. This process is called *energy metabolism* and is described in the next chapter.

Review Questions

1. Define the following terms: *sarcolemma, sarcoplasm, sarcomere, sarcoplasmic reticulum.*
2. Describe the sliding filament theory of muscle contraction.

3. What is the immediate source of energy for muscle contraction?
4. Explain the involvement of calcium, troponin and myosin ATPase activity in muscle contraction.
5. What is an action potential?

References

1. Hoyle, G. How is muscle turned on and off? *Scientific American,* 1970, **222:**84–93.
2. Huxley, A. F. Review lecture: Muscular contraction. *Journal of Physiology, (London),* 1974, **243:**1–43.
3. Huxley, H. E. The structural basis of muscular contraction. *Proceedings of the Royal Society of Medicine,* 1971, **178:** 131–149.
4. Huxley, H. E., and J. Hanson. Changes in the cross-striations of muscle during contraction and stretch, and their structural interpretation. *Nature,* 1954, **173:**973–976.

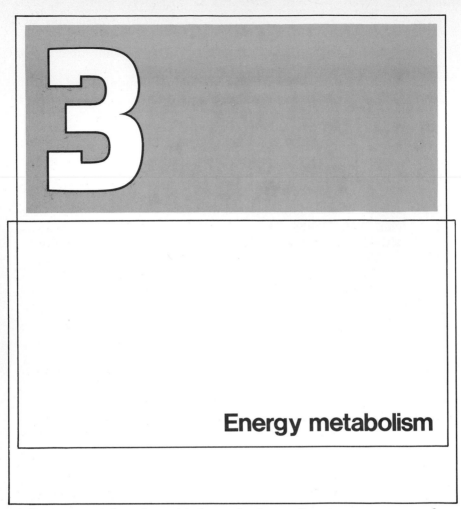

3

Energy metabolism

Adenosine triphosphate is the only immediate energy source for muscle contraction; without ATP, actin filaments do not slide over myosin filaments. Therefore, the body must somehow be able to rebuild ATP as fast as it is broken down if muscle contraction is to continue. This ATP rebuilding means that energy must be obtained from reserve fuels in the muscle to make adenosine diphosphate recombine with phosphate (P) as follows:

$$ADP + P + \text{Energy from Reserve Fuel} \rightarrow ATP.$$

It is important to remember that stored fuels such as carbohydrate and fat *are not changed into ATP molecules.* Rather, a portion of the energy stored in the chemical bonds of the stored fuel molecules is released from those molecules, and that liberated energy then causes adenosine diphosphate (ADP) to combine with phosphate (P) to form adenosine triphosphate (ATP). In general, fuel molecules with larger

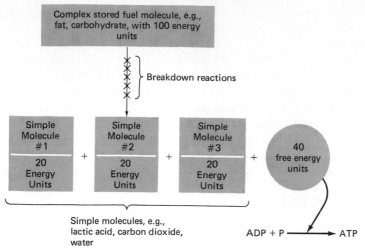

Figure 3.1. Release of energy from stored fuels to produce ATP.

amounts of energy stored in their chemical bonds are broken down into molecules with lesser amounts of energy in their bonds, and the excess energy is used to produce ATP from ADP + P. (See Fig. 3.1.) The first fuel reserve to be called upon when ATP is being used up is a molecule called *creatine phosphate* (or phosphocreatine), which is stored in the muscle fibers.

THE PRIMARY FUEL RESERVE—CREATINE PHOSPHATE

Almost instantaneously as ATP is broken down to ADP + P during muscle contraction, the ATP is resynthesized at the expense of creatine phosphate. In this process creatine phosphate donates its phosphate to ADP as follows:

Creatine phosphate + ADP → Creatine + ATP.

In this reaction, energy stored in the chemical bonds of creatine phosphate is used to cause the coupling of its phosphate to ADP to form ATP; therefore, the creatine molecule that remains contains less energy than the creatine phosphate molecule. This resynthesis or rebuilding of ATP at the expense of creatine phosphate is especially important when extremely heavy exercise, such as sprinting, pushing an automobile or pedaling a bicycle ergometer rapidly against heavy resistance, is sustained for less than 30 seconds. At lesser, more prolonged workloads, creatine phosphate is not depleted as rapidly as with short bursts of severe work.

The breakdown of creatine phosphate does not require the presence of oxygen delivered by the blood; therefore, it is said to be an *anaerobic* process as opposed to an *aerobic* (oxygen-requiring) process. The use of creatine phosphate for ATP resynthesis is one of only two common anaerobic means of releasing energy for ATP production; the other is the breakdown of sugar (glucose) to lactic acid. The series of chemical reactions that causes glucose to be catabolized or broken down to lactic acid is called *anaerobic glycolysis*.

ANAEROBIC GLYCOLYSIS

Glucose can be made available in the muscle cells for breakdown to lactic acid principally by two means: 1) the glucose molecules may pass from the blood through the sarcolemma into the cell interior or 2) the glucose can be split from glycogen stores in the muscle cell itself in a process called *glycogenolysis* (glycogen breakdown).

Glycogen molecules are nothing more than clusters of glucose sugar molecules that are attached to each other in complex chains. (Each glucose molecule has a backbone of six carbon atoms.) The process of breaking the complex glycogen molecules down involves the removal of glucose molecules one at a time from the chain links or bonds in the glycogen molecule.

Anaerobic glycolysis consists of breaking down the six-carbon glucose molecules, which have a great deal of energy stored in their chemical bonds, into two lactic acid molecules, each having three carbons and a combined total of chemical energy less than that found in the more complex glucose molecule. Some of this difference in free energy is used to cause ADP and P to form ATP as follows:

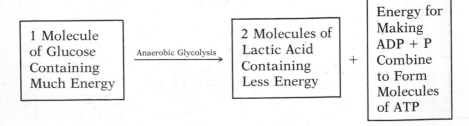

How much ATP can be produced with the energy liberated by the anaerobic breakdown of glycogen or glucose? Examine Fig. 3.2, and you will note that ATP is produced in reactions *F* and *G*, and ATP is

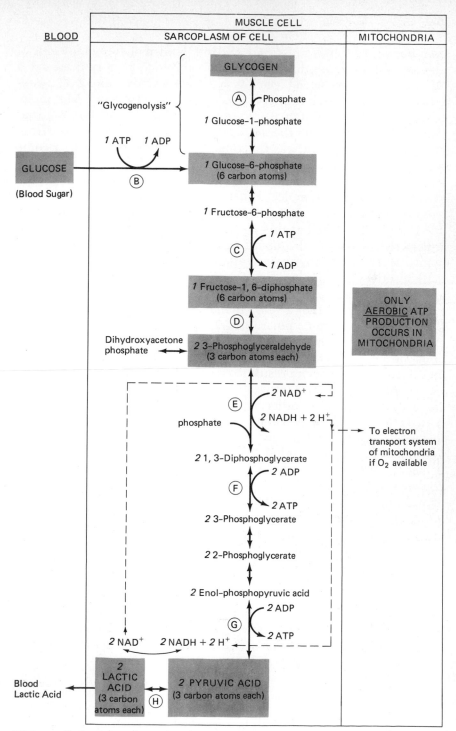

Figure 3.2 Anaerobic glycolysis—the breakdown of glycogen or glucose to lactic acid when oxygen supply is deficient.

used up in reactions *B* and *C*. For the breakdown of every molecule of glucose–6–phosphate that originated from blood glucose there are 4 ATP molecules produced (2 each in reactions *F* and *G*) and 2 ATP molecules used up (1 each in reactions *B* and *C*) for a *net* of 2 ATP molecules produced. Although it may not be evident from Fig. 3.2 that reaction *B* is involved in the derivation of glucose–6–phosphate from glycogen, the glycogen was first made from glucose that had come from the blood and undergone reaction *B* of Fig. 3.2. Therefore, in future calculations we will assume that the anaerobic breakdown of a glucose–6–phosphate molecule derived from either blood glucose or from muscle glycogen results in a *net* production of 2 ATP molecules.

It should be noted at this point that lactic acid and pyruvic acid still have a substantial amount of energy stored in their chemical bonds. Much of this energy is available for ATP production and is released in the breakdown of lactic or pyruvic acid to carbon dioxide and water in *aerobic glycolysis*, as will be discussed later. Thus, anaerobic glycolysis is not a very efficient way to produce ATP because there is so much more potential ATP-producing energy left in the chemical bonds of lactic acid. As will be shown, the *aerobic* breakdown of the lactic acid left at the end of the anaerobic glycolysis of one glucose molecule can result in enough energy to produce an additional 36 molecules of ATP.

There are several other important aspects of glycolysis illustrated in Fig. 3.2 that need to be considered. First, note that the chemical reactions of glycolysis occur entirely in the sarcoplasm of the cell and not in the mitochondria. The reason for this is that all the enzymes that catalyze the reactions of glycolysis are located in the sarcoplasm. The enzymes for *aerobic* ATP production, on the other hand, are all located in the mitochondria.

Second, observe that reaction *D* in Fig. 3.2 is the reaction in which a molecule with six carbon atoms is first broken down into two molecules with three carbon atoms each.

Third, in reactions *E* and *H* of Fig. 3.2, molecules of NAD are involved. The letters NAD stand for the coenzyme, *nicotinamide adenine dinucleotide*, an important molecule whose structure includes the B complex vitamin, nicotinic acid (niacin). A *coenzyme* is a nonprotein molecule necessary for the activity of an enzyme. NAD is important because it acts as an *electron acceptor* in many *oxidation* reactions of energy metabolism and an *electron donor* in *reduction* reactions. *An oxidation reaction need not directly involve oxygen* if an electron acceptor like NAD is available to substitute for oxygen. (Oxygen is eventually required by animals because it is the *final electron acceptor* of metabolism as will be discussed later.) *An oxidation reaction is one in which a compound loses electrons.* In biological oxidation reactions, these electrons removed by oxidation are often accompanied by hydrogen ions (H^+). In the form NAD^+, nicotinamide adenine dinucleotide can accept two negatively charged electrons ($^-$) and one hydrogen ion (H^+) as follows:

$$NAD^+ + 2(^-) + 2\ (H^+) \rightarrow NADH + H^+.$$

Conversely, in a *reduction* reaction (in which a compound gains electrons) NADH can donate two electrons as follows:

$$NADH \rightarrow NAD^+ + 2(^-) + H^+.$$

Referring again to Fig. 3.2, observe that in reaction E NAD^+ is changed to NADH. This means that NAD is accepting electrons in reaction E and, therefore, 3–phosphoglyceraldehyde is being oxidized (losing electrons). On the other hand, in reaction H of Fig. 3.2, as pyruvic acid is changed to lactic acid, NADH *loses* electrons to become NAD^+. Therefore, in H pyruvic acid is *reduced* (gains electrons) to form lactic acid, and the electrons required are donated by NADH.

Without the oxidation reaction E of Fig. 3.2, the reactions that produce ATP (F and G) could not occur. Thus, it is important to have an adequate supply of NAD^+ for reaction E to occur. As NAD^+ is used up in E, it becomes NADH. It is shown by the dotted lines that the NADH produced in E can be transformed to NAD^+ in reaction H, the production of lactic acid from pyruvic acid. This regenerated NAD^+ from reaction H can then be recycled through reaction E. Thus, the production of lactic acid is probably a *beneficial* step in anaerobic metabolism that regenerates the NAD^+ required for ATP production. It seems likely that a person deficient in the capacity to change pyruvic acid to lactic acid would have a lower than normal capacity to produce ATP by anaerobic glycolysis.

A fourth consideration in Fig. 3.2 is that the enzymes that catalyze reactions A and C, *phosphorylase* and *phosphofructokinase*, respectively, seem to be the principal enzymes that determine the maximal rate of glycogen breakdown. Effects of physical training on the capacity of these enzymes will be discussed later in the text.

A final point to consider about Fig. 3.2 is that nearly all of the reactions presented are reversible either directly or indirectly, that is, lactic acid or pyruvic acid under the appropriate conditions can be changed back to glycogen. In particular, reaction H is reversible so that when oxygen supply is adequate, lactic acid can be changed to pyruvic acid, which can then be further broken down to carbon dioxide and water by aerobic metabolism.

AEROBIC CARBOHYDRATE BREAKDOWN

Anaerobic glycolysis can produce a large amount of ATP rapidly to help meet ATP requirements during severe exercise; however, high rates of ATP production by anaerobic glycolysis cannot be sustained very long, and the severity of the exercise must be reduced if the exercise is to be continued. We are not certain why anaerobic glycolysis cannot keep the muscles working longer, but there is substantial evidence that excess acid accumulation in the muscles inactivates phosphorylase and phosphofructokinase so that glycolysis is depressed if the workload remains intense (3). We do know that when exercise is continued for more than about 40–60 seconds, oxygen must be supplied by the blood to the working muscles for *aerobic ATP* production in the mitochondria of those muscles. In the presence of adequate supplies of oxygen the mitochondria of the cells can produce energy from carbohydrate, fat or protein sources. Let us first consider how ATP can be produced at the expense of aerobic carbohydrate breakdown.

When oxygen supply is plentiful and the muscles are not working strenuously, the breakdown of glycogen or glucose starts in the same way as shown in Fig. 3.2 for anaerobic glycolysis. However, under aerobic conditions the pyruvic acid molecules are not converted to lactic acid, but pass instead from the sarcoplasm into the mitochondria, where a series of reactions breaks down each three-carbon pyruvic acid molecule into three molecules of carbon dioxide (CO_2) and three water (H_2O) molecules. (See Fig. 3.3.) As a result of breaking the more complex pyruvic acid molecules into simpler CO_2 and H_2O molecules, which have less energy stored in their bonds, energy is released to form 36 ATP molecules in addition to those found in the anaerobic glycolysis reactions of Fig. 3.2. This overall process is summarized in Fig. 3.3.

The breakdown of pyruvic acid to carbon dioxide and water in the mitochondria is a fairly complex matter, but a general knowledge of what occurs in the mitochondria should help to clarify many points in exercise physiology that will occur later in the text. Therefore, a brief explanation of aerobic carbohydrate catabolism in the mitochondria will be presented now.

First, when oxygen supply is adequate, the pyruvic acid molecules produced in the first phase of glycolysis (Fig. 3.2) diffuse from the sarcoplasm across the mitochondrial membrane to the interior of the mitochondria, where each pyruvic acid molecule loses one carbon atom and two oxygen atoms as CO_2. (See *A*, Fig. 3.4.) At the same time, each pyruvic acid molecule is oxidized in the presence of NAD^+; that is, each pyruvic acid molecule loses two electrons and two hy-

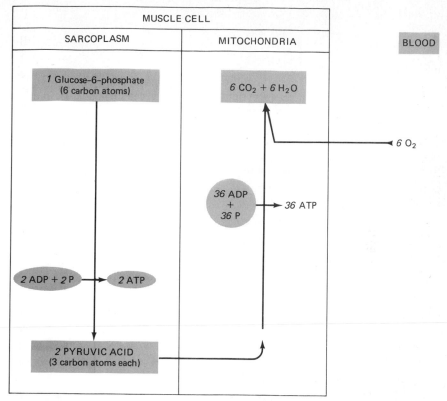

Figure 3.3. Aerobic glycolysis—the complete breakdown of glucose to carbon dioxide and water in the presence of oxygen.

drogen ions. (Fig. 3.4.) These electrons are very important to ATP production as will be described later in this section.

The two-carbon molecule that is left after each pyruvic acid molecule loses its CO_2, electrons and hydrogen ions is called an *acetyl* group. This acetyl group next combines with a molecule called *coenzyme A* (*CoA*) to form *acetyl CoA* (reaction A, Fig. 3.4). Each acetyl CoA molecule then enters a cyclical series of reactions called the *Krebs Cycle* (Citric Acid Cycle), shown in Fig. 3.4.

At the top of the Krebs Cycle diagram, it can be seen that acetyl CoA combines with oxaloacetic acid and loses the coenzyme A molecule, with a molecule of citric acid resulting from this reaction. Citric acid is converted to cis-aconitic acid, which in turn is changed to isocitric acid. In reaction *B*, isocitric acid is oxidized (with the aid of the electron carrier, NAD^+) to oxalosuccinic acid. In reaction *C*, oxalosuccinic acid loses a carbon dioxide (CO_2) molecule and becomes alpha-ketoglutaric acid. The loss of a CO_2 molecule in reaction *C*

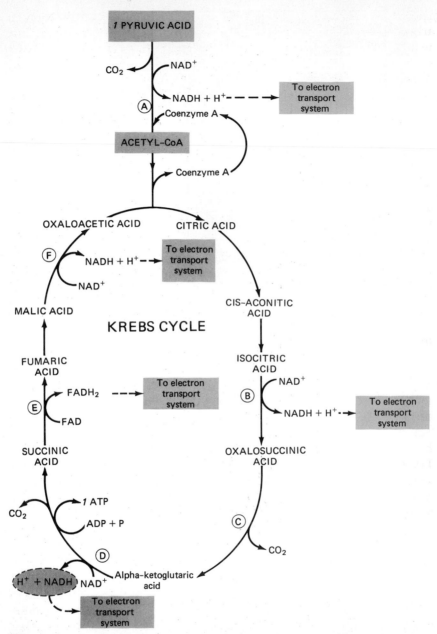

Figure 3.4. Breakdown of a single pyruvic acid molecule to carbon dioxide (CO_2), electrons, and hydrogen ions (H^+) in the Krebs Cycle.

means that we can now consider that only one of the original three carbon atoms of the pyruvic acid molecule remains. (Remember that the first carbon was lost as CO_2 in A of Fig. 3.4.) This last carbon is lost as CO_2 in the complex reaction D in which alpha-ketoglutaric acid undergoes oxidation (with NAD^+) and loss of CO_2 while producing one molecule of ATP. This is the only molecule of ATP actually produced in the Krebs Cycle for *each* acetyl–CoA molecule that travels through the cycle.

After reaction D we can consider that there are no longer any of the original carbons left from pyruvic acid, and it remains only to remove four additional electrons and hydrogen ions in reactions E and F. In reaction E the electron carrier is not the usual NAD^+ molecule but, rather, a molecule called *flavin adenine dinucleotide* (FAD). In reaction F oxaloacetic acid is regenerated so that the cycle can begin anew. To produce larger amounts of ATP from the aerobic breakdown of pyruvic acid, the electrons and hydrogen ions released to the electron carriers, NAD and FAD, must be transported to oxygen by way of the *electron transport system* which is discussed in the following paragraphs.

The Electron Transport System

In the electron transport system (Fig. 3.5), as electrons and hydrogen ions are transferred from one compound to the next, chemical energy is given up at three steps (A, D, F) to provide energy for the formation of ATP from ADP and phosphate groups. That is, the loss of electrons (oxidation) that the various compounds undergo is responsible for the binding of phosphate (phosphorylation) to ADP to form ATP. Thus, the production of ATP in the mitochondria that is associated with the oxidation of successive molecules in the electron transport system is known as *oxidative phosphorylation*. It is this process that provides exercising man with his greatest source of ATP for muscle contraction. Notice that the first molecule to be oxidized (reaction A) is nicotinamide adenine dinucleotide (NADH). In reaction B the flavin adenine dinucleotide ($FADH_2$) that was reduced in A now undergoes oxidation to FAD. From this point on to step G, only electrons are transferred between compounds, whereas the two hydrogen ions (H^+) that had been bound to $FADH_2$ now pass into solution and can be used again in step G, the final oxidation-reduction reaction, where oxygen from the blood accepts two electrons from compound 5 (cytochrome oxidase) and combines with two dissolved hydrogen ions (H^+) to form water (H_2O).

In this scheme of electron transport it can be seen that for every two electrons (or hydrogen atoms) that pass all the way from $NADH + H^+$ to H_2O, three molecules of ATP are produced (at reac-

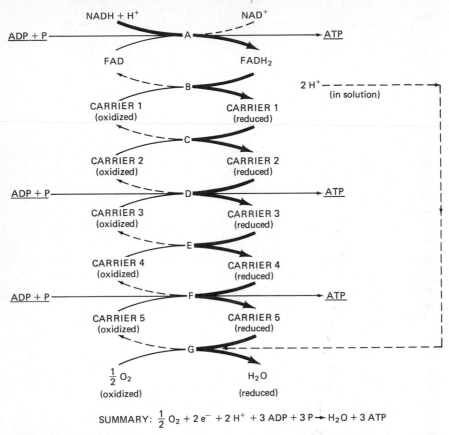

Figure 3.5. Schematic diagram of the electron transport system. CAR-RIER 1 is cytochrome b, CARRIER 2 is coenzyme Q, CARRIER 3 is cytochrome C, CARRIER 4 is cytochrome A, and CARRIER 5 is cytochrome oxidase. The bold lines in the diagram show the path of electrons.

tions A, D, F). Thus, in the aerobic breakdown of glucose or glycogen to carbon dioxide and water, every molecule of NADH that enters the electron transport system potentially can result in the production of three molecules of ATP. On the other hand, a molecule of $FADH_2$ that enters the electron transport system from the Krebs Cycle (reaction E, Fig. 3.4) bypasses the first ATP-producing reaction (A in Fig. 3.5), and therefore results in the production of only two ATP molecules.

Total ATP Production During Aerobic Carbohydrate Breakdown

We are now in a position to determine how many molecules of ATP can be obtained from the aerobic breakdown of a molecule of glucose and where in the cell these ATP molecules are produced. If we know this, we can more easily understand the possible nature of muscle fatigue, the ways in which the body can adapt to physical training by developing its ATP-producing machinery and many other aspects of exercise physiology.

First, refer to Fig. 3.2, the scheme of anaerobic glycolysis. As in the anaerobic breakdown of glucose, aerobic glucose breakdown still results in the production of two ATP molecules in each of two reactions (F and G of Fig. 3.2), and the expenditure of one or two ATP molecules in reactions C and B of Fig. 3.2, depending on whether glucose–6–phosphate comes from stored muscle glycogen or blood glucose, respectively. However, if oxygen is available, the two NADH molecules produced in reaction E of Fig. 3.2 are now able to transfer their electrons and hydrogen ions to the electron transport system of the mitochondria. Since three ATP molecules can be produced for every NADH molecule, a total of six ATP molecules can result from the breakdown of one glucose molecule in reaction E of Fig. 3.2. Thus, rather than the two or three ATP molecules of anaerobic glycolysis, we have shown how six more ATP molecules (a total so far of eight or nine) could result from partial aerobic glycolysis.

But this is only the beginning. Next consult Fig. 3.4, reaction A. For each of the two pyruvic acid molecules that can be derived from one glucose molecule, one NADH and, therefore, three ATP molecules can be produced for a total of six additional ATP molecules. In a similar fashion two NADH and thus six ATP molecules are produced in reactions B, D and F of Fig. 3.4 for another 18 ATP molecules. In reaction E of Fig. 3.4, two molecules of $FADH_2$ can be sent to the electron transport system for an additional four molecules of ATP. (Remember that $FADH_2$ bypasses the first ATP production site in the electron transport system.) Finally, for each pyruvic acid molecule entering the Krebs Cycle, 1 ATP is produced directly at reaction D of Fig. 3.4 for a total of two more ATP molecules from one glucose molecule. A grand total of 38 ATP molecules is produced aerobically. All of this is summarized on page 38.

It should now be obvious that the production of energy (ATP) for exercise is much more efficient (from the standpoint of glucose utilization) when glucose is catabolized aerobically rather than anaerobically. As a matter of fact, the aerobic breakdown of glucose results in 19 times more ATP production per glucose molecule than does anaerobic glycosis (38 ATP vs. 2 ATP). With adequate oxygen but a limited food supply, an organism would obviously be more apt to survive if provided with a biochemical control system that limited its ability to catabolize glucose anaerobically and increased its potential for using the more efficient aerobic process. Such a control system does exist in most higher forms of life, and without oxygen these orga-

The Production of ATP Due to Energy Released by the
Aerobic Breakdown of One Molecule of Glucose-6-Phosphate

Sarcoplasm	Glycolysis (Fig. 3.2, reactions B, C, F, G: $-1 - 1 + 2 + 2 = 2$)	2 ATP
Mitochondria	Krebs Cycle (Fig. 3.4, reaction D: $2 \times 1 = 2$)	2 ATP
	Electron Transport System (Oxidative Phosphorylation)	
	Oxidation of $FADH_2$ (Fig. 3.4, reaction E: $2 \times 2 = 4$)	4 ATP
	Oxidation of NADH (Fig. 3.2, reaction E: Fig. 3.4, reactions A, B, D, F: 3 ATP per NADH or [$10 \times 3 = 30$])	30 ATP
	Total Energy/Glucose-6-phosphate =	38 ATP

nisms can survive at rest for no more than a few minutes and can endure heavy exercise for even less time (40–60 seconds for man).
Although this natural emphasis on aerobic metabolism has undoubtedly helped early man survive prolonged periods of food deprivation
and does favor his capacity for prolonged labor or athletic performance at moderate rates of energy expenditure without the need to
stop for more food, it does not favor man's capacity to perform
extremely heavy muscular labor for prolonged periods or his capacity to perform strenuous athletic feats such as all-out sprinting for
more than a few seconds. Thus, in conditioning an athlete or laborer
for *maximal* rates of work where aerobic energy production cannot be
increased, one must attempt to produce a physiological adaptation
that will result in an ability to continue anaerobic ATP production
beyond the normal limits. On the other hand, for prolonged work at
lower rates of energy expenditure (for example, a marathon run or
cross-country skiing), an adaptation should be produced that results
in higher rates of efficient aerobic ATP production and less anaerobic
glycolysis.

Adaptations of carbohydrate metabolism for various work tasks
will be considered in more detail in later sections of this text. For a
more thorough analysis of energy metabolism during exercise, we
must now turn to the use of two other foodstuffs, fat and protein, for
ATP production.

AEROBIC ATP PRODUCTION FROM FAT (LIPID)

Body fat may look ugly or beautiful depending upon the amount
and where it is distributed, but no matter how it looks, it is an excel-

lent reserve source of fuel for energy production both at rest and during exercise. In fact, one of the physiological adaptations that occurs when a person trains for long–distance running, cycling, or skiing is that fat tends to be used preferentially for ATP production during submaximal exercise while carbohydrate (glucose and glycogen) is spared. The process whereby the energy stored in the chemical bonds of fat molecules is gradually released to cause phosphate (P) and adenosine diphosphate (ADP) to combine into adenosine triphosphate (ATP) is described in the following paragraphs.

Triglycerides

Most of the fat (lipid) that is eaten and stored by man is in the form of triglyceride, a four-part molecule made up of one molecule of glycerol and three molecules of fatty acids as follows:

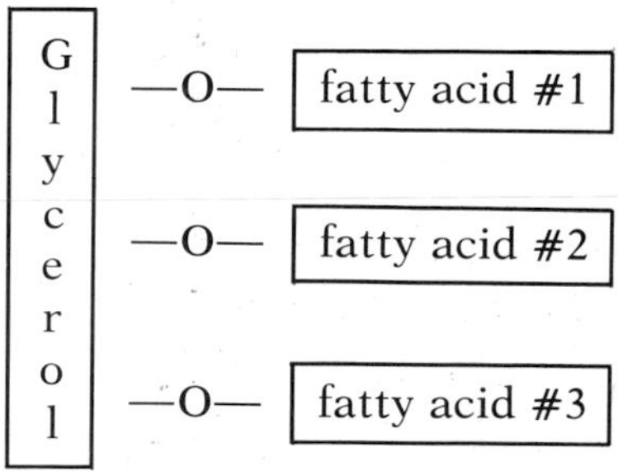

$$
\begin{array}{l}
\text{G} \\
\text{l} \\
\text{y} \quad \text{—O—} \quad \boxed{\text{fatty acid \#1}} \\
\text{c} \\
\text{e} \quad \text{—O—} \quad \boxed{\text{fatty acid \#2}} \\
\text{r} \\
\text{o} \quad \text{—O—} \quad \boxed{\text{fatty acid \#3}} \\
\text{l}
\end{array}
$$

The bulk of the ATP production from fat catabolism comes at the expense of fatty acid molecules that are split off from stored triglyceride molecules, transported by the blood to the muscles, and broken down by the muscles for energy. Therefore, this discussion will be restricted to ATP production from fatty acids, a process called *beta oxidation of fatty acids*. This process occurs exclusively in the mitochondria of the cells.

Oxidation of Fatty Acids

Fatty acids are long chains of carbon (C) atoms that have hydrogen (H) atoms attached to them. In man most of these fatty acids have 16 or 18 carbon atoms. Stearic acid has 18 carbon atoms as follows:

$$HOOC-CH_2-CH_2-CH_2-CH_2-CH_2-CH_2-CH_2-CH_2$$
$$-CH_2-CH_2-CH_2-CH_2-CH_2-CH_2-CH_2-CH_2-CH_3.$$

There is a great deal of energy stored in all of the bonds of stearic

acid, and that energy can be released only if the molecule is first activated or made more chemically reactive by a reaction with molecules
of ATP and coenzyme A as indicated in reaction A of Fig. 3.6. As ATP is
split into adenosine monophosphate (AMP) and two phosphate
groups (PP), energy is released to bring about reaction A. In reaction
B, the activated fatty acid is oxidized with flavin adenine dinucleotide
(FAD) serving as the electron and hydrogen ion acceptor. In reaction
C, another oxidation reaction occurs, this time with the aid of NAD^+.

In reaction D of Fig. 3.6 a two-carbon acetyl unit is split away
from the long chain of carbons and is combined with a second
coenzyme-A molecule to form a molecule of acetyl-CoA. This molecule of acetyl-CoA is indistinguishable from acetyl-CoA derived from
aerobic glycolysis and thus may undergo further breakdown in the
Krebs Cycle (Fig. 3.4). The remaining activated fatty acid molecule
now is two carbon atoms shorter than it was initially and may begin
the beta oxidation cycle anew at reaction B. Reaction A is required

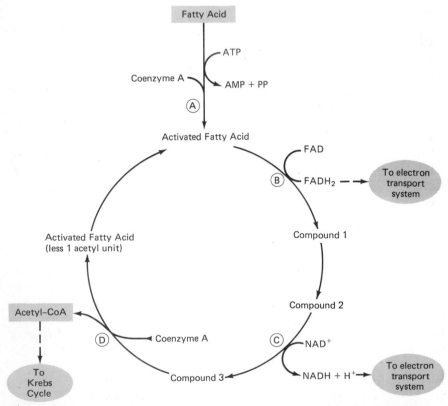

Figure 3.6. Oxidation of a fatty acid. Compound 1 is fatty acyl-CoA, compound 2 is β-hydroxyl acyl-CoA, compound 3 is β-keto acyl-CoA.

only for the first trip through the cycle. For each cycle, two more carbon atoms are split from the fatty acid and changed to acetyl-CoA.

ATP Produced with Fatty Acid Oxidation

Let us now show how much ATP could be produced as the result of the complete breakdown of one molecule of stearic acid, which has 18 carbon atoms in its chain. In the first passage through the fatty acid oxidation cycle, one ATP is used up in activation step A of Fig. 3.6. In reaction B one molecule of $FADH_2$ is formed which, upon passage through the electron transport system, results in the production of two ATP molecules. In reaction C of Fig. 3.6, a molecule of NADH is produced which can, via the electron transport system, cause three ATP molecules to be formed. Finally, in reaction D of Fig. 3.6, an acetyl-CoA molecule is liberated which, by way of the Krebs Cycle and the electron transport system, can be used for energy to produce 12 ATP molecules. (See Figs. 3.4, 3.5 for review.) Thus, in the first cycle of the fatty acid oxidation pathway, 17 ATP molecules are produced and one is expended for a *net* of 16 ATP molecules.

Since stearic acid (18 carbons) has nine acetyl units (nine pairs of carbon atoms), it can be recycled through the oxidation cycle eight times. (On the eighth cycle, two molecules of acetyl-CoA are produced from the remaining four carbon atoms so a ninth cycle is not required.) For each cycle a two-carbon acetyl unit will be split from the fatty acid chain. Because only the first passage through fatty acid oxidation requires the loss of one ATP in reaction A, each of the next six passes through the oxidation cycle can result in the production of 17 ATP molecules. On the eighth and last passage an additional 12 ATP molecules are produced from the extra acetyl-CoA. The grand total of ATP molecules produced with the complete oxidation of stearic acid to CO_2 and H_2O thus becomes

$$16 + (6 \times 17) + 29 = 147.$$

To attempt a comparison between ATP production from carbohydrates and that from fat is a little like comparing a glass of milk and a bottle of beer—each is better under certain conditions. First, let us compare the energy produced per carbon atom. For the aerobic breakdown of a six-carbon glucose molecule, 38 molecules of ATP can be obtained, whereas 147 ATP molecules are produced from the breakdown of an 18-carbon fatty acid molecule. Therefore, on the basis of ATP produced per carbon atom, fat comes out ahead—8.2 to 6.3, or 30 per cent more than carbohydrate. Fat also is the winner over carbohydrate if the comparison is made between energy stored per unit of weight; a pound of fat can supply more than twice the

ATP that can be produced at the expense of a pound of carbohydrate. Fat wins once again if the question concerns the supply of energy for a long duration of exercise or physical labor. The body reserves of carbohydrate are too small to sustain work for prolonged periods, but there is almost always (unfortunately for many) an overabundance of fat that can be called upon.

However, in a very important comparison—the ATP produced per unit of oxygen consumed—carbohydrate is the victor over fat. For example, 6 O_2 molecules are required to produce 38 ATP molecules during the aerobic breakdown of a molecule of glucose, whereas 26 O_2 molecules are used in the combustion of stearic acid to produce 147 ATP molecules. In this comparison carbohydrate is about 12 per cent more efficient in terms of oxygen consumed per ATP molecule produced, and in situations where maximal performance is to a great extent limited by oxygen supply (for example, in long–distance running, cycling or skiing), it is important to oxidize carbohydrate as long as the carbohydrate supply, especially muscle glycogen, lasts.

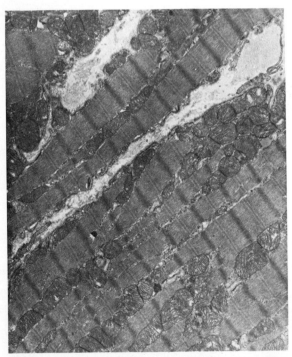

Figure 3.7. Electron micrograph of cardiac myofibrils showing rich supply of globular shaped mitochondria (magnification ×7,500). (Courtesy of G. Colin Budd, Physiology Department, Medical College of Ohio, Toledo, Ohio.)

In summary, both carbohydrates and fat are useful and important sources of reserve energy for exercise. Carbohydrate is a somewhat more efficient fuel in terms of ATP produced per molecule of oxygen consumed, but those persons engaged in long–duration physical labor or athletic events must rely also on fat in order to conserve the rather limited body reserves of carbohydrates.

AEROBIC ATP PRODUCTION FROM PROTEIN

Although many athletic coaches continue to provide their athletes with expensive pre–event meals high in protein hoping to increase their "energy supplies," it has been widely recognized by physiologists for many years that protein makes only minor contributions to ATP production during exercise unless the person who is exercising is also starving (1). This is not to say that protein cannot be used for energy (at rest, protein contributes about 5–10 per cent of the body's energy), but under normal conditions, protein is mostly used for building lean body tissue and is largely spared from energy metabolism as long as fat and carbohydrates are available. It is unusual to find any significant increase in protein use for energy during exercise when compared to rest.

Proteins are complex chains of amino acids, that is, acids that have an amino ($-NH_2$) group attached to one of their carbon atoms. Some of these amino acids are, with the exception of the amino groups, almost identical to compounds that we have seen in our studies of carbohydrate metabolism. For example, the amino acids alanine, serine and cysteine can be converted quite easily to pyruvic acid, which can then be oxidized by the Krebs Cycle (Fig. 3.4) with the consequent production of ATP. Other amino acids can be converted into molecules that occur in the Krebs Cycle and can, therefore, enter the Krebs Cycle and be oxidized to CO_2 and H_2O. Thus, although it is quite possible for proteins to be used for ATP production, the body sees fit to spare most proteins from this fate and uses them instead for the construction of new cells, including skeletal muscle cells. For all practical purposes, therefore, fat and carbohydrates are the main reserve energy sources for man during physical activity; protein is used only under desperate circumstances.

Review Questions

1. How is the catabolism of stored fuels related to the production of ATP?

2. Why is creatine phosphate called the primary fuel reserve?
3. What are two common means of replenishing ATP anaerobically?
4. In which part of the muscle cell does anaerobic metabolism of carbohydrate take place? Why?
5. Explain the importance of nicotinamide adenine dinucleotide (NAD) in oxidation–reduction reactions of energy metabolism.
6. Define oxidative phosphorylation.
7. Contrast the efficiency of aerobic ATP production from carbohydrate with anaerobic energy production. What are some implications of these differences in efficiency for exercise?
8. Explain in your own words how ATP is produced from the breakdown of fatty acids.
9. Compare the production of ATP from carbohydrate with the production of ATP from fat in terms of: 1) ATP per carbon atom, 2) ATP per gram of stored fuel, 3) ATP per liter of oxygen consumed, 4) involvement in various types of physical activity.
10. Describe how proteins can be used to generate ATP.

References

1. Astrand, P-O., and K. Rodahl. *Textbook of Work Physiology.* New York: McGraw-Hill, 1970, p. 456.
2. Gollnick, P. D., and D. W. King. Energy release in the muscle cell. *Medicine and Science in Sports,* 1969, **1:**23–31.
3. Gollnick, P. D., and L. Hermansen. Biochemical adaptations to exercise: anaerobic metabolism. In J. H. Wilmore (Ed.). *Exercise and Sport Sciences Reviews,* 1973, **1:**1–43.
4. McGilvery, R. W. The use of fuels for muscular work. In H. Howald and J. R. Poortmans (Eds.), *Metabolic Adaptation to Prolonged Physical Exercise.* Basel: Birkhauser Verlag, 1975, pp. 12–30.

4

Muscle fiber types and fuels for exercise

In the previous three chapters we have discussed the means by which a skeletal muscle obtains its energy for contraction and replenishes that energy supply at the expense of carbohydrates, fat and, infrequently, protein. We will make use of this background to describe important differences in fuel utilization for a variety of physical activities. But first, let us review the metabolic characteristics of fast- and slow-twitch muscles that, in part, determine which fuels are used during exercise.

MUSCLE FIBER TYPES

All skeletal muscle fibers are not entirely alike. One characteristic that has been used to distinguish two types of fibers in humans is the twitch contraction time of the fiber. If a fiber completes a contraction rapidly, it is a *fast twitch fiber;* if slowly, a *slow twitch fiber.* Fast twitch fibers are most important in activities requiring short, powerful bursts of contraction: the jumps, weight events, and sprints in track and field, the sprints in swimming, and rapid movements in hockey, soccer, basketball, and other team sports (7). The slow twitch fibers, on the other hand, are better adapted for endurance events that require repetitive contractions over a prolonged time period (12, 13, 14). These events are represented by distance running and swimming, canoeing, rowing, cycling, cross-country skiing, and most of the running action of team sports such as basketball and soccer.

As you may have guessed by now, the reason why fast twitch muscle fibers are especially adapted to short, explosive bursts of contraction and slow twitch fibers are used more for submaximal contractions is that these fiber types have different degrees of activity of some of the important enzymes that control energy metabolism. (See Table 4.1.) For example, fast twitch fibers have high levels of myosin ATPase activity in comparison to the slow twitch fibers. Recall that myosin ATPase activity is responsible for splitting ATP to release en-

Table 4.1.   Some Characteristics of Fast and Slow Twitch Muscle Fibers*

Characteristic	Fast	Slow
Myosin ATPase Activity	Greater	Less
Activities of Enzymes for Anaerobic Glycogen and Glucose Breakdown	Greater	Less
No. of Mitochondria	Less	Greater
Activities of Enzymes of Krebs Cycle, Electron Transport System	Less	Greater
No. of Capillaries per Fiber	Less	Greater
Activities of Enzymes for Fatty Acid breakdown	Less	Greater
Recruitment During Short Duration, Maximal Exercise	Greater	Less
Recruitment During Submaximal Exercise	Less	Greater

* It should be recognized that there is a continuum of metabolic profiles of fibers present in skeletal muscle, with many of the characteristics of some fast twitch fibers approaching those of slow fibers. The gross distinction between slow and fast fibers is designed to simplify the discussion.

ergy for the sliding of actin filaments past myosin filaments, and you can understand how greater myosin ATPase activity could result in faster contraction times.

Another important example of differences between enzyme characteristics of fast- and slow-twitch fibers is that fast twitch fibers have greater activities of *glycogen phosphorylase* and *phosphofructokinase*, enzymes that control the breakdown of muscle glycogen and glucose to lactic acid. Since glycogen and glucose breakdown are important for anaerobic ATP production, these fast twitch fibers are well-suited to contraction under conditions where oxygen supply is limited (such as strong, sustained contractions that shut off blood vessels), or where aerobic ATP production is inadequate to meet all the ATP demands of the contracting muscles (during a maximal sprint, for example.)

Slow twitch fibers are better adapted to long-duration exercise because they contain significantly greater amounts of mitochondrial enzymes, that is, the enzymes of the Krebs Cycle, the fatty acid oxidation cycle, and the electron transport system, that are responsible for aerobic ATP production. Slow twitch fibers also tend to have greater stores of intracellular fat that can be called upon for energy during long duration exercise. Finally, slow twitch fibers have a more extensive capillary network that can deliver oxygen, glucose and fatty acids to the fibers more rapidly than is true for fast twitch fibers.

Although fast twitch fibers tend to be used most frequently with explosive, short duration bursts of activity and slow twitch fibers, more often with longer duration activities, both fiber types become fatigued with prolonged heavy exercise, such as a maximal 10 kilometer run (14). Thus, slow twitch fibers are used preferentially in heavy long duration exercise, but as these fibers become exhausted, the fast twitch fibers are also called into play.

Fiber Type and Athletic Performance

Human skeletal muscles have a mixture of fiber types, fast twitch and slow twitch fibers being contained in the same muscle. There is a wide range of mixtures of the two types with ranges from 13–60 per cent slow twitch and 40–87 per cent fast twitch having been reported (11). The average percentage of slow twitch fibers in untrained subjects is about 36 and 46 per cent for thigh and shoulder muscles, respectively. Several studies of champion athletes have shown striking relationships between specific athletic abilities and certain peculiarities of fiber type populations (10, 11). Champion distance runners, for example, are characterized by extremely high percentages (up to 75 per cent) of slow twitch fibers in their leg muscles, whereas world class sprinters tend to possess a much higher than normal proportion (up to 74 per cent) of fast twitch fibers in their muscles. Likewise, cyclists, swimmers, and canoeists tend to have a high percentage of slow twitch fibers in their shoulder muscles compared to untrained subjects.

Do these studies mean that someone who is born with high percentages of fast- or slow-twitch fibers in his legs is bound to be an outstanding sprinter or distance runner? Of course not! There are too many other important factors that go into producing championship performances, such as motivation, skill, body build and dedication, that can mask an apparent physiological advantage such as fiber type population in skeletal muscles. However, it does seem to be true that muscle fiber composition plays an important role in determining championship performance, and that such performances are not likely to be observed in those who are not well-suited to a particular event by an advantageous distribution of fiber types in their muscles.

Heredity Versus Training in the Determination of Fiber Populations

If it is true that a high proportion of a particular fiber type is essential to championship performance, an important question is whether or not one can change his inherited fiber population by diet, training, or some other environmental change.

Early studies on laboratory animals produced evidence that suggested the possibility that a program of endurance training could bring about a greater proportion of slow twitch fibers in the trained animals (4, 8). Further work, however, seems to have demonstrated that only the *capacities* and not the contraction times of fibers can be changed (2, 10, 11). That is, with endurance training, both slow twitch and fast twitch fibers become better adapted to produce ATP for endurance exercise, but fast twitch fibers remain fast twitch fibers and are not converted into slow twitch fibers by training. Endurance training stimulates the production of mitochondrial enzymes for greater aerobic ATP production in both fast and slow twitch fibers, but the fiber types can still be distinguished on the basis of twitch contraction times.

Research on humans supports the idea that training does not bring about changes in the proportions of fast twitch and slow twitch fibers in a muscle (10). Therefore, it is unlikely that one who is born with an average proportion of slow twitch fibers in his leg muscles can ever become a world-class distance runner, no matter how great his dedication to training. As techniques for determining fiber types become more routine, it is possible that coaches will be able to more readily determine which athletes have the greatest potential for becoming champions.* Also, when a coach is puzzled by the poor response to training an athlete seems to experience, the coach might consider the possibility that the athlete in question has already obtained the maximum from his genetic potential. Both coach and athlete might be more satisfied if the athlete would train for another event or sport to which he may be better adapted by birth.

The considerations of heredity and muscle fiber populations discussed in the previous paragraph are probably of minor importance for low level competition. As most of us have observed in adolescent and preadolescent competition, some very unlikely candidates can become champions because of some peculiar combination of luck, fortitude, dedication, and training. It is only at the national and international levels of competition that inheritance of fiber types probably plays a major role in determining championship performance.

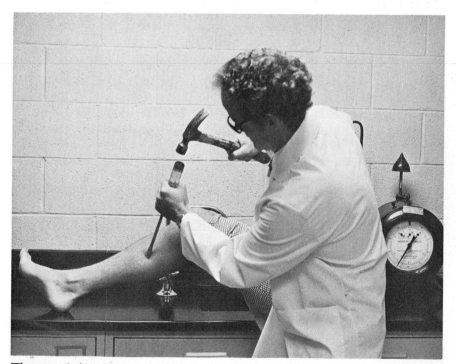

Figure 4.1. Author performing sophisticated biopsy of gastrocnemius muscle. (Photo courtesy of Joseph Conrad.)

* Currently, fiber typing requires that a small portion of muscle be removed with a large biopsy needle, quick frozen, thinly sliced, stained, and examined under a laboratory microscope.

FUELS FOR DIFFERENT TYPES OF EXERCISE

As may be apparent by now, the fuel used for a specific type of exercise is dependent to some extent upon the type of fiber involved in the exercise.

Fast twitch fibers tend to rely on creatine phosphate and the anaerobic breakdown of muscle glycogen and blood glucose for the replenishment of ATP, whereas slow twitch fibers are more apt to burn fat, glycogen and glucose aerobically because of their greater amounts of mitochondrial enzymes and greater supply of oxygen from a more extensive blood supply. These theoretical predictions of energy sources that are based on the anatomical and biochemical properties of muscle fiber types are shown to be quite accurate by direct measurements of the depletion of the various energy stores from muscle biopsies of men who participated in various types of physical activity.

Maximal, Short Bursts of Exercise

When subjects pedal a bicycle ergometer at heavy loads that can be maintained for no more than one or two minutes, nearly 40 per cent of muscle creatine phosphate stores are depleted after only 10 seconds, 50 per cent after 20 seconds, and 70 per cent after 60 seconds (19). Only very small changes in glycogen occur with such heavy work, and no significant change would be expected in blood glucose or fat stores. Nearly all the glycogen that is used is broken down anaerobically to lactic acid. A similar pattern of results would occur with any competitive athletic event lasting less than one or two minutes. The major fuels for such activities are stored ATP, creatine phosphate, and muscle glycogen (19). Thus, throwing, jumping and vaulting in track and field; sprints up to 800 meters; swims to 200 meters; cycling sprints; many individual gymnastics routines including apparatus routines; and weightlifting competitions would be examples of maximal, short bursts of activity that are performed chiefly at the expense of ATP, creatine phosphate and glycogen stores. Examples from physical labor in industry would include heavy lifting activities and activities where a vigorous contraction is sustained with little movement of the joints, such as, holding a heavy portable drill for brief periods (static contraction).

If maximal bursts of activity are repeated many times with intervening rest pauses, there will be some replenishment of ATP and creatine phosphate during the rest periods, and there will eventually be a fall in muscle glycogen levels, but the decrease will be no greater than approximately one-fourth of the glycogen value at rest (9, 19).

There may also be some use of fatty acids from the blood. It seems that ATP and creatine phosphate are replenished during the rest pauses at the expense of glycogen, and to some extent of blood glucose and fatty acids also. Only creatine phosphate, however, is likely to be severely depleted during such repeated work-rest intervals (19). Examples of work-rest intervals that would be accompanied by progressive decreases in ATP, creatine phosphate and muscle glycogen would include football competition, repeated sprints, fast-break basketball play and repeated swim sprints.

There is a rather straightforward relationship between the rate of creatine phosphate utilization and the degree of severity of the exercise. The heavier and more vigorous the activity in relation to one's capacity, the more creatine phosphate will be called upon to provide the energy necessary to replenish ATP supplies in the muscle. Creatine phosphate is always used to some degree at the beginning of any exercise, whether the work load is heavy or light for an individual; but as the loads become lighter and blood supply to the slow twitch fibers increases, less creatine phosphate and more glycogen, blood glucose and fatty acids are utilized for energy as the slow twitch fibers take over more of the work load (19). Thus, the relative intensity of the exercise, which, in turn, determines how long one can persist at an activity, is an extremely important factor in the allocation of fuel.

Heavy Exercise for Less Than 40 Minutes

When a person exercises as hard as possible for longer than one minute, but less than approximately 40 minutes, both creatine phosphate and a substantial amount of muscle glycogen are broken down for energy. The glycogen is catabolized both anaerobically and aerobically. There is still no danger of running out of glycogen in this type of activity, for example, in a 1,500–10,000 meter run or 400–2,000 meter swim, and fat would contribute probably less than 10 per cent of the energy cost of the exercise (19).

One rather conclusive bit of evidence that glycogen is an important fuel in this type of heavy exercise for a brief to moderate period is that subjects who have a genetic absence of glycogen phosphorylase, one of the enzymes necessary for glycogen breakdown, are unable to perform this type of exercise.

Heavy Exercise for 40–120 Minutes

Although the anaerobic breakdown of glycogen and creatine phosphate is important at the beginning of longer heavy exercise periods, a much greater total energy contribution is made by the aerobic breakdown of glycogen, glucose and fatty acids under these conditions. About one-fourth of the energy supply for exercise that results in exhaustion within 120 minutes may be derived from the oxidation of fatty acids, whereas most of the remaining energy is supplied by the aerobic breakdown of muscle glycogen and blood glucose (20). In long periods of heavy exercise, for example in soccer competition, distance running, swimming and cycling, muscle glycogen may be almost totally used up and is thought to be the major limiting factor in these activities (20). Exercise physiologists have found a nearly perfect correlation between the amount of glycogen stored in muscles prior to heavy exercise and one's ability to sustain the exercise for long periods. If muscle glycogen levels are increased by eating a diet high in carbohydrates, endurance also increases; with a fat diet, which lowers glycogen levels, endurance decreases (5, 20).

Heavy Exercise for More Than 120 Minutes

As hard work is prolonged, for example in a marathon race, a greater and greater contribution of the fuel for exercise comes from fat stored in the muscle cells and from fatty acids in the blood (1, 3, 6, 12, 16–22). This increased use of fat is a gradual process but may account for 20 per cent of the energy demands after one hour of exhaustive work and more than 50 per cent after four hours. Blood glucose is also increasingly used as exercise progresses beyond 120 minutes and is thought by many physiologists to be a possible limiting factor in such prolonged, heavy work. The answer to whether blood glucose or muscle glycogen is a more likely limiting factor in prolonged exercise may depend on the capacity of a given athlete to work for a long time at a high intensity. Accordingly, a well-trained athlete who can continue near maximum work for two or three hours probably depletes his muscle glycogen stores; this then limits his ability to continue working at the same high rate. However, a poorly trained subject may have to work at a lesser intensity in order to sustain the work for a long time, and he may suffer from a reduction in blood glucose, and not muscle glycogen.

Light Exercise

With light exercise there is a much greater activation of slow twitch fibers relative to fast twitch fibers, so that nearly all the energy for ATP replenishment is released by the *aerobic* breakdown of fat, glycogen and glucose. As the duration of light exercise increases, so too does the role played by the combustion of free fatty acids for energy. For example, one who walks continuously or works at a machine in industry for eight hours may supply up to 90 per cent of his

Table 4.2. Degree of Depletion of Fuel Reserves with Various Types of Exercise

Fuel	Maximal, Short Bursts, Static Contractions	Heavy Intermittent	Heavy, Less Than 40 Min.	Heavy, 40–120 Min.	Heavy, Over 120 Min.	Light
Creatine Phosphate	Great	Very Great	Moderate	Moderate	Moderate	Negligible
Muscle Glycogen	Slight	Moderate	Moderate	Very Great	Very Great	Negligible
Blood Glucose & Liver Glycogen	Negligible	Slight	Slight	Moderate to Great	Great to Very Great	Slight
Fatty Acids From Blood & Intracellular Triglyceride Stores	Negligible	Slight	Negligible	Negligible	Slight	Slight

energy needs by the aerobic breakdown of fatty acids at the end of the eight hours, but only 25–50 per cent during the first four hours of the work (1, 16, 19). This suggests an increasing recruitment of slow twitch fibers and an increasing activation of the enzymes involved in fatty acid breakdown as exercise is prolonged.

There is usually no severe depletion of fat, carbohydrate, or protein with prolonged light exercise, but occasionally blood glucose values begin to decline (Table 4.2) (17, 19). That muscle glycogen breakdown is not essential to prolonged light exercise is demonstrated by the normal endurance of such exercise by subjects who are unable to break down glycogen.

FUEL STORAGE DEPOTS—ALTERATIONS BY DIET AND EXERCISE

There are four generally recognized major compartments of the body where carbohydrates and fat can be stored. First, within the muscle cells themselves are found stores of glycogen and fat. Second, the blood contains circulating glucose and fatty acids. Third, the liver stores glycogen, which can be broken down to glucose and released into the blood to keep blood glucose levels high as exercise progresses. Finally, many cells of the body besides muscle cells store fat or triglyceride, and as fat is broken down in these cells, free fatty acids are made available to the blood for transport to the working tissues.

In previous discussions of the fuels used for different types of physical activity, it has been stated that with heavy, prolonged exercise muscle glycogen or blood glucose may decrease so much that they could cause one to stop or at least slow down his exercise. Therefore, it is of interest to know the extent to which diet can affect the levels of muscle glycogen, blood glucose and liver glycogen, the principal source of blood glucose. There is no need to consider the effects of diet on fat stores because it is widely accepted that even after severe, prolonged exercise there is a substantial amount of intramuscular triglyceride, fatty acids in the blood and triglyceride in extramuscular fat depots that remain to be used. As a matter of fact, at least one report showed that endurance decreased with greater pre–exercise intramuscular triglyceride stores (20). For most persons too much fat is a far greater problem than too little for exercise purposes.

CARBOHYDRATE STORES AND DIET

Carbohydrate stores, that is, muscle and liver glycogen and blood glucose, can be markedly affected by diet.

Liver Glycogen

In studies of men subjected to liver biopsies after 24 hours on high fat and protein diets, liver glycogen was nearly 90 per cent depleted, but after two days on a carbohydrate rich diet, liver glycogen stores were about 100 per cent greater than normal, resting values (Fig. 4.2) (19). Since prolonged, heavy exercise such as a marathon race can result in a severe depletion of liver glycogen and blood glucose stores, a sound practice would be to eat a fat and protein diet for several days, and then to consume a diet rich in carbohydrates for three or four days prior to competition.

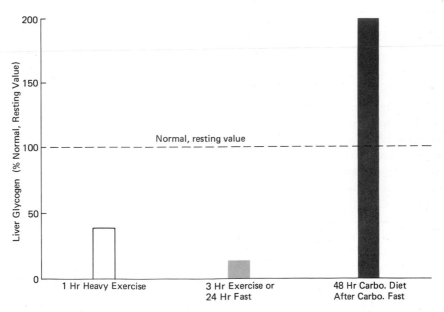

Figure 4.2. Effects of alterations in diet and exercise on liver glycogen. Data from reference 19.

Blood Glucose

Blood glucose stores can be elevated by eating a carbohydrate rich meal, but this high blood glucose level quickly stimulates the pancreas to secrete extra insulin that helps transport the glucose from the blood into the cells of the body tissues, thereby lowering the

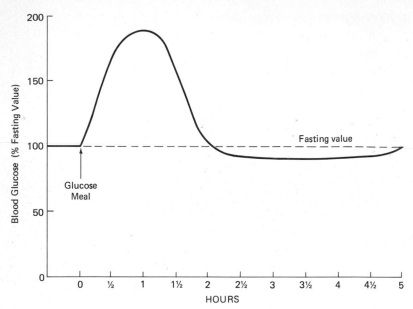

Figure 4.3. **Blood glucose levels following ingestion of 50 grams of glucose.**

blood glucose to below normal values (Fig. 4.3). Therefore, if one were preparing to compete in an intense three– or four–hour activity, he would have to weigh the possible value of consuming a carbohydrate diet an hour before the event with the likelihood that by the end of the race, when it was most needed, the glucose level would have been returned to lower levels by the action of insulin. Another consideration is the possible uncomfortable feeling caused by the ingestion of food one hour before competition. For most persons it seems likely that concentrating on filling liver and muscle glycogen stores for two or three days prior to competition would be a more effective regimen than consuming a carbohydrate meal just prior to the event. The effect of diet on liver glycogen stores has been described in previous paragraphs, and the filling of muscle glycogen stores is discussed next.

Filling of Muscle Glycogen Stores—Diet and Exercise

One's ability to persevere at heavy exercise for about 40 to 120 minutes seems to be limited chiefly by the amount of glycogen stored in the working muscles prior to exercise (5, 19). Therefore, for this type of work, it is important to know how best to increase muscle glycogen stores during the training period. Two factors seem to be important in this regard: diet and exercise.

Research based on biopsy samples of human thigh muscles suggests that maximal filling of muscle glycogen stores occurs only after the muscles have been previously depleted of their glycogen by means of exercise coupled with a low carbohydrate diet (5, 19). With a low carbohydrate diet alone for two days, it is possible to reduce glycogen levels of resting muscle by about 30 per cent, and if this reduction is followed by three or four days of a high carbohydrate diet, the resting glycogen levels will be increased to about 50 per cent over normal values. However, when a low carbohydrate diet is accompanied by exhaustive exercise for approximately 90 minutes, glycogen is almost totally depleted from the muscles. With a subsequent high-carbohydrate diet for three or four days, the glycogen then overshoots normal resting levels by 100–200 per cent (Fig. 4.4) (5, 19).

Thus, to maximally fill muscle glycogen stores, it is sometimes suggested that an athlete consume a low carbohydrate diet (just enough carbohydrate to make the food palatable) for 2–3 days about

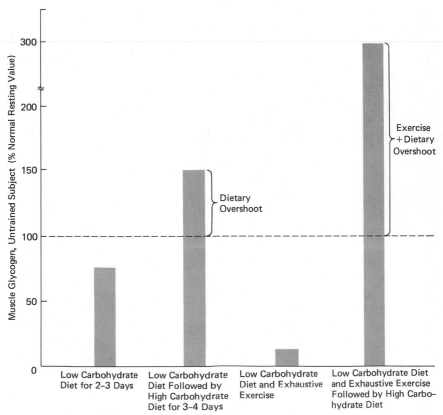

Figure 4.4. Glycogen overshoot in untrained subject following manipulation of diet and exercise.

6–7 days prior to competition. Then, about 3–4 days before competition, the athlete should work to exhaustion to totally deplete glycogen stores. This should be followed by 3–4 days of light workouts and a diet rich in carbohydrates (5).

Although many athletes have given testimonial evidence that this recommended diet-exercise regimen produces good performance results, it should be brought to the reader's attention that athletes who are well trained probably do not experience the glycogen "supercompensation" or "overshoot" phenomenon because their glycogen levels are already high because of their training. Another way to describe this is: Trained athletes may have double the normal resting values of glycogen that are found in untrained subjects so they already have "supercompensated" glycogen values at rest; an extra bout of exercise or extra carbohydrate in the diet does not seem to raise this already high level of glycogen. For well-trained athletes, therefore, it is probably sufficient to regularly consume a high carbohydrate diet to maintain high resting levels of glycogen.

Review Questions

1. Fast twitch muscle fibers are most involved in what sort of exercise?
2. Contrast the enzyme characteristics of fast and slow twitch muscle fibers. Explain the implications for performance of these differences.
3. List two nonenzymatic characteristics of slow twitch fibers that make them well suited for long duration exercise.
4. Describe the effects of physical training on muscle fiber types. Does it seem to be true that fast twitch fibers are changed into slow twitch fibers?
5. Which energy sources are used for a 1-minute maximal burst of exercise? Compare that energy metabolism with the energy sources for a maximal 30-minute exercise bout.
6. Explain the effect of a fat diet on one's ability to sustain heavy exercise for 1–2 hours.
7. What is the effect on blood glucose levels of a high-carbohydrate meal one hour prior to exercise?
8. Outline a diet-exercise program designed to increase muscle glycogen stores.

References

1. Ahlborg, G., P. Felig, L. Hagenfeldt, R. Hendler and J. Wahren. Substrate turnover during prolonged exercise in man. Splanchnic and leg metabolism of glucose, free fatty acids, and amino acids. *Journal of Clinical Investigation*, 1974, **53:**1080–1090.

2. Baldwin, K. M., G. H. Klinkerfuss, R. L. Terjung, P. A. Molé, and J. O. Holloszy. Respiratory capacity of white, red, and intermediate muscle: Adaptative response to exercise. *American Journal of Physiology*, 1972, **222:**373–378.

3. Baldwin, K. M., J. S. Reitman, R. L. Terjung, W. W. Winder and J. O. Holloszy. Substrate depletion in different types of muscle and in liver during prolonged running. *American Journal of Physiology*, 1973, **225:**1045–1050.

4. Barnard, R. J., V. R. Edgerton, and J. B. Peter. Effects of exercise on skeletal muscle. I. Biochemical and histochemical properties. *Journal of Applied Physiology.* 1970, **28:**762–766.

5. Bergstrom, J. and E. Hultman. Nutrition for maximal sports performance. *Journal of the American Medical Association,* 1972, **221:**999–1006.

6. Brooke, J. D., G. J. Davies and L. F. Green. Nutrition during severe prolonged exercise in trained cyclists. *Proceedings of the Nutrition Society,* 1972, **31:**93A.

7. Edgerton, V. R., B. Essen, B. Saltin, and D. R. Simpson. Glycogen depletion in specific types of human skeletal muscle fibers in intermittent and continuous exercise. In H. Howald and J. R. Poortmans (Eds.), *Metabolic Adaptation to Prolonged Physical Exercise,* Basel: Birkhauser Verlag, 1975, pp. 402–415.

8. Edgerton, V. R., L. Gerchman, and R. Carrow. Histochemical changes in rat skeletal muscle after exercise. *Experimental Neurology,* 1969, **24:**110–123.

9. Fox, E. L., S. Robinson and D. L. Wiegman. Metabolic energy sources during continuous and interval running. *Journal of Applied Physiology,* 1969, **27:**174–178.

10. Gollnick, P. D., R. B. Armstrong, B. Saltin, C. W. Saubert IV, W. L. Sembrowich, and R. E. Shepherd. Effect of training on enzyme activity and fiber composition of human skeletal muscle. *Journal of Applied Physiology,* 1973, **34:**107–111.

11. Gollnick, P. D., R. B. Armstrong, C. W. Saubert IV, K. Piehl, and B. Saltin. Enzyme activity and fiber composition in skeletal muscle of untrained and trained men. *Journal of Applied Physiology,* 1972, **33:**312–319.

12. Gollnick, P., R. B. Armstrong, C. W. Saubert IV, W. L. Semb-

rowich, and R. E. Shepherd. Glycogen depletion patterns in human skeletal muscle fibers during prolonged work. *Pflugers Archives*, 1973, **344:**1–12.

13. Gollnick, P., R. B. Armstrong, W. L. Sembrowich, R. E. Shepherd and B. Saltin. Glycogen depletion pattern in human skeletal muscle fibers after heavy exercise. *Journal of Applied Physiology*, 1973, **34:**615–618.

14. Gollnick, P. D., K. Piehl, J. Karlsson, and B. Saltin. Glycogen depletion patterns in human skeletal muscle fibers after varying types and intensities of exercise. In H. Howald and J. R. Poortmans (Eds.), *Metabolic Adaptation to Prolonged Physical Exercise*. Basel: Birkhauser Verlag, 1975, pp. 416–421.

15. Gollnick, P., K. Piehl, C. W. Saubert IV, R. B. Armstrong and B. Saltin. Diet, exercise and glycogen changes in human muscle fibers. *Journal of Applied Physiology*, 1972, **33:**421–425.

16. Hagenfeldt, L. and J. Wahren. Human forearm metabolism during exercise. VII: FFA uptake and oxidation at different work intensities. *Scandinavian Journal of Clinical Laboratory Investigation*, 1972, **30:**429–436.

17. Keul, J., G. Haralambie, T. Arnold and W. Schumann. Heart rate and energy-yielding substrates in blood during long–lasting running. *European Journal of Applied Physiology*, 1974, **32:**279–289.

18. Keul, J., G. Haralambie and G. Frittin. Intermittent exercise: Arterial lipid substrates and arteriovenous differences. *Journal of Applied Physiology*, 1974, **36:**159–162.

19. Pernow, B. and B. Saltin (Eds.). *Muscle Metabolism During Exercise*. New York: Plenum Press, 1971.

20. Reitman, J., K. M. Baldwin and J. O. Holloszy. Intramuscular triglyceride utilization by red, white, and intermediate skeletal muscle and heart during exhausting exercise. *Proceedings of the Society for Experimental Biology and Medicine*, 1973, **142:**628–631.

21. Therriault, D. G., G. A. Beller, J. A. Smoake and L. H. Hartley. Intramuscular energy sources in dogs during physical work. *Journal of Lipid Research*, 1973, **14:**54–60.

22. Wahren, J., P. Felig, G. Ahlborg and L. Jorfeldt. Glucose metabolism during leg exercise in man. *The Journal of Clinical Investigation*, 1971, **50:**2715–2725.

5

Nutrition and athletic performance

There is historical evidence that as early as 532 B.C., some people recognized that optimal nutrition was important for athletic performance. For example, legend has it that Milo of Croton, who won wrestling events at seven straight Olympic Games, consumed each day 20 pounds of bread, 20 pounds of meat and 18 pints of wine. It is also said that he once carried a four-year-old bull on his shoulders around the stadium at Olympia, killed it with a single blow of his fist, and then ate the whole animal in a single day (2).

Thus, for many centuries athletes, coaches, trainers, and physicians have passed down many radical ideas on nutrition for optimal athletic performance. Some of the more absurd ideas that held sway for many years include the practice of letting blood with leeches to remove "toxic substances" from the blood and totally restricting water intake to provide "training discipline." Most of the "wonder" diets for athletes that have been proposed over the years have no sound basis and only serve to make the athlete's life more grueling than it need be. It is unfortunate that so many coaches and athletes are poorly informed on the nutrition of athletes, because this ignorance makes them susceptible to misleading advertising claims and overblown testimonials from equally uninformed coaches and athletes about the value of some special dietary manipulation. It is the purpose of this section of the text, therefore, to cast some light into the shadows of athletic nutrition so that the reader will be better equipped to evaluate new ideas in this field and perhaps save himself, his athletes or his athletic budget needless expense on useless dietary supplements.

KNOWN NUTRITIONAL REQUIREMENTS OF ATHLETES

It is easy to discuss the minimal nutritional requirements that are known to exist for normal persons. Unfortunately, relatively few investigations of nutritional requirements for athletes have been carried out. Also, it is likely that there are unknown nutritional factors important to *optimal* athletic performance. Therefore, the following discussion is incomplete to some extent because of a lack of information regarding these unrecognized nutritional factors.

Total Caloric Requirements for Athletes

The generally accepted common expression of energy units for human energy intake and expenditure is the large calorie (kilocalorie or Calorie) which is the energy required to raise the temperature of one kilogram of water by one degree Celsius under certain conditions. For most persons the average caloric intake required to maintain body weight during normal daily activities ranges between 1700–3000 kcal per day with smaller, older women requiring substantially fewer calories than larger, younger, more active males. Depending on the type of training and competition, athletes require an additional 400–2000 kcal per day to maintain body weight during training, with athletes such as sprinters and field events specialists requiring a few extra kcal and distance runners, swimmers and cyclists requiring perhaps twice the energy that an average adult needs (2).

Protein Requirements for Athletes

One of the most discussed topics among athletes and coaches is the value of high protein diets in athletic nutrition. There are two basic reasons why some believe that a high protein diet is essential to quality performance. First, some still believe that protein is "energy food" that supplies energy for muscle contraction. This belief may stem from early ideas that muscle was "burned" during exercise and that protein was needed to rebuild this muscle tissue during recovery periods. However, it has been known for many years that protein is not a significant fuel during exercise unless the athlete has been starved (2, 3). Therefore, if a coach provides pregame steak for athletes because he hopes to improve their fuel reserves, that coach is wasting money. The provision of such meals for psychological benefits, however, may be another matter. If an athlete believes that eating meat makes him more "virile," the pregame steak may be worth the money.

The second reason why supplemental protein is often considered important for athletes is that the extra protein is supposed to be valuable for building up growing muscles and bones. It is true, of course, that a daily intake of proteins is necessary for building enzymes and tissue cells, including muscle and bone. Proteins are constantly undergoing a dynamic process of being built up and broken down. When proteins are degraded, some of the nitrogen constituents of the protein are lost in the urine. These nitrogenous products can be replaced only by the dietary intake of more protein—the body cannot manufacture nitrogen. Consequently, in order to maintain body protein stores, protein must be included in the diet. The important questions are how much protein is needed daily, and to what extent can additional protein be used by the body for building extra muscle tissue?

The standard rule of thumb for protein intake is that every day a person should consume about one gram of protein for every kilogram of body weight. According to this rule, since a kilogram is about 2.2 pounds, a person who weighs 154 pounds or 70 kilograms should need about 70 grams of protein intake each day to meet the demands of tissue maintenance and growth. Although experts disagree on precisely how much protein is needed daily, very few would maintain that more than one gram of protein per kilogram of body weight is needed every day. As a matter of fact, the one gram per kilogram rule has a built-in safety factor, and most authorities believe that about half that amount would satisfy the needs of most adults. There is some evidence to support the view that a greater protein intake can increase the production of muscle in weightlifters, field events specialists and wrestlers; but most of the extra protein is simply broken down, its nitrogen is lost in the urine and sweat, and the remainder of the protein molecule is converted to fat. On the other hand, as long as other nutrients are not slighted, there is no known risk (other than financial) in consuming extra protein. If one is determined to have protein supplements, he should simply eat more ordinary fish, meats and vegetables and avoid paying premium prices for such concoc-

Table 5.1.   Protein Food Sources

Food Serving (Weight In Grams)	Water (%)	kcal	Fat (%)	Carbohydrate (%)	Protein (%)	Approximate Amount Needed To Supply 70 Grams Protein
Chicken, fried drumstick without bone (38 grams)	55	90	10.5	Trace	31.5	6 drumsticks
Lamb, chop, broiled without bone (112 grams)	47	400	29.5	0	22.3	3 chops
Ham (85 grams)	54	245	22.4	0	21.2	4 servings
Pork chop, without bone (66 grams)	42	260	31.8	0	24.2	4½ chops
Bologna, 4 slices (114 grams)	56	345	27.3	1	11.8	20 slices
Frankfurter, one (51 grams)	58	155	27.5	2	12.0	11½ franks
Tuna fish, canned (85 grams)	61	170	8.2	0	28.2	3 servings (1½ cans)
Hamburger (85 grams)	54	245	20.0	Trace	24.7	3½ servings
Steak, broiled (85 grams)	44	330	31.8	0	23.5	3½ servings

Food					
Navy beans, 1 cup (261 grams)	68	310	0.4	23	6.1	4 cups
Green beans, 1 cup (239 grams)	94	45	Trace	3.0	0.8	36½ cups
Green peas, 1 cup (160 grams)	82	115	0.6	11.9	5.6	8 cups
Peanut butter, 1 tbsp. (16 grams)	2	95	50.0	18.8	25.0	½ lb.
White bread, slice (23 grams)	36	60	4.4	50.0	8.7	35 slices
Cheese pizza, 14 inch (600 grams)	45	1480	8.0	36.0	9.3	1¼ pizzas
Skim milk, 1 cup (246 grams)	90	90	Trace	5.3	3.7	7½ cups
Yogurt, 1 cup (246 grams)	89	120	1.6	5.3	3.3	9 cups
Egg, boiled (50 grams)	74	80	12.0	2.0	13.0	11 eggs
Potato chips, 10 (20 grams)	2	115	40.0	50.0	5.0	700 chips
Watermelon, 2 lbs. (925 grams)	93	115	0.1	2.9	0.2	66 pounds
Beer, 12–oz. can (360 grams)	92	150	0.0	3.8	0.4	49 cans
Cola drink, 8 oz. (240 grams)	90	95	0.0	10.0	0.0	9,684 bottles

tions as "proteins from the sea," "high protein candy bars," "dessicated liver protein flakes," and the like. A list of protein food sources is shown in Table 5.1.

One further concept about dietary protein that should be discussed is the need for "high quality" proteins in the diet. In order for a human protein to be synthesized, the diet must supply all of the amino acids that are components of that protein; if one or more of these "essential" amino acids is missing from the diet, none of the protein can be synthesized. In general, protein from animal sources tends to be "high quality" protein and contains all the essential amino acids, whereas protein derived from vegetables and other foods may be deficient in one or more of these amino acids. The effects on growth of feeding various protein sources to laboratory animals are shown in Fig. 5.1. From the graph it is apparent that feeding a great deal of low quality protein can retard growth much more severely than the feeding of insufficient amounts of high quality protein. It should be noted here that just because a diet is lacking in animal protein it does not mean the diet has inadequate proteins; mixtures of proteins from different vegetables and grains can supply all the essential amino acids (5). That is why vegetarians do not always show signs of protein malnutrition.

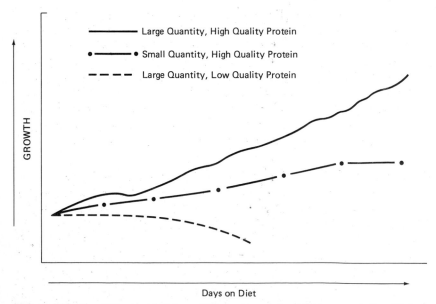

Figure 5.1.   Effects of three different protein diets on growth of laboratory animals.

Fat Requirements for Athletes

Some fat in foods makes food more palatable to most persons, so that a total lack of fat in the diet can lead to inadequate intake of other nutrients because of poor appetite. A total lack of fat would also make adequate calorie intake very difficult for an endurance athlete because of the extremely large quantities of carbohydrates and protein that would be required to supply up to four or five thousand kcal per day. Otherwise, the principal requirement for fat arises from the need for a fatty acid called linoleic acid, which, if absent from the diet, results in symptoms such as weight loss and dry, scaly skin. Only a prolonged, nonfat diet would be apt to result in linoleic acid deficiency because there is such a large store of linoleic acid in the fat depots of the body. In summary, as long as an athlete maintains his optimal weight and does not live on a fat-free diet, there is little danger of his experiencing fat deficiency. On the contrary, a common problem is an excessive intake of fat that leads to obesity and may eventually lead to an increased risk of developing cardiovascular disease.

Carbohydrate Requirements for Athletes

For optimal growth there exists only a small requirement for carbohydrates since many of the body's carbohydrates can be synthesized from protein sources. It would be very difficult for a sedentary person to devise a carbohydrate deficient diet that could be tolerated for long periods because there is a small amount of carbohydrate in nearly all but pure fat foods (for example, corn oil or soybean oil). However, it takes time for the body to adapt to a low carbohydrate diet and in that time period the dieter might experience unpleasant symptoms, including lack of energy. Also, anyone who performs heavy work or prolonged light work needs more than the minimal amounts of carbohydrate for optimal performance. This need for extra carbohydrates is shown in studies of the effects of diet on endurance; a high carbohydrate diet nearly always increases one's endurance to prolonged heavy exercise (6). As a matter of fact, the consumption of a high carbohydrate diet, especially in the days just prior to competition in heavy exercise that lasts for about 40 minutes or longer, is one of the few dietary manipulations for athletes that is supported by solid laboratory and field research evidence (1).

It should be recalled from previous discussions in this chapter that the feeding of extra carbohydrates should not be expected to improve performance in events lasting less than 30–40 minutes, because in these events there is at most only a moderate depletion of muscle glycogen reserves. Unfortunately, there is no known dietary regimen that has been proven to increase the muscle stores of creatine phosphate. Consequently, from an energy point of view, it probably makes little difference whether a javelin thrower eats a normal diet, a high protein diet or a case of bananas every day; none of these will have much effect on his ATP and creatine phosphate stores.

A list of various foods with their caloric values and nutritional composition is shown in Appendix A. If a high carbohydrate diet is desired, a selection of foods should be compiled that 1) has a total caloric content sufficient to maintain optimal body weight for the individual in question and 2) consists of 7–10 per cent high quality protein, about 10 per cent fat, and the remainder carbohydrate.

Vitamin Requirements for Athletes

One of the biggest gold mines for unscrupulous promoters is the sale of millions of dollars worth of unnecessary and sometimes harmful vitamin supplements. This is not to say that no one needs vitamin supplements, only that most people probably do not. The actions of many of the vitamins are required for ATP production, so many athletes and coaches are willing to try out massive doses of vitamins in the hope that more vitamins will help produce more energy.

How are vitamins used in energy metabolism? Recall in our discussions of fuel reserves how often we referred to NAD (nicotinamide adenine dinucleotide), FAD (flavin adenine dinucleotide) and coenzyme A. The basic ingredients of these compounds are the vitamins niacin (nicotinic acid), riboflavin (B_2) and pantothenic acid, respectively. Without these and other vitamins, ATP production would come to a halt. These vitamins and others serve as coenzymes that are required for the proper function of enzymes.

A list of suggested vitamin intakes is shown in Table 5.2. However, it should be noted that there are some difficulties in establishing daily vitamin and mineral allowances that are optimal for everyone. First, there is usually some variability in requirements depending on body weight, age, and metabolic peculiarities, and almost nothing is known about the effects of *severe* athletic training on vitamin levels in the body. Second, daily allowances are sometimes developed on the basis of whether or not some clinical symptom (hair loss, skin discoloration, and so on) appears with less than the recommended daily allowance; however, it may be that subclinical signs, such as changes in enzyme activities or hormone levels, occur in the absence of clinical evidence of vitamin deficiency. Consequently, recommended daily allowances may not be optimal allowances. Since the most important functions of many vitamins are not clearly understood, it is

Table 5.2. Food and Nutrition Board, National Academy of Sciences–National Research Council Recommended Daily Dietary Allowances,[1] Revised 1974. Designed for the maintenance of good nutrition of practically all healthy people in the U.S.A.

	Age (years)	Weight (kg)	Weight (lb)	Height (cm)	Height (in)	Protein (gm)	Energy (kcal)[2]	Vitamin A Activity (RE)[3]	Vitamin A Activity (IU)	Vitamin D (IU)	Vitamin E Activity[5] (IU)	Ascorbic Acid (mg)	Folacin[6] (µg)	Niacin[7] (mg)	Riboflavin (mg)	Thiamin (mg)	Vitamin B6 (mg)	Vitamin B12 (µg)	Calcium (mg)	Phosphorus (mg)	Iodine (µg)	Iron (mg)	Magnesium (mg)	Zinc (mg)
Infants	0.0–0.5	6	14	60	24	kg × 2.2	kg × 117	420[4]	1400	400	4	35	50	5	0.4	0.3	0.3	0.3	360	240	35	10	60	3
	0.5–1.0	9	20	71	28	kg × 2.0	kg × 108	400	2000	400	5	35	50	8	0.6	0.5	0.4	0.3	540	400	45	15	70	5
Children	1–3	13	28	86	34	23	1300	400	2000	400	7	40	100	9	0.8	0.7	0.6	1.0	800	800	60	15	150	10
	4–6	20	44	110	44	30	1800	500	2500	400	9	40	200	12	1.1	0.9	0.9	1.5	800	800	80	10	200	10
	7–10	30	66	135	54	36	2400	700	3300	400	10	40	300	16	1.2	1.2	1.2	2.0	800	800	110	10	250	10
Males	11–14	44	97	158	63	44	2800	1000	5000	400	12	45	400	18	1.5	1.4	1.6	3.0	1200	1200	130	18	350	15
	15–18	61	134	172	69	54	3000	1000	5000	400	15	45	400	20	1.8	1.5	2.0	3.0	1200	1200	150	18	400	15
	19–22	67	147	172	69	54	3000	1000	5000	400	15	45	400	20	1.8	1.5	2.0	3.0	800	800	140	10	350	15
	23–50	70	154	172	69	56	2700	1000	5000		15	45	400	18	1.6	1.4	2.0	3.0	800	800	130	10	350	15
	51+	70	154	172	69	56	2400	1000	5000		15	45	400	16	1.5	1.2	2.0	3.0	800	800	110	10	350	15
Females	11–14	44	97	155	62	44	2400	800	4000	400	12	45	400	16	1.3	1.2	1.6	3.0	1200	1200	115	18	300	15
	15–18	54	119	162	65	48	2100	800	4000	400	12	45	400	14	1.4	1.1	2.0	3.0	1200	1200	115	18	300	15
	19–22	58	128	162	65	46	2100	800	4000	400	12	45	400	14	1.4	1.1	2.0	3.0	800	800	100	18	300	15
	23–50	58	128	162	65	46	2000	800	4000		12	45	400	13	1.2	1.0	2.0	3.0	800	800	100	18	300	15
	51+	58	128	162	65	46	1800	800	4000		12	45	400	12	1.1	1.0	2.0	3.0	800	800	80	10	300	15
Pregnant						+30	+300	1000	5000	400	15	60	800	+2	+0.3	+0.3	2.5	4.0	1200	1200	125	18+[8]	450	20
Lactating						+20	+500	1200	6000	400	15	80	600	+4	+0.5	+0.3	2.5	4.0	1200	1200	150	18	450	25

[1] The allowances are intended to provide for individual variations among most normal persons as they live in the United States under usual environmental stresses. Diets should be based on a variety of common foods in order to provide other nutrients for which human requirements have been less well defined. See text for more-detailed discussion of allowances and of nutrients not tabulated.

[2] Kilojoules (KJ) = 4.2 × kcal.

[3] Retinol equivalents.

[4] Assumed to be all as retinol in milk during the first six months of life. All subsequent intakes are assumed to be one-half as retinol and one-half as β-carotene when calculated from international units. As retinol equivalents, three-fourths are as retinol and one-fourth as β-carotene.

[5] Total vitamin E activity, estimated to be 80 per cent as α-tocopherol and 20 percent other tocopherols. See text for variation in allowances.

[6] The folacin allowances refer to dietary sources as determined by Lactobacillus casei assay. Pure forms of folacin may be effective in doses less than one-fourth of the Recommended Dietary Allowances.

[7] Although allowances are expressesd as niacin, it is recognized that on the average 1 mg of niacin is derived from each 60 mg of dietary tryptophan.

[8] This increased requirement cannot be met by ordinary diets, therefore the use of supplemental iron is recommended.

very difficult to determine optimal levels of intake for the entire population.

In spite of the difficulties present in accurately determining optimal vitamin doses, most nationally recognized figures in nutrition research maintain that nearly all Americans who consume a reasonably well-balanced diet obtain adequate vitamin intake in their foods and that athletes, too, get adequate vitamins because they eat more food and thus get more vitamins than the ordinary person. Let us take a slightly different approach and simply state that there is no unequivocal evidence that any vitamin supplement will enhance athletic performance, but some contradictory evidence concerning at least three vitamins, B_1, C and E, does exist. Let us consider these three first.

Thiamine (B_1). From a biochemical standpoint, thiamine is involved in the reaction by which carbon dioxide is removed from pyruvic acid before pyruvic acid enters the Krebs Cycle; therefore, thiamine is especially important for the breakdown of carbohydrates and fats for energy. Although the most thorough studies in the 1940's showed no effect of thiamine supplementation on work performance, a few others have appeared in the research literature that suggest a beneficial effect of thiamine supplementation on endurance (4). Consequently, there remains a possibility that B_1 supplements might aid performance under certain conditions, but since thiamine is rapidly excreted in the urine as soon as its concentration surpasses a threshold level in the body fluids, it seems unlikely that anyone on a well-balanced diet will benefit from thiamine supplements. There certainly is no clinical evidence, such as painful nerves, heart failure or constipation, that physical training produces thiamine deficiency. There is also no evidence that thiamine supplements are harmful since the excess simply enriches the urine.

Ascorbic Acid (C). Clinical signs of vitamin C deficiency do not occur until after about seven weeks on diets that contain no vitamin C. These signs include hemorrhage beneath the skin after inflation of a blood pressure cuff around the upper arm, slow healing of wounds, and bleeding of the gums. Some believe, though, that these clinical signs only show the late stages of deficiency, and that up to 5 or 10 grams of ascorbic acid per day is required for optimal functioning of the body. Most authorities suggest that 30–60 milligrams of ascorbic acid per day are adequate. Unfortunately, the exact function of ascorbic acid is unknown, so that the argument about how much is needed each day is difficult to resolve.

Because it is suspected that ascorbic acid is involved in the production of hormones from the adrenal glands that are important for exercise, the use of ascorbic acid supplementation as an agent for improving work performance has been studied quite often. As with thiamine, however, the results of this research are contradictory with the vast majority of studies showing no evidence of a beneficial effect of ascorbic acid supplementation on performance (2). Although there is no proven harmful effect of consuming large quantities of vitamin C regularly, many individuals do experience nausea and diarrhea-like symptoms when this is done, and a few recent studies suggest that more damaging effects may occur with habitually high intakes of vitamin C. There is also some evidence that the body acquires a tolerance for large doses of vitamin C, so that continued maintenance of high doses is needed to maintain body stores of the vitamin.

Alpha–tocopherol (E). Because a severe deficiency of vitamin E causes muscular weakness and a reduction of creatine in the muscles, some persons believe that vitamin E supplements should increase strength and creatine concentrations in the muscles, thereby benefiting muscular performance. Once again, however, most of the literature on the effects of vitamin E supplementation on exercise capacity does not point in this direction (2, 4). The more authoritative studies have not provided any evidence that extra quantities of vitamin E can benefit strength or endurance. Therefore, an athlete should not be led to believe that vitamin E supplements supplied in wheat germ, for example, will improve his performance.

Usually, but not always, any meaningful effect of a food supplement will be shown in nearly all the studies in which the effect has been tested. It is most likely that any beneficial effect of supplementary vitamins B_1, C, or E on athletic performance is a small effect that can easily be obscured by more important performance factors, such as training intensity and motivation.

Other Vitamins and Performance. There is no general support for the view that the supplementary intake of any vitamins can benefit athletic performance (2). Some vitamins, for example, A and D, are stored to such a great extent that deficiency symptoms would not occur for months or years with a diet totally lacking in those vitamins. In fact, excessive supplements of A and D have been known to cause toxic side effects including nausea, headaches, diarrhea and even death.

The daily requirements of other vitamins (for example, B_{12}, folic acid, inositol, pantothenic acid and biotin) appear to be so small that the occurrence of deficiencies during exercise or training is highly improbable. If a coach suspects that an athlete has a vitamin-poor diet and has no success in improving that diet, a prudent approach would be to supply the athlete with multiple vitamin capsules on a one per day basis. This approach should minimize not only the expense but also the possible toxic side effects of large dose, "fad" vitamin therapy that is unwarranted according to our present state of knowledge and is perhaps dangerous.

Mineral Requirements for Athletes

Another aspect of athletic nutrition that is sometimes exploited by commercial interests, and may be relied upon by individual athletes and coaches to give a "performance edge," is the use of mineral supplements in the diet. The underlying reason why some people believe that extra minerals might benefit athletic performance is that many minerals such as magnesium, manganese, and calcium are undeniably important cofactors for the proper activity of the enzymes that are involved in energy metabolism, that is, in the production of ATP. Suggested daily mineral allowances are listed in Table 5.2.

Although there are no proven benefits of mineral supplementation for athletic performance, it is conceivable that individual athletes may have slight deficiencies in one or more minerals, depending on their training routines and diets. For individuals on diets that restrict the intake of dairy foods, for example, calcium intake may be inadequate since about 75 per cent of dietary calcium usually comes from daily products. Also, iron supplements may be beneficial for some young adult females whose dietary intake of iron is inadequate to replace the iron lost in the menstrual blood flow. However, it is extremely unlikely that well-fed males would benefit from iron supplementation, since the liver stores substantial amounts of iron that can provide iron stores for months on an iron free diet. Excess iron, cobalt or molybdenum supplementation can, as with some vitamins, cause toxic effects.

Deficiencies in other minerals are extremely rare in normal Americans, so it is highly improbable that mineral supplements will improve athletic performance. Extra salt and fluid intake can be important during prolonged work in the heat, and will be discussed in the chapter on temperature regulation during exercise.

PRE-EVENT MEALS

Most athletes learn what they know about pre-event nutrition from their coaches, who learned it from their own coaches when they were in training, and many times, but certainly not always, the knowledge handed down from coach to athlete is either completely erroneous or unsubstantiated by any physiological facts. It is not uncommon, for example, to hear condemned the eating of perfectly good, high carbohydrate foods such as spaghetti, macaroni and pastries, when eating high carbohydrate meals is nearly the only dietary manipulation that has been shown to be potentially effective in improving performance in high intensity, long duration events. The truth is that the main benefit of the pre-event meal is mostly a psychological one—if the athlete believes that what he is eating will benefit his performance, there is a good chance it might. On the other hand, if the athlete thinks his pre-event meal will hurt his performance, it makes little difference whether he has consumed a well-balanced meal; his performance may be subpar.

Nearly every study of the effects of the composition of pre-event meals, the absence of a meal, or the timing of a meal before competition has failed to provide evidence of any significant beneficial or adverse effect on athletic performance. Therefore, in the absence of a proven effective routine, it is recommended that the athletic coach make the following suggestions to his athletes regarding pre-event nutrition:

1. To avoid a feeling of fullness in the stomach, eat about 4 hours prior to competition. (Most food has left the stomach after 4½ hours and the small intestine after 9 hours. Total gastrointestinal transit time ranges from about 18–48 hours.)
2. Competitors in events lasting longer than about 30 minutes should eat a meal that has 80–90 per cent of its calories in the form of carbohydrates.
3. It is highly unlikely that competitors in events lasting less than 30 minutes will derive any physiological benefit from any particular composition of the pre-event meal. Thus, they should eat whatever they like as long as their experience with that food has not produced discomfort. Although most individuals would prefer not to have baked beans, cabbage and tamales before competition, if one's long experience with such foods has never produced discomfort, it is unlikely that performance will be adversely affected by such a meal.
4. Avoid eating such great quantities of food that discomfort results.
5. Sometimes, the unexpected emotional impact of forthcoming competition makes digestion uncomfortable. An athlete who feels a high level of anticipation is advised to eat only small portions of food in which he has great confidence.
6. Do not worry about the "digestibility" of foods because little or none of the pre-event meal will be used for the immediate

competition, and because a substantial portion of any meal (with the possible exception of liquid diets) will still be in the gut at the time of competition, regardless of its digestibility.

7. Although eating a glucose (dextrose) tablet or two just prior to competition is probably harmless, the intake of large amounts of sugar just before exercise can delay stomach emptying and can cause insulin to lower blood sugar levels to below normal values.

8. Protein is not a significant energy source during exercise and is not recommended as a superior energy food.

9. Remember that superior performance depends on superior ability and superior training. A last minute meal or pill cannot counteract the effects of inadequate training.

Review Questions

1. Describe the protein requirements of different types of athletes.
2. Explain why not all proteins are equally good from the standpoint of nutrition.
3. Review the role of carbohydrate diets in athletic performance.
4. Compare the vitamin and mineral requirements of athletes and nonathletes.
5. What pre-event nutrition plan would you recommend to various types of athletes?

References

1. Bergstrom, J., and E. Hultman. Nutrition for maximal sports performance. *Journal of the American Medical Association,* 1972, **221:**999–1006.
2. Bourne, G. H. Nutrition and exercise. In H. B. Falls (Ed.), *Exercise Physiology.* New York: Academic Press, 1968, pp. 155–171.
3. Consolazio, C. F., H. L. Johnson, R. A. Nelson, J. G. Dramise, and J. H. Skala. Protein metabolism during intensive physical training in the young adult. *American Journal of Clinical Nutrition,* 1975, **28:**29–35.
4. Entenman, C., J. A. Coughlin, and P. D. Ackerman. Substrate utilization and maximum swimming ability in rats and guinea pigs fed wheat germ oil. *Proceedings of the Society for Experimental Biology and Medicine,* 1972, **141:**43–46.

5. Kofranyi, E., F. Jekat, and H. Muller-Wecker. The minimum protein requirements of humans, tested with mixtures of whole egg plus potato and maize plus beans. *Hoppe-Seyler's Zeitschrift für Physiologische Chemie*, 1970, **351**:1485–1493.

6. Pernow, B., and B. Saltin, (Eds.), *Muscle Metabolism During Exercise*. New York: Plenum Press, 1971.

6

Estimation of aerobic and anaerobic energy expenditure during exercise

Knowledge of the energy expended in various physical activities is very important for precise prescription of exercise in weight control, for the prescription of exercise used in the rehabilitation of heart disease patients, for the provision of reasonable systematic training regimens for normal subjects, and for planning sensible conditioning programs for athletes. As will be described in this chapter, the usual method of determining energy expenditure also provides information about the relative contributions of anaerobic and aerobic energy production for the exercise activity and about the type of fuel metabolized during exercise.

In studies of biological energy intake and expenditure, the most common expression of energy units is the large *calorie* or *kilocalorie* (kcal), which is the amount of heat required to raise the temperature of 1 kilogram of water from 14.5°C. to 15.5°C. at normal atmospheric pressure. It is possible, but very difficult and costly, to directly measure the energy expended by a subject as he exercises inside a closed chamber which has walls specifically designed to absorb and measure the heat produced. However, it is much simpler to estimate that energy indirectly by measuring the amount of oxygen consumed by the subject. Oxygen consumption (oxygen uptake) is the difference between the volume of oxygen inspired and that expired, and represents the oxygen used in the electron transport system of the mitochondria.

Because energy expenditure is due to the breakdown of ATP, and because that ATP is replenished as the result of oxygen utilization in the mitochondria either during exercise or during recovery, there is a direct relationship between oxygen consumption and energy expenditure. Accurate measurements of the kilocalories of heat produced as the result of oxygen utilization show that normal subjects on a mixed diet of fat, carbohydrate, and protein expend about 5 kcal of energy for each liter of oxygen they consume. Therefore, if it were known that the gallant Slavic knight, Sir Lykziz Bierlotz, consumed 15 liters of oxygen while fighting a dragon to save a beautiful princess, one could calculate that the brave fellow expended $15 \times 5 = 75$ kcal of energy.

CALCULATION OF OXYGEN UPTAKE AND CARBON DIOXIDE PRODUCTION

To calculate oxygen uptake (V_{O_2}) during a period of exercise or rest, one must subtract the volume of oxygen expired during that time period from the volume of oxygen inspired during the same time. Calculation of these two volumes requires knowledge of a) the volume of inspired and expired air during the test period and b) the concentration of oxygen in inspired and expired air. Thus,

V_{O_2} = Volume $O_{2_{inspired}}$ − Volume $O_{2_{expired}}$,
 Volume $O_{2_{inspired}}$ = Volume $Air_{inspired}$ × Concentration $O_{2_{inspired}}$,
 and Volume $O_{2_{expired}}$ = Volume $Air_{expired}$ × Concentration $O_{2_{expired}}$

By substitution of terms,

V_{O_2} = (Vol Air_{insp} × Conc $O_{2_{insp}}$) − (Vol Air_{exp} × Conc $O_{2_{exp}}$).

The concentration of O_2 in inspired air at sea level is a very constant 20.93% or .2093 liter O_2 per liter of air. The concentration of O_2 in a sample of the expired air must be measured in the laboratory with an oxygen analyzer.

Either the inspired or the expired air volume can be determined if the other is measured and if the concentration of nitrogen (N_2) in the expired air is analyzed. This calculation of one volume from knowledge of the other volume is made possible because the concentration of nitrogen in inspired air is a constant 79.04% or .7904 liter N_2 per liter of air and because volume of N_2 inspired is unchanged in the body and is therefore equal to the volume of N_2 expired. For example,

$$\text{Vol Air}_{exp} \times \text{Conc N}_{2\,exp} = \text{Vol Air}_{insp} \times \text{Conc N}_{2\,insp} \text{ . Thus,}$$

$$\text{Vol Air}_{exp} = \frac{\text{Vol Air}_{insp} \times .7904}{\text{Conc N}_{2\,exp}} \text{, and}$$

$$\text{Vol Air}_{insp} = \frac{\text{Vol Air}_{exp} \times \text{Conc N}_{2\,exp}}{.7904} .$$

Therefore, if the volume of *inspired* air is measured,

$$V_{O_2} = (\text{Vol Air}_{insp} \times .2093) - \left[\left(\frac{\text{Vol Air}_{insp} \times .7904}{\text{Conc N}_{2\,exp}} \right) \times \text{Conc O}_{2\,exp} \right] ;$$

but if the volume of *expired* air is measured,

$$V_{O_2} = \left[\left(\frac{\text{Vol Air}_{exp} \times \text{Conc N}_{2\,exp}}{.7904} \right) \times .2093 \right] - (\text{Vol Air}_{exp} \times \text{Conc O}_{2\,exp})$$

For example, if the volume of air inspired during 5 minutes of exercise were 200 liters, and the concentrations of O_2 and N_2 in a sample of the expired air were .1700 (17%) and .7800 (78%), respectively,

$$V_{O_2} = (200 \times .2093) - \left[\left(\frac{200 \times .7904}{.7800} \right) \times .1700 \right] = 7.41 \text{ liters}$$

in 5 minutes or 1.48 liters per minute. If, on the other hand, the volume of air expired during 1 minute of exercise was determined to be 100 liters and the concentrations of O_2 and N_2 in a sample of the expired air were .1600 (16%) and .7850 (78.5%), respectively,

$$V_{O_2} = \left[\left(\frac{100 \times .7850}{.7904} \right) \times .2093 \right] - (100 \times .1600)$$

$$= 4.79 \text{ liters per minute.}$$

The production of carbon dioxide (V_{CO_2}) is calculated in much the same way as V_{O_2}, that is,

$$V_{CO_2} = (\text{Vol Air}_{exp} \times \text{Conc CO}_{2\,exp}) - (\text{Vol Air}_{insp} \times \text{Conc CO}_{2\,insp}).$$

Because the concentration of CO_2 in inspired air is only .0003 (0.03%)

and is usually ignored, the equation for carbon dioxide production then becomes V_{CO_2} = Vol $Air_{exp} \times$ Conc CO_{2exp} and is easily computed if the volume of expired air is measured. If the volume of *inspired* air is measured rather than expired air,

$$V_{CO_2} = \left(\frac{\text{Vol Air}_{insp} \times .7904}{\text{Conc N}_{2exp}} \right) \times \text{Conc CO}_{2exp}.$$

The concentration of N_2 in expired air is usually found by subtracting the sum of the analyzed O_{2exp} and CO_{2exp} from 1.00 since there are only tiny amounts of gasses other than N_2, O_2 and CO_2 in ordinary air. Accordingly, if O_{2exp} and CO_{2exp} were analyzed as .1800 (18.00%) and .0300 (3.00%), respectively, N_{2exp} would be $1.00 - (.18 + .03) = .79$ (79 %).

OXYGEN DEFICIT AND OXYGEN DEBT

As stated in the preceding discussion, ATP replenishment is ultimately the result of oxygen consumption in the electron transport system of the mitochondria of the body's cells. But during the first few seconds of light exercise and for all of short–duration heavy exercise, ATP is produced primarily as a result of *anaerobic* (without oxygen) mechanisms, that is, mostly by the breakdown of creatine phosphate and muscle glycogen or glucose. Extra oxygen is then used *after the activity has been concluded* to make up for the initial anaerobic production of ATP. There are three reasons why aerobic energy generation makes only a small contribution during heavy work and during the first part of submaximal work. First, it takes a few seconds for the circulation to deliver the required extra oxygen to the working muscles. Second, aerobic metabolism is sparked by the presence of excess ADP in the mitochondria that acts as an acceptor of phosphate to produce ATP (that is, ADP + P = ATP). Until such ADP accumulates as the result of ATP breakdown, rapid oxygen consumption and ATP production by the mitochondria do not begin (3). Accordingly, ATP must be generated by anaerobic means until the aerobic production of ATP in the mitochondria can catch up. Finally, in heavy work the rate of demand for ATP is simply too great to be met solely by aerobic energy production during exercise; the breakdown of creatine phosphate and glycogen must occur to meet the high rate of energy use by the muscle.

The inadequacy of aerobic energy production to meet the total energy needs of the body, especially at the beginning of an exercise period, is known as the *oxygen deficit*, and the tendency of the body to repay this aerobic energy deficit by consuming more than usual amounts of oxygen during the period of recovery after the exercise is part of what is known as the oxygen debt (Fig. 6.1). *Operationally, the oxygen deficit is defined as the difference between the total energy cost of the work (expressed as units of oxygen) and the measured portion of the total energy cost that was met during the exercise period by aerobic energy production, that is, by oxygen consumption during the exercise period. Oxygen debt, on the other hand, is the oxygen consumed during recovery that is in excess of the amounts that normally would have been consumed at rest during an equivalent time period.* To better understand these concepts, inspect Fig. 6.1 carefully. Observe the area "O₂ Consumed at Rest" at the base of the graph. This rectangle represents the resting rate of oxygen uptake, in this case 0.25 *l*/min., that would have occurred even if the exericse had *not* taken place. Next, observe the unshaded area under the curve between the start and finish of exercise. The area represents the *net* or excess oxygen consumption during exercise, that is, the portion of the total aerobic energy cost (above that which would have occurred during a similar period of rest) that was met during the exercise period itself. The area shaded with gray at the left of the diagram represents that portion of the total energy cost that could not be met aerobically during exercise. In other words, *this oxygen deficit portion of the energy cost of exercise was met by replenishing ATP supplies anaerobically, chiefly by the breakdown of creatine phosphate, muscle glycogen, and blood glucose.*

The horizontal line drawn in Fig. 6.1 at 3.0 liters of oxygen up-

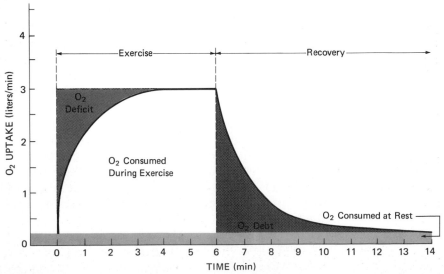

Figure 6.1. Energy expenditure during exercise (in terms of oxygen uptake).

take per minute represents the rate of total energy expenditure (in terms of oxygen) that was needed to perform this particular exercise. Notice that only during the last 3 minutes of exercise was the exerciser able to meet the total energy costs aerobically (by the uptake of oxygen). Accordingly, the oxygen deficit in this case occurred only during the first 3 minutes of exercise. For any given minute, one need only subtract the amount of oxygen consumed from the total energy expenditure to obtain the oxygen deficit for that minute. For example, for the first minute of exercise shown in Fig. 6.1, oxygen consumption was on the average about 1.6 liters (ranging from 0.25–2.20 l.), whereas the total energy use was 3.0 liters; therefore, the oxygen deficit for the first minute of work was $3.0 - 1.6 = 1.4$ liters of oxygen. For the sixth minute of exercise, on the other hand, the oxygen uptake and the energy cost were the same, 3.0 liters, so there was no additional oxygen deficit contracted during that minute.

In Fig. 6.1, the darkly shaded area shown in the recovery period illustrates the oxygen uptake after exercise that is above the normal resting level of oxygen uptake. This excess oxygen uptake during recovery is called the *oxygen debt*. Oxygen debt can be measured if one knows the total oxygen consumed during recovery and the rate of oxygen consumption that normally occurs during rest.

Estimation of Oxygen Cost, Caloric Cost, Oxygen Deficit and Oxygen Debt

For *steady-state* work (work that can be maintained for a long period with aerobic energy production and only a brief period of anaerobic energy production at the start of the exercise bout) only oxygen uptake need be measured during rest, exercise, and recovery to enable one to estimate total energy cost, oxygen deficit and oxygen debt in terms of oxygen units. For example, assume that a person worked as in Fig. 6.1 for 6 minutes and recovered for 8 minutes, and that the measured oxygen uptake values were as follows:

Rest: 0.25 l/min
Exercise: 1st min = 1.6 l, 2nd min = 2.5 l, 3rd min = 2.8 l, 4th, 5th, & 6th min = 3.0 l.
Recovery: 1st min = 2.0 l, 2nd min = 1.0 l, 3rd min = 0.7 l, 4th min = 0.5 l, 5th min = 0.4 l, 6th min = 0.3 l, 7th min = 0.27 l, 8th min = 0.26 l.

This example will be used to show how the following equations can be used to help determine the various portions of energy expenditure as a result of exercise.

Net O₂ Cost of Exercise is the total oxygen consumed during both exercise and recovery less the oxygen that would have been consumed during the same period had the subject been at rest.

$$\text{NET } O_2 \text{ COST OF EXERCISE} = \text{Exercise } V_{O_2} + \text{Recovery } V_{O_2}$$
$$- (\text{Rest } \dot{V}_{O_2} \times \text{Total Exercise \& Recovery Time})$$

It should be noted that the symbol V refers to a volume, whereas $\dot{V}$ represents a volume per unit of time, usually per minute. In the example, Exercise $V_{O_2} = 1.6 + 2.5 + 2.8 + 3.0 + 3.0 + 3.0 = 15.9$ l, Recovery $V_{O_2} = 2.0 + 1.0 + 0.7 + 0.5 + 0.4 + 0.3 + 0.27 + 0.26 = 5.43\ l$, Rest $\dot{V}_{O_2} = 0.25\ l/min$, and Total Exercise & Recovery Time = 14 min. Therefore,

$$\text{NET } O_2 \text{ COST OF EXERCISE} = 15.9 + 5.43 - (0.25 \times 14)$$
$$= 21.33 - 3.5 = 17.83\ l\ O_2$$

Net Caloric Cost of Exercise is the total caloric cost of both exercise and recovery less the calories that would have been expended during the same period had the subject been at rest. This caloric cost is determined indirectly on the basis of measured oxygen consumption. Depending upon foodstuffs being used for energy, each liter of oxygen consumed is associated with a specific number of expended calories, the *caloric equivalent* of a liter of oxygen (usually about 5 kcal per liter).

$$\text{NET CALORIC COST OF EXERCISE}$$
$$= \text{Net } O_2 \text{ Cost of Exercise } (l)$$
$$\times \text{ Caloric Equivalent of a Liter of } O_2$$

In the example, net oxygen cost was 17.83 liters, and the caloric equivalent was 5.0 kcal per liter. Therefore,

$$\text{NET CALORIC COST OF EXERCISE} = 17.83 \times 5.0 = 89.15 \text{ kcal.}$$

Oxygen Deficit in Steady State Exercise is the difference between the theoretical oxygen cost of the exercise had steady state oxygen uptake been reached instantaneously at the start of exercise and the actual oxygen uptake observed during the exercise period. In the example shown in Fig. 6.1, the steady state level of oxygen uptake was not reached until the third minute at 3.0 l/min. Accordingly, during the first 3 minutes the subject was replenishing ATP anaerobically and contracting an oxygen deficit.

$$\text{OXYGEN DEFICIT IN STEADY STATE EXERCISE}$$
$$= (\text{Steady State Exercise } \dot{V}_{O_2} \times \text{Exercise Time}) - \text{Exercise } V_{O_2}$$

In the example of Fig. 6.1, Steady State Exercise $\dot{V}_{O_2}$ = 3.0 l/min, Exercise Time = 6 min, and the exercise V_{O_2} = 15.9 l. Accordingly,

OXYGEN DEFICIT = (3.0 × 6) − 15.9 = 18.0 − 15.9 = 2.1 liters.

Oxygen Deficit in Non-steady State Exercise is technically more difficult to measure accurately because the oxygen uptake during exercise never reaches a steady plateau, so that an estimated "steady-state" level of oxygen uptake must be computed. In severe exercise that can be maintained for only a few minutes, oxygen debt is much greater than oxygen deficit (2) and, thus, cannot be used to accurately assess oxygen deficit. Because of the technical difficulties involved, the estimation of oxygen deficit in nonsteady state exercise will be described only in Appendix B.

Oxygen Debt is the difference between the oxygen consumed during recovery after exercise and the oxygen that would have been consumed during the same time interval had the subject remained at rest. In Fig. 6.1, the total oxygen consumed during 8 minutes of recovery was 5.43 l, and the resting rate of oxygen uptake was 0.25 l/min. Therefore, assuming the subject would have consumed 0.25 × 8 = 2.0 l of oxygen during 8 minutes had he remained at rest, the oxygen debt shown in Fig. 6.1 was 5.43 − 2.0 = 3.43 l.

OXYGEN DEBT = Recovery V_{O_2} − Resting $\dot{V}_{O_2}$ × Min. of Recovery)

DETERMINATION OF THE CALORIC EQUIVALENT OF OXYGEN CONSUMED

In exercise of short duration where a relatively small volume of oxygen is consumed, it is usually satisfactory to assume that each liter of oxygen consumed is equivalent to about 5.0 kcal. But when exercise is prolonged for an hour or more, this value could be up to 6% in error. Such an error is negligible in most situations, but if greater accuracy is needed, such as, to determine energy balance over a 24-hour period, a more exact caloric equivalent must be determined. This determination involves measuring the urinary nitrogen excreted, the oxygen consumed, and the carbon dioxide produced during rest, steady state exercise and recovery, so that a *nonprotein respiratory-exchange ratio* (R) or *respiratory quotient* (RQ) may be computed.

Respiratory-Exchange Ratio

As oxygen is consumed in the mitochondria in the process of catabolizing a particular foodstuff, for example, fat, carbohydrate or protein, the oxygen consumption is associated with a certain amount of carbon dioxide production, especially in reactions of the Krebs Cycle. Each type of food broken down gives a particular ratio of the volume of CO_2 produced to the volume of O_2 consumed. This ratio, V_{CO_2}/V_{O_2}, is known as the respiratory–exchange ratio (R) or the respiratory quotient (RQ). For example, when glucose is completely oxidized $(C_6H_{12}O_6 + 6O_2 \rightarrow 6CO_2 + 6H_2O)$, each volume of oxygen consumed is associated with the same volume of carbon dioxide production, so the R or RQ for glucose is $6CO_2/6O_2 = 1.0$. It takes relatively more oxygen, though, to combust a typical fat molecule $(2C_{51}H_{98}O_6 + 145O_2 \rightarrow 102CO_2 + 98H_2O)$, and the R for pure fat is about $102CO_2/145O_2 = 0.70$. The R value for protein is about 0.83.

Because less oxygen must be consumed to produce the same amount of ATP when carbohydrates is catabolized than when fat is being broken down (Chapter 3), the oxygen consumed when carbohydrate is combusted (as indicated by an R value of about 1.0) has a greater energy value or caloric value than does the oxygen consumed when fat is burned at an R value approaching 0.7. Some of the caloric equivalents for different R values are shown in Table 6.1.

Notice that the R values of Table 6.1 are labeled *nonprotein R*. This means that the volume of oxygen consumed, and the volume of

Table 6.1. Calaoric Equivalents for Oxygen, and Foodstuff Contributions to Energy for Various Nonprotein Respiratory Exchange Ratios.

Nonprotein Respiratory- Exchange Ratio (R or RQ)	kcal/Liter O_2	Approximate Contributions to Energy	
		Fat (%)	Carbohydrate (%)
1.00	5.047	0	100
0.98	5.022	6	94
0.96	4.997	12	88
0.94	4.973	19	81
0.92	4.948	26	74
0.90	4.928	32	68
0.88	4.900	38	62
0.86	4.875	47	53
0.84	4.850	53	47
0.82	4.825	62	38
0.80	4.801	68	32
0.78	4.776	74	26
0.76	4.752	81	19
0.74	4.727	88	12
0.72	4.702	94	6
0.70	4.686	100	0

carbon dioxide produced as the result of the metabolism of protein during exercise, must be subtracted from the total oxygen consumption and carbon dioxide production. To find the rather small contribution of protein to these gas volumes, one must measure the urinary nitrogen excreted during the exercise period and compute the amount of protein broken down plus the oxygen consumed and the carbon dioxide produced because of the protein breakdown. With short–duration exercise the contribution of protein metabolism is so small that it can safely be neglected. If R values are to be used at all to determine the exact caloric equivalent of a liter of oxygen consumed, it is best to measure the protein contribution to exercise metabolism. For most practical purposes, however, the use of 5.0 as an assumed caloric equivalent for a liter of oxygen can be justified, so that neither carbon dioxide production nor urinary nitrogen needs to be measured. In many laboratories the possibility of error using an assumed caloric equivalent of 5.0 is much less than the likelihood of error in measuring nitrogen and carbon dioxide.

Precautions Necessary in Interpreting R. Any factor which influences the production of carbon dioxide or the consumption of oxygen, but which is not directly related to the combustion of foodstuffs, can obviously result in a respiratory-exchange ratio that is misleading. In heavy exercise, for example, it is not unusual to observe R values greater than 1.0 during exercise and values less than 0.7 during recovery. Such values for R are not very helpful when one is attempting to determine an accurate caloric equivalent for oxygen consumed because even burning pure glucose or pure fat does not result in R values greater than 1.0 or less than 0.7, respectively.

Two factors that are commonly thought to be linked to erroneous R values are unnecessarily heavy breathing or hyperventilation by an anxious subject, which causes him to exhale too much carbon dioxide and elevate R, and the production of large amounts of lactic acid, which not only tends to make the subject hyperventilate but also causes him to expire considerable carbon dioxide due to a breakdown of carbonic acid in the blood to carbon dioxide and water. After heavy exercise is completed, carbon dioxide tends to be retained in the body to replenish the body stores of bicarbonate that were used to buffer the lactic acid during activity; this retention of carbon dioxide may lower R in the recovery period to less than 0.7 for many minutes or even an hour or more.

Because of the fact that unusual R values are most apt to be observed during heavy, nonsteady state exercise, the determination of R is usually restricted to exercise of a submaximal steady state nature. For heavy exercise a caloric equivalent of 5.0 kilocalories per liter of oxygen can be assumed so that reliance on R values is unnecessary.

DETERMINATION OF THE CONTRIBUTION OF VARIOUS FOODSTUFFS TO ENERGY EXPENDITURE

Physical educators, doctors, coaches, dieters and athletes are often curious about how much fat, carbohydrate or protein is used up in various types of exercise. As was discussed in Chapters 4 and 5, a general explanation is that protein breakdown is insignificant during exercise for a well-fed person, that carbohydrate is utilized most in short duration heavy exercise, and that fat is a major source of fuel for low intensity, long duration exercise. However, a fairly precise estimate of the contributions of fat, carbohydrate and protein to energy expenditure can be obtained from a knowledge of the volume of oxygen consumed, the volume of carbon dioxide produced, and the urinary nitrogen excreted during steady state exercise.

The following equations have been derived for use in the determination of foodstuff contribution to energy expenditure (1):

1. Protein used during activity (g) =

   6.25 × grams of urinary nitrogen excreted during activity

2. Carbohydrate used during activity (g) =

   $4.12 \, V_{CO_2} \, (l) - 2.91 \, V_{O_2} \, (l) - 2.56$ urinary nitrogen (g)

3. Fat used during activity (g) =

   $1.69 \, V_{O_2} \, (l) - 1.69 \, V_{CO_2} \, (l) - 1.94$ urinary nitrogen (g)

4. Energy expended (kcal) =

   $3.78 \, V_{O_2} \, (l) + 1.16 \, V_{CO_2} \, (l) - 2.98$ urinary nitrogen (g)

5. Energy due to protein (kcal) = 4.1 × protein used (g)

6. Energy due to carbohydrate (kcal) = 4.1 × carbohydrate used (g)

7. Energy due to fat (kcal) = 9.3 × fat used (g)

As an illustration of how these equations could be used, suppose that Susie Sweetcheeks wanted to know whether riding her bicycle to school 4 miles each way would have any impact on her massive hulk (100 kg or 220 lbs) if she rode 5 days per week for 40 weeks. Susie asked Dr. Nosemuch, the local, friendly exercise-physiologist, if he would perform the appropriate tests. With the good doctor's help the following data were obtained for a one-way bicycle trip:

$$\text{Urinary nitrogen} = 0.01 \text{ g}, V_{CO_2} = 60 \; l, V_{O_2} = 68 \; l.$$

Thus, on a 4-mile bicycle ride Susie used $6.25 \times 0.01 = .0625$ g protein, $(4.12 \times 60) - (2.91 \times 68) - (2.56 \times 0.01) = 49.29$ g carbohydrate, and $(1.69 \times 68) - (1.69 \times 60) - (1.94 \times 0.01) = 13.50$ g fat, and she expended $(3.78 \times 68) + (1.16 \times 60) - (2.98 \times 0.01) = 327$ kcal of energy. The energy expended because of protein breakdown was $4.1 \times .0625 = 0.26$ kcal, that because of carbohydrate breakdown was $4.1 \times 49.29 = 202.09$ kcal, and that because of fat breakdown was $9.3 \times 13.50 = 125.55$ kcal.

Of the 327 kcal of energy expended on her trip to school, less than 1 per cent was because of protein breakdown, about 62% because of carbohydrate breakdown, and 38 per cent because of fat breakdown. In 400 trips on her bicycle, Susie would expend $400 \times 125.55 = 50,220$ kcal from fat breakdown alone, and a total of $400 \times 327 = 130,800$ kcal from all sources. Although a caloric expenditure of 9300 kcal is required to catabolize a kilogram of pure fat, only about 7700 kcal must be spent to break down a kilogram of fat *tissue*, which contains water and connective tissue in addition to pure fat. (This translates into an expenditure of 3500 kcal per pound of fat tissue.) Accordingly, Susie would lose $50,220/7700 = 6.5$ kilograms (14.3 lbs.) of fat tissue from the use of fat alone in a year of cycling back and forth to school, assuming she did not alter her caloric intake. But since the other degraded foodstuffs, such as glycogen and protein, are preferentially replenished after exercise at the expense of energy derived from further fat breakdown, the actual fat loss would amount to 17 kg (37.4 lbs.) ($130,800/7700$). Such a weight loss would be very admirable and would not require any reduction in food intake. Of course, if Susie were able to reduce her caloric intake as she increased her caloric expenditure by cycling, she could lose weight even more rapidly.

In Table 6.1 are listed the approximate percentage contributions of fat and carbohydrate for various respiratory-exchange ratios. If, for example, an exerciser consumed 20 liters of oxygen in an activity at an average R of 0.90, Table 6.1 shows that each of those liters of oxygen was equivalent to about 4.93 kcal, and that 32 per cent of the total caloric expenditure was the result of fat breakdown, whereas 68 per cent was due to carbohydrate. The total energy expenditure, therefore, was $20 \times 4.93 = 98.6$ kcal, and of this total 32 per cent or 31.6 kcal resulted from fat combustion and 68 per cent or 67.0 kcal from carbohydrate.

Review Questions

1. What is the physiological basis for the estimation of energy expenditure in units of oxygen consumption?
2. Define the following terms both operationally and in terms of how they are related to aerobic and/or anaerobic energy expenditure: oxygen deficit, net oxygen cost of exercise, oxygen debt, net oxygen consumed during exercise.
3. How is the respiratory-exchange ratio used to roughly determine the relative contributions of fat and carbohydrate as fuels for exercise? What is the physiological basis for this technique?
4. If, as a result of an exercise bout, a subject excreted 0.005 grams of urinary nitrogen, consumed 50 liters of oxygen, and produced 45 liters of carbon dioxide, calculate the following: total energy expenditure and energy contributed by protein, fat and carbohydrate breakdown.

References

1. Consolazio, C. F., R. E. Johnson, and L. J. Pecora. *Physiological Measurements of Metabolic Functions in Man*. New York: McGraw-Hill, 1963, p. 316.
2. Hermansen, L. Anaerobic energy release. *Medicine and Science in Sports*, 1969, **1**:32–38.
3. Holloszy, J. O. Long-term metabolic adaptations in muscle to endurance exercise. In J. P. Naughton and H. K. Hellerstein (Eds.), *Exercise Testing and Exercise Training in Coronary Heart Disease*. New York: Academic Press, 1973, pp. 211–222.

7

The physiological basis of muscular strength

It is unfortunate that physical education students sometimes feel defensive about being connected with a profession that is "only interested in muscles." The fact is that muscle contraction not only allows man to move from one place to another, but it is also the only way man has to express his thoughts and emotions. Muscle contraction is necessary for speech, for writing, and even for blinking; in terms of communication the brain is useless dead weight in the absence of muscle contraction. Muscle contraction produces the force we call "muscular strength," and each of us is familiar with some of the basic responses and adaptations associated with muscle strength. For example, muscles contract more forcefully with an appropriate emotional set, and strength training produces larger muscles which, in turn, result in greater strength.

WHAT IS STRENGTH?

The word "strength" has at least 12 definitions in the dictionary and has many uses in the English language. Unfortunately, this has led to rather careless usage of the term in physical education and athletics. Thus, we have all heard the phrases "strong runner" and "strong swimmer" used to describe a distance runner or swimmer with great endurance, "strong fullback" to describe a football player who is difficult to tackle, and "strongman" to describe one who can lift heavy weights. *Muscular strength is best defined operationally as the greatest amount of force that muscles can produce in a single maximal effort.* Therefore, a person who can lift a greater weight than another in a single lift is stronger than the second person, even though the second person may be able to lift more total weight for perhaps ten repetitions. In this case, the second person has greater *muscular endurance.*

Strength is certainly necessary for satisfactory performance in athletic events, such as cycling, swimming, tennis and golf, that are dominated by other factors including endurance, technique or speed. But strength is most important in such events as the shotput, discus, hammer, and javelin throws, wrestling and weightlifting. Strength is not only an important factor in many athletic events, but it is important for at least three other reasons. First, adequate strength is vital to the performance of all common activities such as standing, walking, opening a wooden window that has been swollen by moisture, lifting heavy bags of groceries, and pushing a car out of a snowbank. Second, at least minimal levels of abdominal and shoulder muscle strength are required to help prevent low back pain and excessive spinal curvatures that could lead to discomfort. Finally, strong well-developed muscles give a pleasing appearance to the body, and in our culture, physical beauty makes the establishment of interpersonal relationships much easier, and tends to enhance one's confidence through an improved self-image. Not only do strong muscles often lead to broad shoulders and large chests in males, but they also can enhance the carriage and esthetically pleasing shapes of females. Too often physical educators minimize the motivating power of appearance improvement in trying to "sell" strength training programs. Many people can be motivated to improve strength for the sake of appearance rather than for the purpose of avoiding low back pain, pushing cars out of snowbanks more easily, or winning shotput championships.

In earlier chapters we learned some important details about the structure of skeletal muscle, the way it contracts, and the different means muscles can use to obtain energy to sustain contractions. We are now prepared to learn how the body controls the degree of force produced by muscle contraction and how maximal force can be increased by appropriate overload training. These topics will be taken up in this and subsequent chapters.

TYPES OF CONTRACTION

Static (isometric), isotonic and isokinetic types of strength are produced by static, isotonic and isokinetic contractions, respectively. A *static contraction* is one in which minimal muscle fiber shortening produces force with no change in the angle of a joint, whereas *isotonic contractions* result from muscle fiber shortening that causes a joint to move through some range of motion against a constant resistance, and *isokinetic contractions* occur as muscle fibers shorten to counteract an "accommodating" resistance developed by a device that allows only a constant rate of movement regardless of the force exerted by contracting muscle.

In addition, isotonic and isokinetic contractions may be classified as *concentric* or *eccentric* contractions, depending upon whether the whole active muscles shorten or lengthen, respectively, during the movement. For example, in the upward phase of a pullup or "chin," the elbow flexors (biceps brachii, for example) are shortening, and the angle of the elbow joint is decreasing from 180 degrees to perhaps 15 degrees. Since the active muscles are shortening, this is a *concentric* contraction. On the other hand, during the downward phase of a pullup, whole muscles lengthen as progressively fewer muscle fibers are activated. This contraction causes a gradual increase in the angle of the elbow joint until it is once again 180 degrees. Therefore, the downward phase of a pullup is an example of an *eccentric* contraction. Although during this type of isotonic, eccentric contraction, each elbow flexor muscle as a whole is lengthening, remember that some fibers must be shortening or the subject would drop immediately from the pullup bar. Eventually, the number of active muscle fibers is so small that total contractile force just equals the force required to stretch the connective tissues of the muscle and tendon, but it is not great enough to raise the body from the straight hang position. These few fibers at this time are contracting "isometrically."

In an isokinetic, eccentric contraction, a mechanical device or a human assistant gradually overcomes the contractile force of a muscle group to cause a joint angle to increase at a constant rate. In this instance, muscle fiber shortening is overcome by a more powerful mechanical force which gradually inhibits or stretches more and more fibers. It appears that either muscle fibers are inhibited from contracting by a nerve reflex triggered by the great tension on the muscle (described later in this chapter), or some sarcomeres in the active fibers are being stretched as they attempt to shorten, while others are simultaneously contracting. Exactly how this phenomenon might occur is unknown. Intuitively, it seems that cross bridges in some sarcomeres may be more susceptible to disruption by mechanical forces than others.

NEURAL CONTROL OF MUSCULAR STRENGTH: GRADED CONTRACTIONS

The body has an amazing ability to call forth just the right amount of muscular force to perform an endless variety of tasks— from drawing a fine line on a sheet of paper to lifting a 90-pound barbell. If it were not for this ability to control contractile force, it would be common to see ice cream cones plastered to their owner's foreheads and seamstresses going berserk while attempting to thread needles. There are two ways by which the organism can vary the strength of a muscle contraction: It can vary the total number of motor units recruited in a muscle, or it can vary the frequency with which a given number of motor units is activated.

Motor Units

A motor unit consists of a motor nerve cell (neuron) that originates in the spinal cord and all of the muscle fibers that are supplied by that neuron (Fig. 7.1). The number of muscle fibers innervated by a single motor nerve fiber varies from as few as 5 in some eye muscles, which require fine control, to as many as 1,000 or more in large muscles (such as the gastrocnemius), which do not require a high degree of control. As the name "motor unit" implies, all the muscle fibers within a given motor unit contract or relax nearly simultaneously; that is, it is not possible for some of the muscle fibers of a motor unit to relax while others contract. Also, if the muscle fibers of a motor unit are activated sufficiently by the nerve to contract, those fibers will contract maximally. This is the so-called "all or none" law; under a given set of conditions muscle fibers in a motor unit either contract maximally or they do not contract at all. This is an important concept for understanding graded muscle contractions. Remember that this "all or none" law applies to the muscle fibers of a given motor unit and not to an entire muscle. This application of the law is explained in the following paragraph.

Let us assume that a gastrocnemius muscle is innervated by 300 neurons that are contained in a branch of the sciatic nerve and that each of those 300 neurons supplies from 50 to 2,000 muscle fibers.

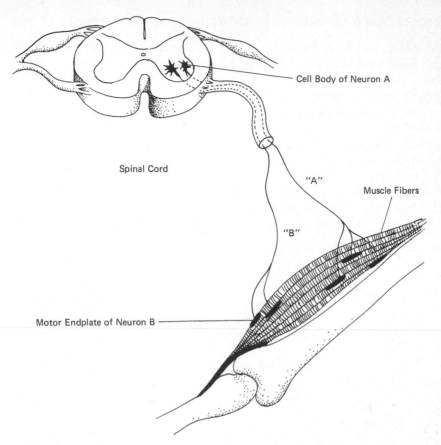

Figure 7.1. Sketch of two motor units. Neuron "A" innervates three muscle fibers, neuron "B" only two.

Thus, this muscle has 300 motor units, each consisting of a neuron and 50–2,000 muscle fibers. Since all the muscle fibers of each of these motor units will contract maximally if the motor units are adequately stimulated, the smallest number of muscle fibers that can contract is 50, the size of the smallest motor unit. If each muscle fiber produces a force of 1 gram, the *minimum* force that this muscle can produce is 50 × 1 = 50 grams, a little less than 2 ounces. The *maximum* amount of force that could be exerted depends on the total number of muscle fibers in the muscle. If we suppose that the average motor unit has 400 muscle fibers, then a total of *300 motor units × 400 fibers per unit × 1 gram force per fiber = 120,000 grams (264 pounds)* of force could be produced by our hypothetical gastrocnemius muscle. Therefore, the muscle could produce almost any degree of force between 50 and 120,000 grams, depending on how many motor units were called into play at one time.

Frequency of Stimulation of Motor Units

All motor units do not fire in unison except under conditions of maximal stimulation. For submaximal contractions some motor units are at rest, while others produce the required force. But the resting and active motor units exchange roles frequently so that fatigue of any one motor unit is avoided. This *asynchronous* contraction of motor units is also responsible for the smooth, nonjerky nature of voluntary contractions. By increasing the frequency with which a given number of motor units is fired (so that rest pauses are shorter), more of these motor units can be active at any given time to give a greater strength of contraction. For example, assume that each of 100 motor units, each having an equal number of muscle fibers, fires every 0.01 second and that, at any one time, there are about 60 motor units active and 40 at rest. Next, assume that each motor unit begins to fire more frequently so that there are 90 active motor units at a given instant with only 10 at rest. According to the "all or none" law, the force exerted when 90 of the motor units are simultaneously active is 50 per cent greater than when only 60 are active. Thus, the same 100 motor units can produce a stronger or weaker contraction when their rate of firing is either increased or decreased, respectively.

Smooth, Voluntary Contractions. When skeletal muscles are stimulated briefly with a massive electric shock, they "twitch" or produce a rapid maximal contraction for a brief instant before returning to

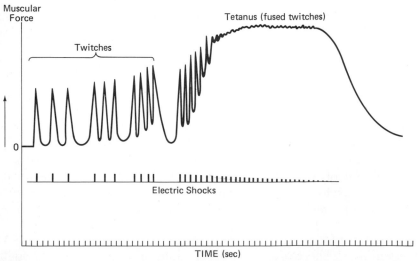

Figure 7.2. Fusion of muscle twitches to form a tetanic contraction.

the rested state. This sort of contraction is not of much use in most physical activity; instead a much smoother, longer acting type of contraction is needed. The smooth contractions that are typical of human movements result from the fusion of asynchronous twitches of fibers from different motor units so that, at any given instant, only the appropriate amount of force is produced.

As a rough illustration of the fusion of asynchronously twitching fibers to produce a smooth movement, assume that a slow, continuous flexion of the index finger requires the force of contraction of 100 muscle fibers (but not the same 100 fibers) during the entire movement. This contractile force could be accomplished by activating different groups of 10 motor units, each with 10 muscle fibers, every 20 milliseconds. Accordingly, twitch contractions of 100 fibers would start the movement and would be immediately succeeded by the twitching of another 100 fibers, which would be followed by twitches of another 100 fibers, and so on. The twitches of the first group of 100 fibers would be smoothly fused into the twitches of successive batches of 100 fibers until the movement was completed.

Tetanic Contractions of Motor Units. It is possible to produce greater force in a smooth voluntary movement by the high-frequency stimulation of individual motor units, so that twitches of muscle fibers in these units fuse into a constant, steady contraction for as long as these motor units are active (only a fraction of a second, except during maximal contractions). These steady contractions are called *tetanic contractions*, and the muscle fibers involved are said to be in a state of tetanus (Fig. 7.2). Tetanus of a certain number of motor units at any one time does not, of course, mean that an entire muscle is in a state of rigid contraction. As more or fewer motor units fire tetanically, a greater or lesser contraction will result, so that a movement such as a pullup can be completed smoothly.

As inspection of Fig. 7.2 shows, a tetanic contraction produces more force than a single twitch. The explanation given for this phenomenon is that during a *twitch* contraction, part of the contractile energy is used to overcome the resistance to change of length of the connective tissue and other components of the muscle. However, in *tetanus*, the muscle is not allowed to return to its resting length, so that resistance of the tissue need not be repeatedly overcome (2). Thus, the contractile energy normally expended in overcoming internal muscle resistance in a twitch can be used to do work in a tetanic contraction. The fact that tetanic contractions produce more force than twitch contractions is not a violation of the "all or none" law because the conditions (length, temperature, etc.) of the muscle fibers prior to stimulation are dissimilar.

NEURAL CONTROL OF MUSCULAR STRENGTH: EXCITATORY AND INHIBITORY NEURONS

In the previous portions of this chapter, reference has often been made to the role of the motor nerve in the activation of muscle fibers. Obviously, the motor nerve or neuron is influenced by stimuli from other nerves that reach the cell body of the motor nerve as it lies in the anterior part of the gray matter of the spinal cord (Fig. 7.3). The biceps muscle of the upper arm will not contract maximally, for example, until the brain sends thousands of stimuli down to the spinal cord to stimulate (facilitate) all the motor neurons of the biceps. In addition to stimuli from the motor areas of the cortex of the brain and from other lower brain areas (such as the basal ganglia, the reticular formation and the cerebellum), reflex stimuli from higher and lower levels of the spinal cord, and from peripheral organs such as muscle spindles, modify the activity of anterior motor neurons and, consequently, are involved in the control of muscle strength (7). A basic understanding of how the activity of the motor neurons is af-

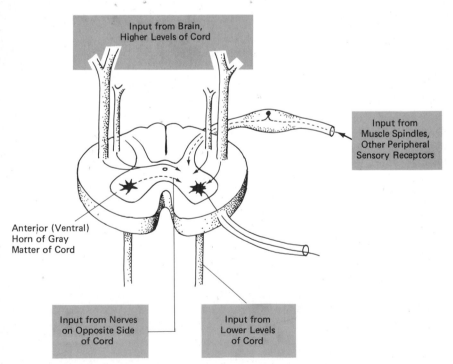

Input from Brain, Higher Levels of Cord

Input from Muscle Spindles, Other Peripheral Sensory Receptors

Anterior (Ventral) Horn of Gray Matter of Cord

Input from Nerves on Opposite Side of Cord

Input from Lower Levels of Cord

Figure 7.3. Schematic diagram of some of the many types of nerve fibers that affect the activity of the lower motor neuron.

fected by other parts of the nervous system is helpful in determining how strength is affected by psychological, emotional, environmental and training phenomena.

All neurons send signals to other neurons by transmitting small amounts of chemicals (*neurotransmitters*) to the other neurons. Some of these neurotransmitters excite a neuron and tend to make it fire, whereas others inhibit the neuron and keep it quiescent. These neurotransmitters are called *excitatory* (*facilitatory*) and *inhibitory* neurotransmitters, respectively. Any given neuron secretes either an excitatory or an inhibitory substance, not both, and is therefore known either as an excitatory neuron or an inhibitory neuron.

Whether or not a motor neuron fires or becomes quiet depends upon the *net* effect of all the excitatory and inhibitory stimuli that arrive at the motor neuron at any instant. Let us assume for illustration purposes that a motor neuron will fire if it has a *net* of 100 *excitatory* neurotransmitter molecules on its cell body at any given time. Now suppose that we measure all the molecules of excitatory and inhibitory chemicals that are on this neuron at time X and find 200 excitatory molecules and 150 inhibitory molecules. The net result of these stimuli is $200 - 150 = 50$ excitatory molecules, and the motor neuron will not fire because its threshold of a net 100 excitatory molecules has not been met. Next, suppose that 150 excitatory molecules and 20 inhibitory molecules are present at a given moment. In this situation a net of $150 - 20 = 130$ excitatory molecules surpasses the firing threshold of 100, and the nerve will now fire. Therefore, there are three ways in which a quiet motor neuron can be stimulated to fire: by increasing the excitatory stimuli while the inhibitory stimuli remain constant, by decreasing the inhibitory stimuli while the excitatory stimuli remain constant, and by a combination of increasing the excitatory and decreasing the inhibitory stimuli. The last method is probably the most common.

There are both excitatory and inhibitory stimuli that descend from lower parts of the brain to the spinal motor nerves. The inhibitory impulses are important in helping man avoid spastic, painful contractions of muscles whenever a violent burst of excitatory impulses reaches the motor neuron from other parts of the nervous system. However, when a person wishes to exert a maximal strength effort, the inhibitory influences from the brain stem may interfere with his ability to call forth all his motor units at once. One explanation of individual differences in strength maintains that a stronger individual is the one who is capable of blocking more of his inhibitory neurons, so that more motor units can reach their firing thresholds (4). Perhaps through strength training, one can learn to reduce the inhibitory output of the brain to the lower motor neurons.

CENTRAL MODIFIERS OF STRENGTH—THE CORTEX, CEREBELLUM, AND LOWER BRAIN CENTERS

Even though complex movements are initiated by the motor areas of the cerebral cortex, these impulses are accompanied by output from other parts of the brain that tend to alter somewhat the eventual movement response (Fig. 7.4). For example, output from the vestibular nuclei adjusts the ultimate motor response to take into account changes in balance or acceleration as sensed by the inner ear,

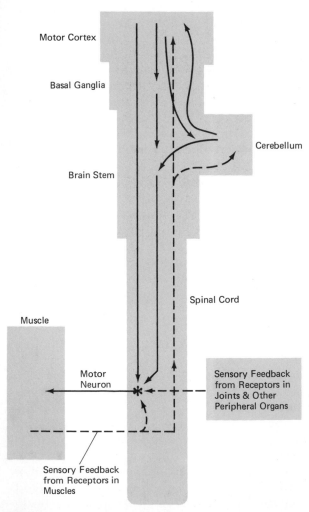

Figure 7.4. Schematic diagram illustrating some modifiers of motor stimuli.

and output from the cerebellum affects the motor response according to the cerebellum's analysis of all the data it receives from both brain centers and peripheral receptors, such as the muscle spindles of the muscles themselves.

It is also apparent that other parts of the brain can generate stimuli that influence motor behavior. Many emotions, for example, arise in the limbic lobe of the cortex and in the hypothalamus, and can influence a wide variety of motor activity from a complete cessation of movement associated with overwhelming fear or shock to the uncontrollable movements associated with rage (9). It takes an exceptionally sensitive teacher or coach to identify emotional influences on movement behavior and to help his students or athletes cope with and hopefully master the emotions. A coach must understand the powerful impact that emotions have on young minds and try to make certain that he does not foster inappropriate emotions ("Kill 'em!" "Hurt 'em!") that could result in physical or psychological injury in the name of winning performances. On the other hand, the appropriate use of "pep talks" can often bring out the best in performance, both on and off the athletic field.

PERIPHERAL MODIFIERS OF STRENGTH—JOINT RECEPTORS, MUSCLE SPINDLES, AND TENDON ORGANS

It would be convenient if there were located in moving limbs some sensors that could determine the extent to which a movement initiated by the brain were accomplishing its goal, and then report that information back to the brain and spinal cord, so that any necessary corrections in the movement could be made. Fortunately, such a movement feedback system is present in muscles and joints. It can report to the brain and cord the status of joint movements, limb positions, muscle force, muscle stretch and speed of muscle stretch.

The ability to judge the appropriateness of a muscle contraction, to judge where limbs are in space in relation to each other, and to know how fast and to what extent joint angles are changing is called the *kinesthetic sense*. This sense is obviously of vital importance in all human movements, but especially those involved in skills such as tumbling, diving, and pole vaulting where a failure of kinesthetic sense could easily result in severe injury or death. The nerve endings or receptors that sense limb and joint position lie in the connective tissues around joint capsules and in ligaments; they are extremely sensitive, and conduct their information back to the spinal cord and brain very rapidly so that corrections in movements may likewise be made quickly.

The role of joint receptors in modifying muscular strength can be illustrated as follows. In executing a pole vault, the joint receptors feed back information on how the body parts are aligned just prior to the "handstand" at the peak of the vault. If the vaulter senses from this information that he must bring himself closer to the pole, he exerts more arm strength to accomplish that goal. If, on the other hand, the vaulter senses that his body is too far ahead of the pole, he can decrease the strength of his arm contractions to correct the faulty position. As another example, consider a weightlifter who, while completing a press, senses that his extended arms are moving behind his head, and makes a rapid decision about what to do with the 200-pound barbell supported above his head by his rapidly tiring arms! Kinesthetic sense has doubtless saved many weightlifters embarrassing falls and serious injuries.

Muscle Spindles, the Stretch Reflex, and the Gamma Motor System

Both the length of muscles and the rate of changes in muscle length are sensed by receptors called *muscle spindles* that are buried in the muscles themselves (Fig. 7.5) (7). These spindles are covered by connective tissue that is interwoven with that surrounding the regular (*extrafusal*) muscle fibers, so that anytime the whole muscle is

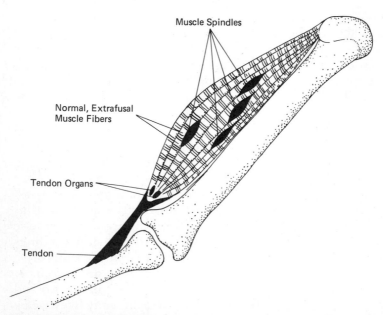

Muscle Spindles

Normal, Extrafusal Muscle Fibers

Tendon Organs

Tendon

Figure 7.5. Schematic diagram illustrating location of muscle spindles and tendon organs.

stretched or shortened, the spindle is also stretched or shortened. The interior of the muscle spindle usually contains 2–12 small, peculiar muscle fibers, called *intrafusal fibers* because of their location inside the *fusiform* (tapering from the middle toward each end) spindle (Fig. 7.5). The larger, extrafusal muscle fibers that surround the spindles are innervated by large *alpha motor neurons* with cell bodies located in the spinal cord (Figs. 7.5, 7.6).

The middle portion of an intrafusal fiber does not contract; this portion of the fiber is stretched whenever the contractile ends of the intrafusal fiber are stimulated to contract by their motor nerves, the small *gamma motor neurons* (Fig. 7.6). Thus, *there are two ways in which the middle, noncontractile part of the intrafusal fibers can be stretched*. First, when the whole muscle (extrafusal fibers) is

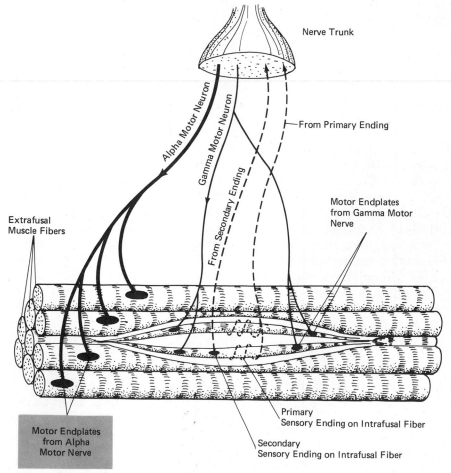

Figure 7.6. **Schematic simplified diagram of muscle spindle anatomy.**

stretched, the stretch is transmitted through the connective tissue to the muscle spindle which then is also stretched. Second, if a motor impulse comes from the spinal cord down the gamma motor nerve, the outer two-thirds of the intrafusal fibers contract and pull on the noncontractile middle third of the fibers thereby causing them to be stretched.

Once the middle portion of an intrafusal fiber is stretched, the stretch is sensed by one or both of two sensory nerve endings attached to this middle part of the intrafusal fiber (Fig. 7.6). The *primary* ending senses not only the stretch of the intrafusal fiber, *but also the velocity* of the stretch, and feeds this information back to the spinal cord and on up to the cerebellum, so that any necessary adjustments can be made in muscle contraction, as will be described in the next section (7). The *secondary* endings sense only the stretch of the intrafusal fibers. Thus, the muscle spindles are responsible for the myotatic or stretch reflex, an important spinal reflex that is involved in nearly all human movements and is especially important in the control of posture.

The Stretch Reflex.   If a muscle is suddenly stretched, for example, by a wrestler who forcefully pulls his opponent's arm in an attempted takedown, the muscle almost instantaneously contracts to resist that stretch. This reflex operates at the level of the spinal cord, that is, it does not require conscious thought by the brain. A simple example of the stretch (myotatic) reflex is the knee jerk reflex that is diagrammed in Fig. 7.7. As the reflex hammer strikes the patellar tendon, the quadriceps muscles are rapidly stretched. This stretch of extrafusal fibers is transmitted via connective tissue to the muscle spindle and its intrafusal fibers. As the central portions of the intrafusal fibers are stretched, the primary and secondary sensory endings are stimulated to send an excitatory impulse to the *alpha motor neurons* in the spinal cord. These large alpha motor neurons then stimulate the extrafusal fibers of the same muscle to contract, thereby relieving the stretch. At the same time inhibitory impulses are transmitted to the antagonistic muscles to cause them to relax.

Whenever muscle length changes, the muscle spindles report the changing conditions back to the brain and spinal cord so that appropriate adjustments in muscle contraction can be made. Note, however, that a muscle jerk does not always occur when a muscle is stretched. Ordinarily, muscle stretch is less rapid than when caused by a tap of the tendon hammer, and other factors, such as the stretch of the antagonists, modify the response to stretch so that a less dramatic response occurs.

It is important to think of the information that comes to the alpha motor neurons from the muscle spindles as only one of many

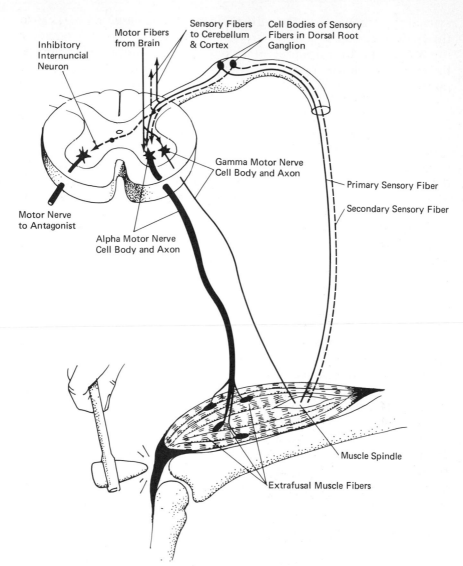

Figure 7.7. Schematic illustration of stretch reflex.

types of information that the motor neurons receive. These neurons are constantly being bombarded with information from the muscles, joints, ligaments, and tendons, from other neurons at the same and different levels of the spinal cord, and from various parts of the brain. Muscle spindles are, however, one of the more important sources of information for movement, because the ability to sense muscle length and speed of length change is obviously important for complex and even simple movement, including the maintenance of an erect posture.

When a person stands erect, gravity tends to pull him forward or backward whenever posture is not perfectly balanced. As gravity pulls one forward, the muscles at the back of the legs are stretched, and the stretch reflex causes these muscles to contract against gravity so that balance is regained. Conversely, if gravity pulls one slightly backward, the muscles in the front of the legs are stretched and are quickly stimulated to contract by the action of muscle spindles and the stretch reflex. Erect posture then can be maintained primarily by a gentle to and fro swaying motion around the point of perfect balance with the aid of irregular stretch reflex activity (2).

The Gamma Motor System and Muscle Strength. The muscle spindles can become especially sensitive to stretch if the intrafusal fibers are slightly contracted by low level, steady (tonic) activity of the gamma motor nerves. This tonic gamma motor stimulation causes a very slight stretch of the middle portions of the intrafusal fibers so that the smallest additional stretch of the extrafusal fibers activates the primary and secondary endings of the muscle spindles. Such tonic activity of the gamma motor nerves is important for fine control of movement and posture, and can be brought about by excitatory impulses descending to the gamma motor nerves in the spinal cord from nerves originating in the hypothalamus and the reticular formation of the brain stem (7).

It is also apparent that the gamma system operates during most movements of the limbs in order to "reset" muscle spindles that have been shortened by movements of surrounding extrafusal fibers; the spindles are then able to respond to stretch of the now shortened extrafusal fibers (Fig. 7.8) (6). As an illustration of this complex phenomenon, let us imagine that a wrestler is about to contract his gastrocnemius muscle by plantar flexion of the ankle, in order to escape from a particularly troublesome hold by his opponent. Upon shortening the gastrocnemius during plantar flexion, the intrafusal fibers would go slack with little tension at the ends of the fibers were there no gamma activity. If this should happen, any lengthening or stretch of the gastrocnemius from its newly shortened position could not be sensed by the spindles until after the intrafusal fibers had been stretched past their original positions. Thus, without gamma motor activity, the wrestler would be unable to sense muscle stretch until his gastrocnemius had returned to its original length; he might, therefore, be unable to rapidly counteract a move by his opponent that would stretch the gastrocnemius.

This example is similar to that shown in Fig. 7.8. In Fig. 7.8a, the relative lengths of intrafusal and extrafusal fibers are shown before

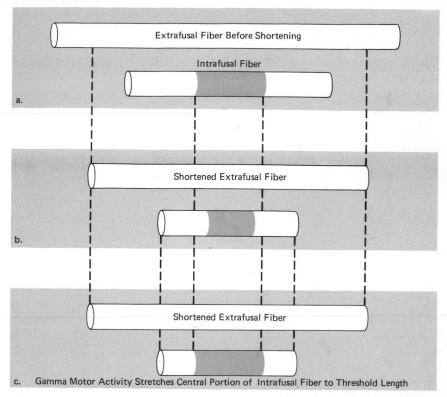

a.

b.

c.

Figure 7.8. Role of gamma motor stimuli in maintaining sensitivity of muscle spindle sensory endings at different lengths of extrafusal muscle fibers. See text for discussion.

contraction of the muscle. In Fig. 7.8b, the diagram shows what might occur if there were *no* tonic gamma motor nerve stimuli to reset the central portions of the intrafusal fibers to their initial stretch-sensitive lengths. Fig. 7.8c shows the effect of gamma activity on maintaining the central portions of the intrafusal fibers at their sensitive lengths, that is, the lengths shown in Fig. 7.8a. Note that in Fig. 7.8c, the *total* intrafusal fiber length is the same as that shown in Fig. 7.8b, but the gamma activity in Fig. 7.8c has shortened the outer contractile portions while stretching the central portions to reset them to their stretch-sensitive lengths.

Research supports the view that under normal circumstances, the initiation of movement is brought about by stimulation of both alpha and gamma motor neurons by the brain (alpha-gamma coactivation) so that muscles are always sensitive to changes in length (6). The increased gamma activity during contraction may also aid the expression of maximal muscle strength by creating extra excitatory stimuli from the primary and secondary sensory endings of the muscle spindles. These stimuli could excite the alpha motor neurons that cause the maximal contractions of the extrafusal fibers (7). It is possible that one reason some persons exhibit great strength is that they have more powerful means of stimulating both alpha and gamma motor neurons simultaneously. Such an ability would maximize excitatory stimuli to alpha motor neurons of the spinal cord and thereby maximize nerve stimuli to the muscles.

Tendon Organ Reflexes and Muscle Strength

In previous paragraphs, we have discussed how stimuli from sensory endings in muscle spindles might aid the expression of strength

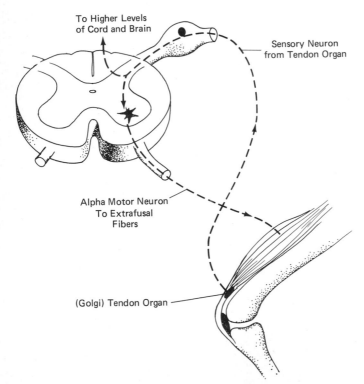

Figure 7.9. Schematic diagram of tendon organ reflex. Contraction or severe stretch of muscle stimulates sensory ending of tendon organ which then sends inhibitory stimuli via sensory nerve to alpha motor nerve. Inhibition of alpha motor nerve reduces muscle contraction, thereby reducing tension on tendon organ.

by exciting alpha motor nerves in the spinal cord. We should also consider the possibility that *fewer inhibitory impulses* delivered to the alpha motor nerves would also tend to increase muscle strength. In an earlier section it was suggested that with strength training, inhibitory influences from the brain may be reduced. We shall now show that peripheral reflexes called tendon organ reflexes also inhibit alpha motor neuron activity as the force of muscle contraction increases. It may be that strength training also leads to a reduction of these inhibitory impulses.

Tendon organs (Golgi tendon organs) are located at the junctions of muscle and tendon (Fig. 7.5) and are sensitive mostly to contractile force, although extreme stretch of a muscle can also cause these receptors to fire. These tendon organs, consequently, report the level of muscle tension being exerted back to the spinal cord and the brain so that any necessary corrections in force can be made (Fig. 7.9). The tendon organ reflex is inhibitory, that is, greater amounts of tension in the muscle cause proportionate increases in inhibitory stimuli to flow from the tendon organ receptors to the alpha motor neurons, so that even greater contraction tends to be inhibited.

Although some authorities see the tendon organ reflex as a safety mechanism that prevents separation of tendon from bone when a contraction becomes too strong, others believe it serves primarily to

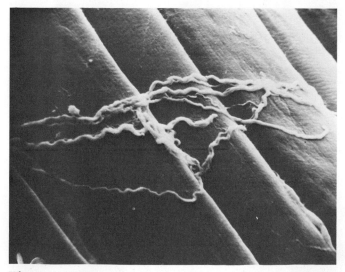

Figure 7.10. Stereo electron micrograph showing white nerve fibrils lying on surfaces of four muscle fibers. (Courtesy of R. E. Carrow, W. W. Heusner and W. D. Van Huss, Michigan State University, E. Lansing, Michigan.)

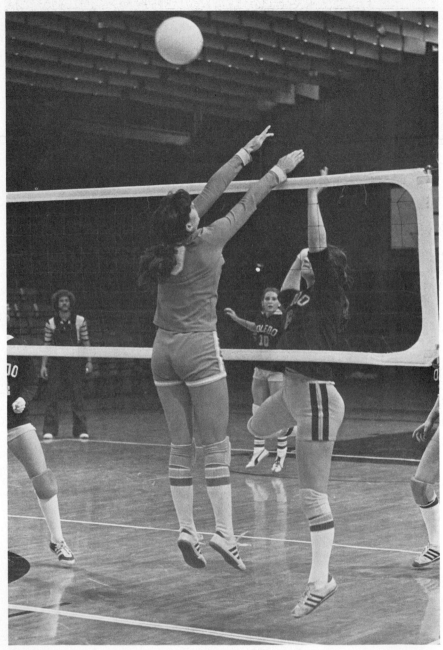

Figure 7.11.   Both central and peripheral inputs to motor neurons are essential to volleyball skills. (Courtesy of Office of Public Information, University of Toledo, Toledo, Ohio.)

feed back data about force levels in the muscle to the central nervous system (7). Regardless of its primary function, its role in the expression of muscular strength is obviously an inhibitory one, and any involvement of this reflex in strength training must include an adaptation, whereby the sensitivity of the organ to high levels of tension is reduced, or reaches a plateau. Such an involvement is highly speculative, and strength improvements may in fact proceed in spite of increased inhibition by tendon organ reflexes.

STRENGTH AND MUSCLE CROSS-SECTIONAL AREA

There is a nearly perfect relationship between the cross-sectional area of an isolated animal muscle in the laboratory and the maximal force that muscle can produce. For each square centimeter of cross-sectional area, various muscles can produce about 1–2 kilograms (2.2–4.4 pounds) of measured force (11). In the intact human being, this relationship between cross-sectional area and muscular strength is still very strong, but as discussed in Chapter 9, increases in strength caused by training are often proportionately greater than increases in muscle size, so that the relationship between muscle size and strength is somewhat weaker in the whole organism than in the isolated muscle preparation. Nevertheless, the single best predictor of the strength of a person's muscles is the cross-sectional area of those muscles.

Cross-sectional area of muscles is, of course, only roughly estimated by measuring the circumference or girth of a limb. Girth measurements include not only muscle, but fat and bone as well. Also, they do not take into account differences in the spatial arrangements of muscle fibers, that is, whether the fibers run parallel or at angles to the long axis of the muscle. Consequently, limb girth is even less closely related to muscle strength than muscle cross-sectional area. Nevertheless, a significant linear relationship does exist between limb girth and strength. Therefore, limb girth measurements can be used to predict muscle strength, albeit not with 100 per cent accuracy.

From the physiological standpoint, why should bigger muscles generally be stronger? The answer seems to be that larger muscles have greater quantities of actin and myosin filaments and, therefore, greater numbers of cross bridges that can be activated to produce muscular force during contraction. The only reason someone with relatively small muscles might possess greater strength than a larger person is that the smaller individual may be able to activate more motor units.

STRENGTH AND ANGLE OF MUSCLE PULL ON BONE

A second important factor in determining the measured strength of a muscle contraction in man is the angle at which the muscle must exert tension on the bone. For elbow flexion, as an illustration, more vertical force is transmitted to the lower part of the arm at about 115 degrees of flexion than at either greater or lesser angles (Fig. 7.12). Therefore, a muscle has its optimum strength (when measured in man) at or near its optimum angle of pull on the bone where resistance is being applied. (Note that the angle of pull of the muscle on the bone is of major importance; the joint angle often, but not always, reflects this angle.) This fact should be remembered when reading the following paragraphs and when developing technique in a particular athletic skill. For example, at the start of a 100 meter dash, the best combination of hip, knee and ankle joint angles should be selected to provide the most explosive first stride away from the starting blocks. Studies of mechanical analysis and applied anatomy are helpful in developing such techniques.

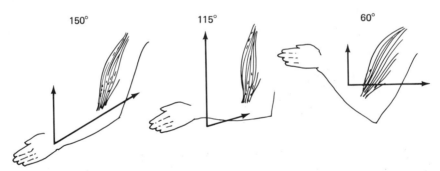

Figure 7.12. Effectiveness of angle of biceps pull on radius during elbow flexion at various elbow angles.

STRENGTH AND MUSCLE LENGTH

According to the sliding filament theory of muscle contraction as described in Chapter 2, there should be an optimal length of a muscle at which the greatest number of cross bridges can be activated to generate force. If a muscle was stretched too far, actin filaments would tend to be pulled away from myosin filaments and cross bridge attachments, whereas if a muscle was shortened too much, it appears that actin filaments might interfere with each other in making cross bridges effective for contraction (Fig. 7.13) (11). These concepts seem to be borne out in electron micrographs of stretched and shortened

A. Optimal Length, 16
effective cross bridges,
maximum strength

B. Too Much Stretch, 12
effective cross bridges,
reduced strength

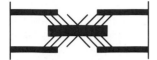

C. Too Much Shortening, 14
effective and 2 antagonistic
cross bridges for net of 12,
reduced strength

Figure 7.13.   **Effect of muscle length on number of
potentially active cross bridges.**

muscles and may explain the relationship between length and active
tension shown in Fig. 7.14. (11). It has also been suggested that shortening of a muscle decreases muscle force by reducing the calcium activation of cross bridges (10).

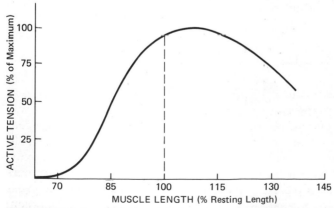

Figure 7.14.   **Relationship between muscle length and
active tension.**

In Fig. 7.14 it can be seen that maximal active tension is produced in a muscle that is stretched just slightly past its normal resting length in the body. To illustrate this concept, it is necessary to select a muscle that, when stretched, will not be at an ineffective angle of pull. The gastrocnemius is such a muscle; it should contract somewhat more forcefully when the angle is first dorsiflexed so that the gastrocnemius is stretched just beyond its normal resting length. Thus, a high jumper could expect to get a stronger plantar flexion on takeoff with a shoe that had a thick sole and a low heel that would place the plantar flexor muscles, including the gastrocnemius, on stretch. Alas, after such a shoe was used successfully by Soviet high jumpers in the early 1960's, it was banned from competition.

There are, however, other examples in athletics where muscles stretched just prior to contraction produce the greatest force. To achieve the greatest distance, the discus thrower must allow his outstretched throwing arm to follow his trunk as he spins around the

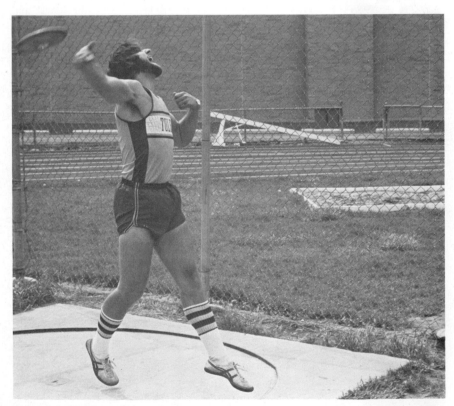

Figure 7.15.   Increasing force in the discus throw by stretching shoulder and arm muscles prior to contraction. (Courtesy of Office of Public Information, University of Toledo, Toledo, Ohio.)

throwing circle prior to the final release of the discus. Likewise, the weightlifter stretches hip and knee extensors as he squats to raise a heavy barbell, and the canoeist stretches his elbow extensors prior to initiating a stroke of his paddle.

As was cautioned in the previous section, one must always consider the most effective angle of pull of a muscle before deciding whether or not a muscle should be stretched prior to contraction. Consider the biceps of the arm, for example. If the biceps were placed on stretch, the elbow would be extended maximally, and most of the contractile force of the biceps would be directed toward pulling the head of the radius toward the humerus at the elbow. As shown in Fig. 7.12, the elbow flexors give maximal force at about 115 degrees of elbow flexion, not at 180 degrees or more. Thus, one must consider many factors when developing techniques in athletics; initial muscle length and angle of muscle pull must be considered together as only two of those factors. In measuring isometric muscular strength one should always document the joint angle at which the measurement is taken.

STRENGTH AND PRE-EXERTION COUNTERMOVEMENT (WINDUP)

In the previous section it was stated that placing the biceps muscle on stretch would not be effective in increasing strength, because of the inefficient angle of attachment of the muscle to the bone when the elbow is extended. This is true when strength is measured isometrically, but if elbow flexion *through the complete range of motion* of the elbow joint is to be made, one can exert a greater force on a dynamometer or lift a heavier weight by first making and then braking a rapid countermovement (in this case, elbow extension) with a resistance such as the weight of the dumbbell to be lifted during the subsequent elbow flexion (1, 3). This countermovement or windup causes the biceps to be stretched as it contracts eccentrically to brake the downward movement of the dumbbell and results in an immediate high level of force during the rapidly ensuing elbow flexion movement. A similar sort of positive effect of countermovement is sought whenever one winds up prior to throwing a javelin, baseball, football or discus; when one winds up with a sledge hammer as he tries to ring the gong at a carnival; or when a woodsman winds up with his ax prior to chopping a tree. The apparent reason why a windup or countermovement aids the expression of strength is that by stretching the elastic muscle and connective tissue during the eccentric contraction phase, energy is stored in these tissues that is immediately released during the first part of the subsequent concentric contraction (3). This stored energy is somewhat similar to that observed when a rubber band is first stretched and then released. When measuring strength, precautions should be taken to either eliminate or standardize windup movements since there will be differences in subjects' skills in performing them.

STRENGTH AND SPEED OF CONTRACTION

A muscle can produce a small force more rapidly than a great force. It is common knowledge that an animal trainer can lift a Baby-lonian butterfly over his head more quickly than he can an Abys-sinian antelope, but the physiological explanation for this phenome-non is not entirely clear. The relationship between contraction speed and the load that must be overcome by contraction is shown in Fig. 7.16. It seems that more time must be required to activate the extra cross bridges that are required to produce greater and greater force, but exactly why this should be is unknown (7).

Notice in Fig. 7.16 that at 100 per cent of maximum tension, the muscle is in a state of isometric contraction, that is, it cannot move the load. Therefore, maximum isometric strength at any joint angle is always greater than dynamic concentric strength at that angle. This does not seem to be the case for eccentric contractions, however. Maximum strength at a given joint angle is greater when the muscle is lengthening (as it attempts to overcome too great a load) than when it is concentrically or isometrically contracting (2). The expla-nation for the greater strength of eccentric contractions is also not

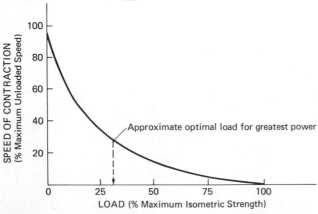

Figure 7.16. **Relationship between load and speed of contraction.**

known, but is probably due in part to the lack of muscle force needed to overcome internal resistance of muscle and connective tissue during an eccentric contraction. The "wasted" force that is used to overcome internal resistance during concentric and isometric contractions can be used to help overcome external resistance in eccentric contractions.

The relationship between load and speed of contraction suggests that Fig. 7.16 might be studied to gain insight into the optimal combinations of speed and load required to provide the greatest possible muscular *power, which is defined as the product of force and speed,* that is, Power = Force × Speed or Force × Distance/Time. Power is particularly important in athletic events such as the shot put, discus throw, high jump, long jump and pole vault. In the shot put and discus throw, muscular strength (force) can be improved to a much greater extent than speed, and since there is no evidence that increases in strength cause decreases in speed (in fact, speed of loaded movements such as a shot put will improve), the athlete simply applies his maximum strength with all the speed he can muster. In the jumps and vaults, on the other hand, some optimal body weight will result in the greatest strength and speed combination. If the jumper loses too much weight, he may also lose strength, but should he get too heavy, extra strength will be of no value.

In an industrial situation an efficiency expert may determine with the aid of Fig. 7.16 that packages weighing about 30 per cent of one's maximal isometric strength will be optimal for the most rapid loading of a truck. Packages heavier or lighter than this would require too long a time to lift the same total weight of the product onto the truck. Of course, other factors such as fatigue and package bulk would have to be considered. It is known that men produce maximum bicycling power when pedaling at about 30 per cent of leg extensor maximal strength (4).

STRENGTH AND WARM-UP

When an isolated muscle in the laboratory is cooled, its strength and speed of contraction and relaxation are reduced, whereas heat increases contractile strength and speed. Nerves also conduct impulses more rapidly, and connective tissues such as ligaments and tendons become more pliable with greater temperature. These enhanced functions are probably the result of greater enzyme activity and less resistance to change of length (lower "viscosity") in the heated tissues. If such effects of warming occur in man, then maximal strength should be somewhat improved by warm-up of the muscle prior to the exertion of muscular force.

There are many types of warmup that different performers have tried in hopes of increasing strength (5). These can be classified as *passive warm-up, active general warm-up,* and *active practice warm-up.* Passive warm-up includes massage and the local or general application of heat by means of infrared lamps, ultrasound, diathermy, steam baths, sauna baths, hot water baths, hot showers and hot packs. Active general warm-up is the use of physical activity such as running or calisthenics to raise body temperature, and active practice warm-up is the practice of all or parts of a movement prior to measurement or competition in that same movement.

Most research on passive warm-up has shown that it is not particularly helpful in the expression of muscular strength, perhaps because many of the warm-up techniques were applied too briefly or without enough intensity to change deep muscle temperature (5). As an example, several studies included the use of hot showers for only a few minutes, probably because of the discomfort of the subjects. Although a brief shower may warm the skin, this warmth is transmitted slowly to the muscles, and the important factor is that muscle temperature must be elevated. Similarly, when only a portion of the body such as an arm or leg is heated, the body very effectively rids itself of the extra heat load by evaporative heat loss through increased sweating, and by greater radiation of heat from the rest of the body surface, so that muscle temperature, even of the heated arm, is little changed; the blood cools the muscle faster than the environment heats it. Massage does not change muscle temperature, and it is therefore not surprising that massage does not affect muscle strength (5).

On the other hand, strength is usually somewhat benefitted by active general warm-up and active practice warm-up. Running, stair stepping, and cycling for 5–30 minutes prior to strength or vertical jump measurements usually improve performance. Similarly, repeated trials with the shot, discus or javelin prior to competition improve performance by 5–50 per cent over the no–warm-up condition. Active warm-up appears to be most effective if practiced for 5 to 30 minutes, and should usually precede testing or competition by no more than 15 minutes (5).

Some or most of the effectiveness of active practice warm-up, such as skill practice, is thought to be due to an activation of the appropriate nerve pathways so that more motor units can be brought into play. One must also consider the likelihood that for some individuals the warm-up effect is partly psychological because most performers have been taught to believe in the value of warm-up. Since there is no evidence that active warm-up of a reasonable duration is detrimental to performance, such warm-up routines should be recommended with a view toward not only an enhancement of strength performance, but also toward the possibility of preventing injury to "cold" muscles and joints. This last assumption on injury prevention is unsupported by experimental research, but it is warranted on the basis of the experiences of many athletes and coaches.

STRENGTH, AGE, AND SEX

It is common knowledge that males are generally stronger than females and that people get stronger as they grow older until they are in their twenties, after which time, strength gradually declines with advancing age. These facts are described in Fig. 7.17, where the average strengths of many muscle groups for males and females from 8–60 years of age are plotted as percentages of the maximum strength of males, which occurs in the middle-to-late twenties (1, 4, 8). As a rule of thumb, it can be said that females after about age sixteen are about two-thirds as strong as males and that muscle strength of boys is only slightly greater than that of girls prior to puberty. At puberty, the strength of males dramatically increases, probably be-

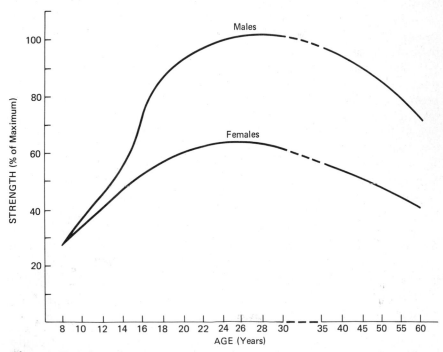

Figure 7.17. Average strength of many muscle groups as a function of age and sex. Data from reference 8.

cause of the influence of testosterone, the chief male sex hormone, which stimulates muscle growth. These sex differences in muscle strength are greater in muscles of the arms, shoulders, and trunk, and smaller in muscles of the legs.

Figure 7.17 simply describes the influence of age and sex on strength. The explanation of *how* these differences develop is not entirely certain, but considerations of muscle size, nervous system maturation and cultural sex roles are thought to be important. Muscle size, for example, increases with age in both sexes and is greater for males than females after puberty. Because we know that strength is related to the cross-sectional area of the muscle (more actin and myosin filaments), it might seem likely that the only explanation needed for the curves of Fig. 7.17 is the effect of muscle size unless the muscles of females have different strengths per unit of the cross-sectional area than males. Indeed, researchers have estimated that females are equally as strong as males when strength is expressed per unit of cross-sectional area of the muscles. Thus, most of the strength differences between the sexes can be explained by differences in muscle size caused by male sex hormones (4, 8). However, muscle size cannot be the sole explanation of strength gains with increasing age, because strength increases faster in both males and females than does muscle size. It seems apparent that the maturation of the nervous system with age must allow older persons (up to about 25 years old), both male and female, to call more motor units into action during strength-related activities.

There is undoubtedly a cultural effect that also plays some role in determining sex differences in strength. Young girls in general have been taught that forceful physical exertion is unfeminine, and consequently, after puberty they usually shy away from activities that would have a training effect on strength. Therefore, comparisons between males and females in strength may be somewhat unfair, since males are likely to be in a more "trained" state than females. In this light it is interesting that leg muscle strength, especially before puberty, is very similar in girls and boys. Perhaps the explanation for this is that young boys and girls tend to have similar amounts of training of these leg muscles because they do similar amounts of walking and running. For muscles of the arms and shoulders, though, boys usually have more training from rope climbing, wrestling, throwing and other "masculine" activities.

Variation in Strength Within Sexes and Age Groups

Although a definite effect of age and sex on muscular strength can be shown if large numbers of subjects are tested, one must not expect every 10-year-old to be stronger than every 8-year-old, or every

15-year-old girl to be weaker than every 15-year-old boy. There is a wide range of strength at a given age or in a given sex. One of the reasons for strength differences within an age group, especially before age 18, is that children mature at different rates, so that it is possible to find two 12-year-olds whose biological or maturation age as determined by x-ray measurements of bones are 10 and 15, respectively (1). The 12-year-old who has not matured as rapidly will probably have smaller muscles, a less highly developed nervous system, and, if males are compared, a lower secretion of male sex hormones. All of these factors will tend to make the less mature person less strong than his more mature counterpart. In the physical education class, therefore, instructors should compare strength performances of children classified according to height or some other estimate of biological age rather than according to chronological age. In like manner, a small immature boy should not be expected to be stronger than larger girls his same age. The physical educator who recognizes the impact of age, sex, maturity and muscle size on strength is better prepared to help reduce potentially harmful peer pressures among children who, in the case of boys, think that weaker classmates are "sissies" or, in the case of girls, think that stronger classmates are "Amazons."

Review Questions

1. Define the following terms: maximal strength, isotonic contraction, isometric contraction, isokinetic contraction, motor unit, tetanic contraction.
2. Explain how the nervous system governs the amount of force generated by skeletal muscles so that the same muscles are capable of smoothly lifting both a piece of paper and a heavy tire. Include in your explanation a discussion of asynchronous twitches of muscle fibers from different motor units.
3. Describe how excitatory and inhibitory stimuli from the central nervous system, and from peripheral receptors, modify the output of the lower motor neurons and thereby modify the contractions of muscles.
4. Diagram and describe the stretch reflex.
5. Define: intrafusal fibers, extrafusal fibers, primary and secondary endings of muscle spindles, the gamma motor system, and alpha motor neuron.
6. Explain how muscle spindles can remain sensitive to stretch of a muscle while the muscle is undergoing changes in length.
7. What is the function of the Golgi tendon organs?

8. Describe and explain the relationships between muscle strength and the following: cross–sectional area of the muscle, angle of muscle pull on bone, muscle length, windup, speed of contraction, warm-up, age, and sex.

References

1. Asmussen, E. Growth in muscular strength and power. In G. L. Rarick (Ed.), *Physical Activity: Human Growth and Development.* New York: Academic Press, 1973, pp. 60–79.
2. Asmussen, E. The neuromuscular system and exercise. In H. B. Falls (Ed.), *Exercise Physiology.* New York: Academic Press, 1968, pp. 3–42.
3. Asmussen, E., and F. Bonde-Petersen. Storage of elastic energy in skeletal muscles in man. *Acta Physiologica Scandinavica,* 1974, **91**:385–392.
4. Astrand, P.-O., and K. Rodahl. *Textbook of Work Physiology.* New York: McGraw-Hill, 1970.
5. Franks, B. D. Physical warm-up. In W. P. Morgan (Ed.), *Ergogenic Aids and Muscular Performance.* New York: Academic Press, 1972, pp. 159–191.
6. Granit, R. Linkage of alpha and gamma motoneurones in voluntary movement. *Nature New Biology.* 1973, **243**:52–53.
7. Henneman, E. Peripheral mechanisms involved in the control of muscle. In V. B. Mountcastle (Ed.), *Medical Physiology,* 13th ed. St. Louis: The C. V. Mosby Co., 1974, pp. 617–635.
8. Hettinger, T.*Physiology of Strength.* Springfield, Ill.: Charles C Thomas, 1961.
9. Ikai, M., and A. H. Steinhaus. Some factors modifying the expression of human strength. *Journal of Applied Physiology,* 1961, **16**:157–163.
10. Ridgeway, E. B., and A. M. Gordon. Muscle activation: effects of small length changes on calcium release in single fibers. *Science,* 1975, **189**:881–884.
11. Zierler, K. L. Mechanism of muscle contraction and its energetics. In V. B. Mountcastle (Ed.), *Medical Physiology,* 13th ed. St. Louis: The C. V. Mosby Co., 1974, pp. 77–120.

8

Evaluation of muscular strength

The evaluation of all aspects of physical fitness, including muscular strength, is important for three principal reasons. First, without tests of physical fitness, it is impossible to accurately assess the need for a given type of fitness training program for a particular individual or group of individuals. Second, results of fitness tests can be used by the physical educator, physician or athletic coach to improve his precision in the prescription of a given training or rehabilitation program. Third, a regular fitness testing and retesting program will help establish the effectiveness or inadequacy of a training program. In this and other chapters of the text, some basic principles of fitness testing will be presented. For greater detail one should consult testing manuals and specific journals for a given test (3).

Testing of muscular strength can be frustrating. For one thing, there is no convenient method to measure all the types of strength that are employed in daily activities and in athletic competition. Also, a test once selected must be used in any retest of strength after a training program, because the type of test used often has a great bearing on whether improvements with a specific training program will seem small or large (1). These and other aspects of strength testing will be discussed in this chapter. As a beginning, the three different ways in which muscular strength are expressed will be described in the next section.

STATIC, ISOTONIC AND ISOKINETIC STRENGTH

Maximal strength is expressed by isometric, isotonic, or isokinetic contractions. Isometric (static) strength is the maximal amount of muscular force one can exert briefly without movement of a joint. For example, one might stand in a doorway and push upwards against the top of the doorframe with all his might. He would ordinarily move neither his elbow joints nor the doorframe in such an exertion. Isometric strength can be measured by instruments called *dynamometers or tensiometers*, and such measurements are usually quite reproducible from one time to the next (2). Isometric strength is called into play when one pushes a car, carries heavy parcels, or pulls on a window that either does not move or moves very slowly. The name "isometric" is derived from the fact that muscle fibers which contract statically have very little change in length *(iso: equal, metric: measure)*.

Maximal isotonic strength is the greatest force that one can briefly exert throughout an entire movement. Thus, strength of forearm flexors is commonly measured by testing how heavy a barbell one can move through a complete range of elbow flexion, whereas hip- and knee-extension strength might be tested with a half or full squat movement with a barbell on the shoulders. There are also various types of commercial machines (such as Universal Gym) which can be used to measure isotonic strength. This type of strength is known as isotonic strength because the same force is produced (*iso:* equal, *tonic:* tone or tension) throughout the movement. *Maximal isotonic strength for a given movement is limited by the greatest muscular force that can be produced at the least effective angle of the joints involved in the movement.* Thus, in elbow flexion, isotonic strength is the force that can be produced at full extension as the movement begins.

When special "accommodating resistance" equipment is available, a type of controlled dynamic strength can be measured. In such contractions there is a constant speed of movement but changing forces throughout the movement. This type of maximal strength is known as isokinetic strength (*iso:* equal, *kinetic:* motion) because the rate of movement is held constant. The accommodating resistance device changes its internal mechanical resistance in proportion to changes in force applied by the subject. Accordingly, as one contracts his muscles more forcefully, the device increases its resistance to the force so that the speed of movement does not increase. Isokinetic strength is not truly isotonic because tension or force varies according to the effectiveness of the muscle contraction at different joint angles. (See Chapter 7 for review.) This type of strength is similar to that expressed during a hotly contested arm wrestling match where the contractions are nearly static, but the force changes as slight "dynamic" movements produce different joint angles and, therefore, more or less forceful contractions.

It should be pointed out that although relatively expensive machinery is needed for accurately measuring isokinetic strength, accommodating resistance for isokinetic *training* can be approximated by having one person actively resist the contractions of another through the range of motion of the joint. For example, one person could resist another's maximal knee extension efforts with his hands and slowly allow the knee extension to be completed (Fig. 8.1).

In Chapter 9, some of the contradictory evidence concerning

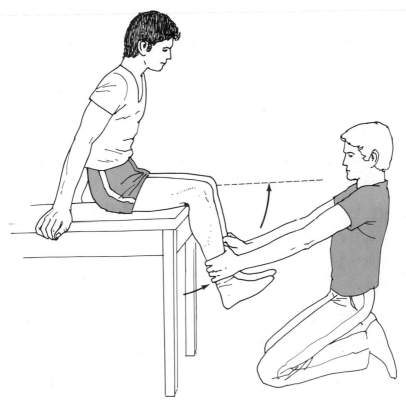

Figure 8.1. "Isokinetic" training.

which type of strength training, such as static, isotonic, or isokinetic, will be discussed. In the next section of this chapter, we will describe the techniques used to measure the three types of strength.

MEASUREMENT OF STRENGTH

Estimates of strength can be obtained with isometric, isotonic or isokinetic contractions. Isometric strength is usually measured with a spring-loaded dynamometer or cable tensiometer; isotonic strength is measured by a person's ability to lift a maximal weight through a complete range of motion; and isokinetic strength is measured with an isokinetic dynamometer (Fig. 8.2 abc).

Isometric Strength

Isometric strength assessment is relatively simple and reproducible, providing 1) the tester has had some experience, 2) he uses a recently calibrated dynamometer, and 3) he uses standardized testing routines to insure that desired limb joint angles are properly maintained and that extraneous contractions of other muscles are minimized (2). Common positions for the measurement of isometric elbow flexion strength and knee extension strength are shown in Fig. 8.3. (2).

Isotonic Strength

Isotonic strength is usually measured as the maximal weight that can be lifted correctly once in a given movement. This weight is known as the 1 R.M. (one repetition maximum). The maximal weight that could be lifted correctly three consecutive times without significant rest would be known as 3 R.M. One might test maximal elbow flexion strength by having the standing subject raise the heaviest barbell possible from his thighs through complete elbow flexion to a position just anterior to his clavicles. The maximal weight that can be lifted properly must be deterimed by trial and error.

Isokinetic Strength

As previously mentioned, isokinetic strength is determined with the aid of an accommodating resistance device that has an accurate indicator of the force exerted. Most of these devices are quite expensive.

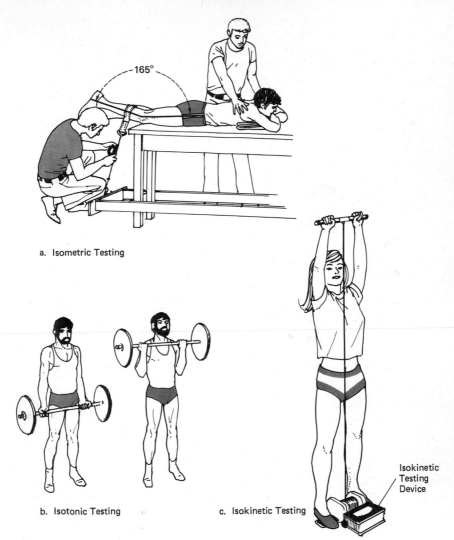

a. Isometric Testing

b. Isotonic Testing

c. Isokinetic Testing

Isokinetic
Testing
Device

Figure 8.2.   Strength evaluation.

CALIBRATION, SENSITIVITY AND REPRODUCIBILITY

In any kind of testing it is extremely important that the *sensitivity* and *reproducibility* of *calibrated* instruments have been recently analyzed so that meaningful measurements are assured. A commercial force-measuring device may have a very fancy "scientific" looking dial or scale that reads from 0–500 pounds, but it may not be sensitive enough to record any force under 100 pounds or distinguish

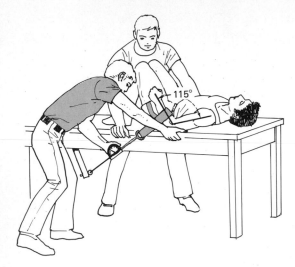

Elbow Flexion Strength

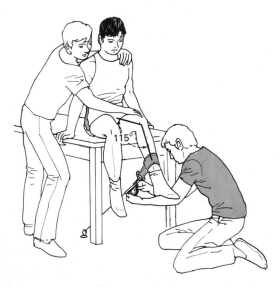

Knee Extension

Figure 8.3. Common positions for isometric testing of elbow flexion and knee extension strength.

between measurements less than 25 pounds apart. Such a device may also have a total lack of reproducibility, that is, it may not register the same reading every time the same force is measured.

Not only are impressive looking instruments subject to gross error, but even the actual mass of simple weight discs designed for barbells may vary 20 per cent or more from the weight stamped into the metal of the disc by the manufacturer. Accordingly, even weight discs should be checked with a scale that is known to be accurate before those weight discs are used in evaluating isotonic strength, or before they are used in the calibration of other force-measuring devices.

It should be pointed out that calibration of instruments and analysis of the sensitivity and reproducibility of one's measurements are important in all types of testing, not just in the testing of strength. It is hoped that the materials on strength testing in this chapter will be found adaptable to the testing of other phenomena in exercise physiology and other areas.

Calibration of Testing Equipment

When one determines the *actual* values corresponding to *observed* measurements or readings on some instrument, he *calibrates* that instrument. After calibration, the operator of a quantitative measuring device can then determine true measurements (within the sensitivity range of the instrument), based upon the readout of the instrument, even if the instrument itself cannot be corrected to give true readings. This can be done by preparing a calibration curve as depicted in Fig. 8.4.

The instrument calibration curve in Fig. 8.4 shows that the instrument in question can be used to record force only between 10 and 60 kilograms and that within that range of sensitivity the instrument registers 10 kilograms less than the actual force being measured. Thus, an instrument reading of 40 kilograms must be corrected to 50 kilograms to reflect the true force. If there were no linear portion of the curve in Fig. 8.4 (that is, the portion between 10–60 kilograms), the instrument could not be used because it would be impossible to extrapolate data between the points given in the curve. For example, an instrument reading of 53 kilograms would have an unknown true value if 53 did not fall on the linear portion of the calibration curve. Fortunately, most instruments have at least some range of linear response, but many are completely insensitive at low and/or high values.

Just about any instrument designed to measure force can be calibrated by loading it with weights that are predetermined to be accurate. This includes devices used to assess isometric and isokinetic

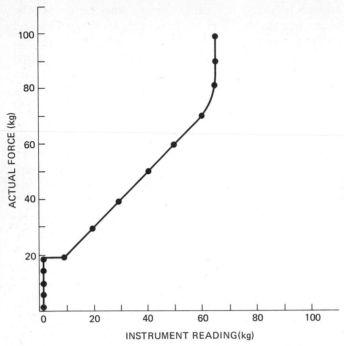

Figure 8.4. Calibration curve constructed by suspending known weights from dynamometer and comparing these weights with instrument readings.

strength. Isotonic strength, of course, should be evaluated by the subject's movement of calibrated weights through a standard range of motion.

Reproducibility of Measurements

Before one can have much confidence in the results of any sort of measurement, including the measurement of strength, he must be sure that his measurement is sensitive and that repeated measurements on the same subject at different times will give similar values. As stated previously, sensitivity is the degree to which the test can distinguish between forces that are similar, and is evaluated by constructing a calibration curve with known weights, with successive weights only slightly heavier than the previous ones. There are three common reasons why a measurement technique may not be reproducible. First, the measuring instrument or procedure used may not be capable of providing reproducible values. Second, the quality being measured may not be reproducible. Just as the taste of Mulligan stew is not reproducible because of the inherent variability of the ingredients, so, too, the measurement of a quality such as strength, conceivably could have poor reproducibility because of varying emotional or physiological factors. Third, a measurement may have inadequate reproducibility because a good technique is used by a poor technician, that is, the tester or testers may not be able to apply a measurement procedure in exactly the same way each time the procedure is administered. (A test which has poor reproducibility when used by a single tester is said to have poor "reliability," whereas a test which is reproducible for one tester, but not for others, has poor "objectivity.")

One simple technique can be used to determine the overall degree of reproducibility of a strength measurement procedure and to isolate the source of any lack of reproducibility in that procedure. The overall reproducibility can be assessed by making perhaps 10 repeated, standardized measurements of strength (allowing for adequate rest between tests) on three subjects of low, medium, and high strength. (It is possible for a procedure to be reproducible only for certain levels of strength.) A common way to express the degree of reproducibility so obtained is by calculating the *coefficient of variation* of the results. The coefficient of variation expresses the variability within a group of numbers (the scores of the repeated tests) as a percentage of the average (mean) of those numbers. If the variability of the measurements is only two or three per cent of the average value, then the measurement procedure has outstanding (almost unbelievable) reproducibility. Variability of 5–10 per cent of the average value is more common, and variability greater than 15 or 20 per cent suggests that better reproducibility needs to be obtained. No matter how good others have found the reproducibility of a given test to be, a tester should always analyze the reproducibility of the test in his hands under the exact situations he will encounter.

The calculation procedure for the coefficient of variation of any group of measurements is as follows.

Step 1: Add the data and arrive at a *total*.

Step 2: Square each number by multiplying it by itself.

Step 3: Add the squared numbers from Step 2 to arrive at a *sum of squares*.

Step 4: Square the *total* obtained in Step 1 to arrive at a *total squared*.

Step 5: Find the *standard deviation* (variability) of the numbers as follows:

    a. Divide the *total squared* from Step 4 by the number of measurements (N). (In this case the number of repeated tests on a subject.)

    b. Subtract the number obtained in Step 5a from the *sum of squares* found in Step 3.

    c. Divide the number obtained in Step 5b by the number of measurements less one (N − 1).

    d. Find the square root of the value obtained in Step 5c. The *standard deviation* thus computed represents about 1/3 of the spread of the scores from the mean. One standard deviation less than the mean, plus one standard deviation greater than the mean, include 2/3 of the scores.

Step 6: Find the average (mean) of the measurements by dividing the *total* obtained in Step 1 by the number of measurements (N).

Step 7: Divide the *standard deviation* obtained in Step 5c by the *mean* found in Step 6. Round off to three decimal places and then multiply by 100 (move the decimal two places to the right). This is the *coefficient of variation* and is expressed as a percentage.

Example:

    Suppose one measured the wing strength of the rare, yellow, tufted flea flicker 10 times and obtained the following data.

Trial	Strength (grams)	Squares	Procedure	
1	1	1	Step 1:	The total of all 10 measures is 16.
2	2	4	Step 2:	The squares are shown to the right of the strength measurements.
3	3	9	Step 3:	The sum of squares is 30.
4	2	4	Step 4:	$16 \times 16 = 256$
5	2	4	Step 5a:	256 divided by 10 is 25.6
6	1	1	Step 5b:	$30 - 25.6 = 4.4$
7	2	4	Step 5c:	4.4 divided by 9 is 0.49
8	1	1	Step 5d:	The square root of 0.49 is 0.7
9	1	1	Step 6:	16 divided by 10 is 1.6, the average strength value
10	1	1	Step 7:	0.7 divided by 1.6 is .438
				$100 \times .438 = 43.8\%$

    In this example, the wing strength measurements averaged 1.6 grams, but there was a substantial variability in these measurements. A coefficient of variation of 43.8 per cent means that the spread of about 2/3 of the strength measures could be expected to fall between 43.8 per cent below the mean and 43.8 per cent above the mean, that is, between 0.7 grams and 2.3 grams in this example. Considering that a perfectly reproducible test would give the same result every time it was administered to the same subject, a coefficient of variation of plus or minus 43.8 per cent suggests that one could have little confidence that a single measure of wing strength in the flea flicker represented the true strength of the wing.

Once the overall reproducibility of a test is determined under conditions similar to those that will occur when the test is administered in practice, that is, with the same tester (s), same instruments, and same standardized instructions and procedures, the exact source of poor reproducibility can be isolated by repeated determinations of the coefficient of variation with progressive elimination of each of the possible sources of poor reproducibility. For instance, if the reproducibility of the force measuring test is satisfactory when known weights are measured repeatedly, but not when a subject's strength is measured repeatedly, it can usually be assumed that the instrument and the testers are not sources of poor reproducibility, but that the expression of strength by the subject is. If results with other subjects show the same intrasubject variability, then another test will have to be used or a different way of exerting force will have to be considered. On the other hand, if reproducibility is good when a single tester is used, but not with several testers, changes in the standardized routines are in order so that all testers administer the test in the same careful manner. Finally, if the coefficient of variation is too high even when a known weight is repeatedly tested, the source of poor reproducibility is probably the instrument itself.

Review Questions

1. Describe and give examples of static, isotonic, and isokinetic strength expression in daily activities or athletic competition.
2. Define the terms *sensitivity* and *reproducibility* as they are used in the text. Define the term *calibration* as used in the text.
3. Compute the coefficient of variation for the following data: 3, 4, 2, 3, 5, 3, 6, 4, 5, 2. What is the significance of this value?

References

1. Clarke, D. H. Adaptations in strength and muscular endurance resulting from exercise. In J. H. Wilmore (Ed.), *Exercise and Sport Sciences Reviews*, 1973, **1**:73–102.
2. Clarke, H. H. *Muscular Strength and Endurance in Man.* Englewood Cliffs, N.J.: Prentice-Hall, Inc., 1966.
3. Clarke, H. H. *Application of Measurement to Health and Physical Education.* Englewood Cliffs, N.J.: Prentice-Hall, Inc., 1967.

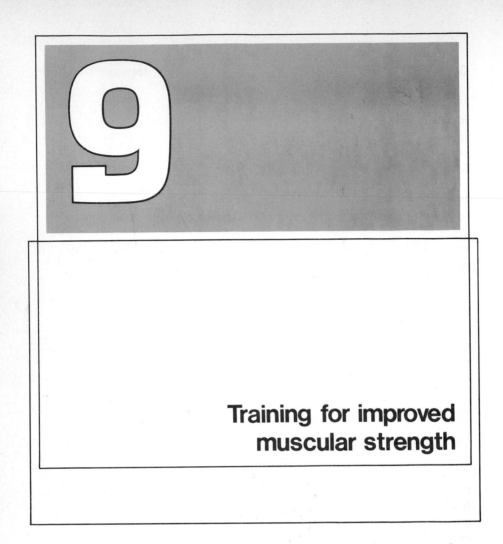

9

Training for improved muscular strength

Anyone who has read popular magazines on strength fitness or has visited a weight-training room in a school or in a commercial health salon knows that every weight-training devotee has his own peculiar ideas about the best ways to gain strength. These ideas include strange dietary concoctions, synthetic hormone shots, special breathing routines, and gorilla-like shouts during a lift. Since gains in strength can be brought about by "psychological/emotional" techniques (13, 21), it is likely that any technique that the trainee firmly believes in will have some beneficial effect on his strength. However, if one analyzes the research on principles for strength training and on various training methods, it becomes apparent that for most individuals certain principles and techniques lead to greater gains in strength than others. These research-based principles and techniques are described in this chapter and should serve as the basis of strength training programs.

GENERAL PRINCIPLES OF STRENGTH TRAINING

Regardless of whether one trains by isometric, isotonic or isokinetic methods, there are four general principles that should be followed to insure that the greatest possible training adaptation and strength gains will occur. These principles are discussed in the following paragraphs.

Principle 1: The training program should provide a progressive heavy overload of the specific muscle groups that are to be strengthened (4). The determination of the specific muscle groups that are to be strengthened can be made in either a simple or a sophisticated manner. Simply, one needs only to slowly perform a movement he wishes to strengthen, and to squeeze or palpate muscles on each side of the joint(s) involved until he finds those muscle groups that become tense and hard to the touch during the movement. The muscles that become tense are the muscles that are responsible for the movement, and these muscles must be trained with heavy resistance if the movement is to be strengthened. For example, if one wishes to improve his vertical jumping ability, he must overload primarily the hip and knee extensors and ankle plantar flexors that become tense and cause the jumping movement. To train these muscles one need only to perform movements of the joints that mimic the joint movements during jumping and to overload those movements with isometric, isotonic or isokinetic resistance. Such activities would include overloaded squats and toe raises. With this simple system of determining the specific muscle groups to be overloaded, one need not know the names of muscles or the names of strength-training exercises; one need only find out by trial and error which muscles become tense during a movement that is to be strengthened and then, again somewhat by trial and error, one must decide how to perform similar movements against heavy resistance.

A more sophisticated approach to the determination of muscle groups that should be overloaded would include the use of mechanical analysis of the movement with cinematography, the use of electromyography, and the application of knowledge gained from a study of applied anatomy. Such sophisticated procedures are beyond the scope of this text, but they are usually described in applied anatomy, kinesiology and biomechanics books. *When in doubt one must remember that one should overload movements that are as similar as possible to those movements that are to be strengthened.*

Once the muscles to be strengthened have been determined and appropriate resistive exercises, either isometric, isotonic or isokinetic, have been selected, *one must perform those exercises with maximal or near maximal resistance to bring forth the greatest strength increments.* The muscles will adapt only to the load placed upon them;

a minimal overload will bring about a minimal strength gain, whereas a maximal overload will bring about a maximal strength gain. To gain the greatest strength one must exercise with few repetitions and heavy resistance.

Not only must heavy loads be placed on the muscles at the start of a strength-training program, but the loads must be progressively increased to keep pace with newly won increments in strength. Thus, heavy resistance is relative to the capacity of the muscle and must increase as the muscle improves its capacity.

Principle 2: Make the training as interesting as possible. One of the chief problems of all physical fitness training programs is simply to maintain the enthusiasm of the trainee so that he does not drop out of the program. A poorly designed strength-training program can be unrelentingly boring. No matter how great a program is in theory, it is useless if no one can stick to it. The maintenance of interest is particularly important in physical training programs for children of elementary school age who have a difficult time understanding the need for fitness programs. If those programs can be disguised as gamelike activities, young children will enjoy becoming fit without having to appreciate fitness intellectually. With older persons, it is important to vary the training routines by rotating the use of isometric, isotonic and isokinetic programs and by varying to some extent the progression of the prescribed exercises.

Principle 3: Exercise large muscle groups before smaller ones. As muscles become fatigued, further training during that period becomes less and less effective and eventually impossible. Most movements become fatiguing as smaller muscle groups involved in those movements are fatigued. Therefore, it is important to exercise the larger muscles involved in the movement first so that the capacities of those muscles can be overloaded before the smaller muscles become fatigued. For example, if one wished to improve his ability to lift a heavy barbell from the floor to a position overhead with elbows extended, he should exercise large leg muscles early in his routines and the smaller elbow extensors later.

Principle 4: Allow adequate recovery of the muscles between individual exercises and between exercise periods. This principle is related to the previous one because underlying it is the idea that strenuous overload of muscles is difficult to achieve when the muscles are tired, sore, or generally have not recovered from previous activity. According to this principle, it is important to arrange a strength-training routine so that successive exercises only minimally involve the same muscle groups. For example, it would not make sense to follow pushups with dips on the parallel bars because both these activities overload the elbow extensors, and relatively few dips could be done immediately after the pushups. A better idea would be to follow the pushups with weighted situps and then perhaps squats before performing the dips. In this way abdominal and thigh muscles would be exercised before returning to the elbow extensors.

This principle also suggests that there is some minimal time period that should intervene between training sessions. Studies have shown that it sometimes takes many hours before muscles respond to exhaustive exercise by increasing their energy reserves and their protein contents to greater than pre-exercise values. It is only logical that the greatest training adaptation should occur when the muscle is best prepared to tolerate the greatest overload, that is, when it has almost fully recovered from a previous training session. From a practical standpoint, most weight trainers find that isotonic workouts about three times per week allow the greatest training adaptation with the least soreness.

Isometric Training: General Principles

Systematic research on different methods of improving muscular strength with isometric exercise routines received its greatest impetus in the 1950's with the publication of numerous studies in Germany. Isometric exercise programs were hailed as the "quick and easy" way to enhanced muscular strength because these studies had effectively demonstrated that very little time was needed to develop substantial levels of strength. Later experience and further research soon showed that isometric strength training was not without its drawbacks, however. Some of these drawbacks will be discussed in later paragraphs, but let us now consider the basic principles of isometric training that most authorities agree will maximize the value of this particular training method (4, 12).

Isometric training should be practiced at several different joint angles because the training effect tends to occur mostly at the angle selected for training (8). If elbow flexion is overloaded at 90 degrees, for example, most of the strength gain will occur at that angle with little or no improvement at angles other than 90 degrees. If a recognized "weak spot" in a particular movement needs specific training, isometric exercise at that angle of the joint(s) involved in the movement may be in order. Otherwise, angles throughout the range of motion of the joint(s) should be selected for training. It often makes sense to concentrate on angles at the extremes of the joint range of motion because the extreme portions of the range of motion are usually the weakest and, therefore, the limiting phases of the movement.

Each contraction should be a maximal voluntary contraction. Although several studies indicate that maximal strength gains can occur with contractions of about 50 percent of maximum, it is usually not feasible to measure the strength of each contraction to make certain that 50 per cent of maximal force is being applied. Also, since some do not respond to this lower level of exertion, a maximal effort should insure that all trainees get a training benefit (12). Finally, by always applying a maximum effort as strength improves, a progressive increase in the training stimulus is assured.

Each maximal contraction should be held for 2–5 seconds. The maximal contraction does not usually fatigue a person until after about 10 seconds, but research has shown that holding the contraction longer than 2–5 seconds does not increase the training effect (12). Since fatigue is usually associated with pain and soreness, there seems to be no good reason to hold the contraction for longer than a few seconds.

The isometric contractions should be repeated 1–5 times during each training session. The training sessions should be held daily unless unusual soreness occurs. Muscles should be allowed 2–3 minutes recovery between maximal efforts. During this recovery period, other muscles can be trained. Because isometric training sessions are usually of brief duration, there is less depletion of energy stores, and usually less soreness than with isotonic or isokinetic exercise. Consequently, the muscles seem to need less time to recover from previous exercise than with other training methods. Training 3–4 times per week will eventually lead to the same strength gains as the daily routines, but progress will be slower (12).

Strength gains achieved with isometric training can be maintained with the normal training session conducted once per week. All categories of physical fitness improvements are more difficult to achieve than to maintain; strength improvements are no exception. Maintenance training once per week is a somewhat conservative suggestion since some authorities have found that a single maximal contraction held for 2 seconds once every 2 weeks is sufficient to maintain strength gains (12). Once again, it seems prudent to provide a somewhat greater than minimal maintenance program to insure that all trainees respond maximally. Without maintenance programs, improved isometric strength regresses toward starting strength levels. Although perhaps 40 per cent of strength gains may be lost in a month or two without a strength maintenance program, some of the strength gain—up to 40 per cent in some studies—seems to be retained for a year or more (4, 12).

Isometric contractions produce extreme rises in blood pressure if held more than a second or two and should be avoided by those afflicted with cardiovascular disease. Although there is a paucity of evidence that patients have actually suffered physical harm with isometrics, the potential for such harm certainly exists, and the prudent course of action is to prohibit cardiac patients from using isometrics until it is demonstrated that isometric exercise is not harmful to those with atherosclerosis, high blood pressure, and other cardiovascular diseases (20).

As with other training programs, isometric training should be made as interesting as possible by varying the routines. Also, large muscle groups should be exercised before smaller ones to minimize early fatigue of the small muscles.

Isotonic Training: General Principles

Isotonic weight training programs have stood the test of time not only in the training of most champion weightlifters, but also in the rehabilitation of muscles grown weak by immobilization in plaster casts or by neuromuscular disease. Any overload of the muscles beyond their normal daily activities will improve muscular strength, but systematic experimentation has shown that certain general principles of isotonic training should be followed if the greatest gains possible with this method are to be achieved.

During each training session, 3–4 sets of each exercise should be performed with the heaviest weight that can be correctly lifted 1–6 times during each set. Another way to express this degree of overload is in terms of *repetitions maximum* (R.M.). One R.M. is the maximum weight that can be lifted correctly one time, 2 R.M. is the maximum weight that can be lifted twice, and so forth. Obviously, the greater the number of R.M., the lighter is the weight that can be lifted. Research suggests that a few repetitions with near maximal weights produce the greatest strength gains (4). The stated principle of 3–4 sets of 1–6 R.M. is broad enough to satisfy the recommendations of most well-conducted research studies. As training goes beyond the level of 6 R.M., it becomes progressively less effective for training muscular strength and better for improving anaerobic muscular endurance.

There seems to be no particular advantage to exercising with eccentric rather than concentric contractions during isotonic training (15). Although eccentric routines subjectively seem easier to accomplish, this benefit may be offset by the greater soreness usually reported with eccentric contractions.

The determination of how much weight can be correctly lifted through a range of motion for a given number of repetitions is made on a trial-and-error basis. To provide for a progressive increase in the overload to the muscle, the determination of 1–6 R.M. should be made about once every two weeks of training. It is important to perform the exercises correctly, without excessive jerking or the use of extra muscle groups. When a trainee lifts improperly as a result of attempting to lift too much, he is in danger of injuring himself.

During an isotonic training session, allow about 5–10 minutes for recovery between sets of the same exercise. Training sessions should be held 3–4 times per week (4). Heavy isotonic training can be extremely fatiguing and may result in a great deal of soreness if adequate recovery time between exercise sets and between training sessions is not allowed. Because isotonic workouts are usually longer than isometric sessions, greater depletion of energy reserves and greater production of lactic acid occurs. Accordingly, somewhat longer recovery periods are needed after isotonic exercise. Depending upon one's training goals, isotonic training sessions normally last 1–2 hours, whereas isometric routines are often completed in 30 minutes or less.

Exercise large muscle groups first. Because isotonic exertions are limited by the strength of the muscle at the weakest point in the range of motion, fatigue of small muscle groups is more likely to limit the overload that can be tolerated in a single isotonic training session than in either isometric or isokinetic types of training. Consequently, exercises such as the bench press, full- or half-squat or inclined press should be performed before dumbbell curls, situps or toe raises (22). Presses and squats stress larger muscle groups than the other exercises.

Strengthening of muscles responsible for a complex movement should be accomplished with exercises designed to incorporate or mimic that movement. Because complex movements such as a baseball throw or a dolphin kick in swimming are acutely dependent upon the nervous system for accuracy, weight training for such movements should simulate as closely as possible the actual movements. This can usually be accomplished fairly satisfactorily with the help of weighted baseballs and bats, and with weights suspended from pulleys anchored to walls, ceilings and floors.

Maintain isotonic strength with two normal workouts per week. With fewer than two workouts per week most trainees find that strength gains are lost after a few months. Two training sessions per week, on the other hand, are usually adequate to maintain, but not to increase, strength gained during prior training (4).

Isokinetic Training: General Principles

Isokinetic strength training programs combine the features of both isometric and isotonic programs in the sense that isokinetic training should be done with maximal exertions (as in isometric training) throughout a complete range of motion (as in isotonic training). In the absence of comprehensive research, the following principles for isokinetic training are recommended:

For the improvement of pure strength 1–5 maximal isokinetic contractions, each lasting 1–3 seconds, should be performed 4–5 times per week. For the improvement of strength in a complex rapid movement each maximal contraction should be completed as rapidly as possible (22). This recommendation is based on the notion that a certain duration of contraction at each point in the range of motion is probably optimal for the greatest strength gains and that this duration should not be so long that the muscle becomes fatigued during the movement. Since maximal static contractions are fatiguing after about 10 seconds, a duration of 3 seconds should be appropriate for movements with a great range of motion, whereas 1 second seems adequate for movements such as toe raises which have a shorter range of motion. For a rapid complex movement such as a baseball throw, however, it seems logical that the isokinetic device should be set for a faster controlled speed to better train the nervous system for strength coupled with speed. Research suggests that training with fast contractions somehow develops strength better than training with slower contractions, even when testing is done with slow contractions (23).

Because the slower maximal contractions approach isometric training, it appears that a total work time shorter than that required for isotonic training is in order. Since there is less work done during each training session with isokinetic techniques, more frequent sessions than suggested for isotonic programs are probably acceptable because a shorter recovery time between isokinetic sessions is thought to be required. Recovery time between repetitions of the same movement should range from 2–5 minutes.

Adequate maintenance of isokinetic strength gains can probably be achieved with 1–2 normal training sessions per week. This recommendation is a compromise between the suggested maintenance programs for isometric and isotonic strength.

CHOICE OF TRAINING METHODS

As is perhaps obvious by now, each method of strength training has its advantages and drawbacks. It should be emphasized that *any method of training that overloads the muscles will result in strength gains*. It is extremely important that the trainee uses a method in which he has confidence and which will maintain his interest for the months required to develop substantial strength. Rigorous adherence to a particular type of program is probably far more important than which type of program is selected.

Advantages often ascribed to isometric training are: It takes little time; requires no expensive equipment; can be performed anywhere; usually causes little soreness; and is easy to maintain. Disadvantages of this technique are: 1) that strength is not developed well throughout the range of motion unless so many angles within the range are strengthened that the time advantage is lost, 2) that training of the nervous system in a movement does not occur, 3) that progress is difficult to assess without a tensiometer or dynamometer so that the training becomes boring, 4) that isometric contractions produce high systolic and diastolic blood pressure, and 5) that isotonic or isokinetic methods generally seem to produce greater strength gains than isometric training (4, 23).

Isotonic training is the most common method of strength training used by specialists in the strength business—weightlifters. Isotonic training builds strength throughout a range of motion and provides some training of the nervous system as well as the muscles. Progress is easy to follow as more weight is added with newly gained strength, so isotonic training tends to be less boring than isometric training. This type of training can be adapted to many different kinds of athletic movements with the aid of weighted implements (balls, disci, shots, and so on) and pulleys. However, isotonic training can be relatively expensive, depending on the sophistication of equipment desired. It also often results in soreness and injury due to the possibility of selecting a weight that is too heavy for the lifter's capacity. If this weight cannot be handled in a weak part of the range of motion, the lifter must either risk muscle injury by excessive straining or risk injury from a falling barbell. Isotonic training takes 1–2 hours per session, and it becomes frustrating to continually have to change weights on barbells and dumbbells for different exercises unless several bars and extra weight discs are purchased. Finally, most of the strength gained in isotonic training occurs at the weakest points of the range of motion so that the entire range is not maximally trained.

Isokinetic training is a relatively new system and has not been as thoroughly tested as the other techniques. It does seem to provide a good combination of the attributes of both isometric and isotonic training with few of their disadvantages. Isokinetic training provides maximal resistance to the muscles at all points in the range of motion, requires less time than isotonic programs, can be performed at different speeds, and is said to cause less injury and soreness than isotonic training (22). A few isokinetic devices are similar in cost to a good set of barbells and dumbbells and offer the advantage that no changes of weights or turning of knobs is required to switch from one exercise to another or from one trainee to another; the same device can be used to train the little finger or the powerful leg muscles. Isokinetic devices that provide a force readout or recorder can be used to provide motivation and to assess whether or not the trainee is giving the effort required for best results.

Most of the isokinetic training equipment, however, tends to be very expensive and more suitable for a physical rehabilitation ward in a hospital than for the high school gymnasium or for the home.

Also, some believe that a scale reading on an isokinetic training device does not provide as good a motivation as the weight added to a barbell as strength improves. More field testing of isokinetic devices is required before this contention can be verified.

One factor that should not be overlooked when comparing strength-training methods is the procedure used to evaluate strength. If isometric contractions are used to test strength, isometric or isokinetic training is likely to provide the best training stimulus, whereas both isotonic and isokinetic training should provide similar results when tested isotonically, because both methods provide heavy overload to the weakest point in the range of motion of the tested movement. Likewise, it seems logical that isokinetic training would be the best method to use if isokinetic evaluation were employed, because only isokinetic training can provide maximal resistance through the entire range of motion. One well-designed study that compared strength increments produced by two isokinetic programs and one isotonic training program used isometric, isotonic and isokinetic testing methods (23). Both isokinetic programs re-

Table 9.1.   Summary of Advantages of Isokinetic, Isotonic, and Isometric Training Methods. A Rating of 1 Is Superior; 2, Intermediate; and 3, Inferior

Criterion	Type of Training		
	Isokinetic	Isotonic	Isometric
Rate of Strength Gain	1	2	3
Strength Gain Throughout Range of Motion	Excellent	Good	Poor
Time per Training Session	2	3	1
Expense	2–3	2	1
Ease of Performance	2	3	1
Ease of Progress Assessment	Expensive Equipment Required	Excellent	Dynamometer Required
Adaptability to Specific Movement	1	2	3
Probability of Soreness	Little Soreness	Much Soreness	Little Soreness
Probability of Musculo-skeletal Injury	Slight	Moderate	Slight
Cardiac Risk	Some	Slight	Moderate
Skill Improvement	Some	Slight	None

sulted in greater strength gains than the isotonic regime, and the high-speed isokinetic routine was more effective than the low-speed program (23). A summary of the relative advantages of isokinetic, isotonic and isometric training is shown in Table 9.1.

RESPONSE TO STRENGTH TRAINING: EFFECTS OF AGE AND SEX

The influence of muscle size, nervous system maturation, male sex hormone and cultural sex-roles is apparent in the relationship between age and sex and strength gains with training as described in Fig. 9.1 (12). In this graph, strength gains of males who are about 25 years old are taken as 100 per cent because the greatest strength increments with training occur at this age. (This does not mean that muscular strength improves by 100 per cent at this age. Maximum strength gains, expressed as a percentage of initial strength, vary from small to large depending on which muscle group is tested.)

Inspection of the upper curve of Fig. 9.1 suggests that much of the male's greater ability to gain strength with training is because of the

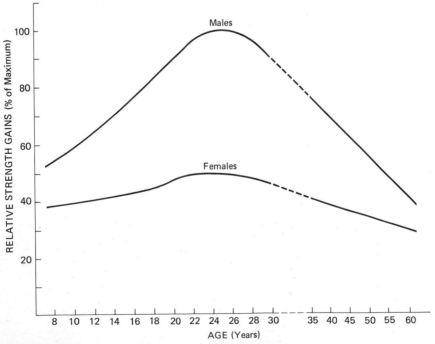

Figure 9.1. Response to strength training: effects of age and sex.

presence of male sex hormones since the male graph begins to move sharply upward at puberty, the time of great increases in testosterone secretion, and moves downward after age 30 when testosterone levels in males begin to decline with advancing age.

Muscle size differences between sexes and ages also seem to affect the trainability of muscles, probably because the greatest strength increases are found in larger muscles which in everyday life are not stressed to as great an extent in respect to their capacities as are smaller muscles (12). Thus, much greater percentage increases in strength can be achieved by the large leg muscles than by muscles of the fingers. Since males at a given age have larger muscles than females, it is only natural that they should have a relatively greater responsiveness to strength training.

The same holds true for the effect of muscle size on strength at various age classifications; older subjects have larger muscles and, consequently, greater responsiveness to training. However, trainability increases more rapidly than muscle size, so it is likely that nervous system maturation also plays a role in the greater responsiveness of older subjects up to about age 30.

Examples of Training Effects on Muscular Strength

With isometric training of nonathletic adult males for about 10 weeks, strength of the wrist flexors (handgrip muscles) might increase by about 9 per cent, the elbow flexors by about 18 per cent, elbow extensors by 2 per cent, hip extensors by 35 per cent and plantar flexors of the lower leg by 50 per cent (12). With isotonic weightlifting routines for 10 weeks, the elbow extensor and chest muscles used in the bench press may improve their maximum strength by 7–10 per cent, and the hip and knee extensors used in the squat may gain 4–5 per cent in strength (22). After 8 weeks of isokinetic training, it has been shown that 15–25 per cent gains in strength of most muscle groups might be expected, with strength in some movements increasing by up to 96 per cent. (23).

It should also be pointed out that with large muscle groups, strength increases are usually slow to begin but then accelerate rapidly for a few weeks and reach a plateau or slow down their rates of gain after the muscles have become quite strong. In other words, a greater percentage of improvements in strength should be expected in persons who begin with very low levels of strength. Although strength gains are more difficult to obtain as training progresses, serious weightlifters can keep improving strength significantly for several years.

At least some of the sex and age differences in strength trainability may also occur because of differences in willingness to stress the muscles. Because of the social reluctance of some females and older males to "train like a bunch of athletes," such persons are unwilling to train strenuously. Recent changes in cultural norms for sex roles may alter this presumed effect on strength trainability.

Physical educators and coaches, especially of female classes or teams, should become familiar with the differences in strength-training responsiveness between sexes and age groups, so that they do not expect the same responses of all ages and both sexes. Once again it should be emphasized that there is a great variability in responsiveness within sexes and age groups. The wise physical education instructor or coach is the one who can detect these individual differences and adapt his programs to best suit the individuals whom he is trying to develop.

PHYSIOLOGICAL MECHANISMS UNDERLYING STRENGTH IMPROVEMENT

There are two basic ways in which training with overload could enhance the maximal strength of muscles—more motor units could be called into action, or individual motor units could exert more force. The first of these possibilities would implicate the nervous system in the strength adaptation, whereas the second would involve an adaptation in the muscles themselves.

Adaptations of the Nervous System to Strength Training

Although the precise nature of neural adaptations to strength training is obscure, there is substantial evidence that such adaptations do occur.

One line of evidence that links nervous system changes to strength increases is that strength in a limb can be increased dramatically in one training session before any major changes in muscle size can occur, even when the limb on the opposite side of the body is the only one to undergo training (4). For example, suppose that both right and left maximal knee-extension strengths were found to be 100 pounds prior to training, and that 30 repetitions of right knee extension with 60 pounds of resistance were then performed over a 20 minute period. After 20 minutes of training with the right leg only, it might be found that upon maximum exertion *both right and left* knee extension strengths increased by 20 pounds. Because there is no known way that the muscle structure could be changed to bring about a greater number of active cross bridges in such a short period (especially in the untrained limb), most authorities conclude that the nervous system has in this time "learned" to either increase its excitatory influence, or decrease its inhibitory influence on the alpha motor neurons of the spinal cord so that more motor units could be called into play. Whether such changes are central or peripheral is completely unknown, but it seems reasonable that these adaptations could be enhanced by a long-term program of strength training.

A second type of experiment implicates the central nervous system in muscle strength changes. In these experiments strength increases are shown when a subject shouts during exertion, or when a pistol shot is fired near the subject a few seconds before strength testing (13). Similar strength increases are sometimes found when a subject is given hypnotic suggestions of increased strength, whereas strength decrements are often shown after hypnotic suggestion of decreased strength (21). The strength enhancement results are usually interpreted to mean that the brain under hypnosis has either increased its flow of excitatory stimuli or decreased the flow of inhibitory stimuli to the motor neurons of the spinal cord.

A third argument in support of nervous system involvement in the expression of strength includes evidence from electrical stimulation experiments; this evidence usually shows that a voluntary maximal contraction in man is not as forceful as a contraction brought on by electrical stimulation of the muscles in question (14, 25). The interpretation given to these results is that man does not voluntarily send enough excitatory stimuli from his brain to the motor neurons of the spinal cord to counteract inhibitory stimuli sufficiently for excitation of all motor units. The extended logic is that by training he can "learn" to either increase excitatory output from the brain or decrease inhibitory output and thereby increase strength.

Although electrical stimulation usually causes a greater expression of strength than does a maximal voluntary exertion, muscular *training* by electrical stimulation of the nerve supplying a muscle does *not* result in as great a strength increase as does training by voluntary contractions of the same muscle (18). Again, this fourth kind of evidence supports the idea that some of the strength increments brought on by voluntary training must rely on changes in the nervous system that do not occur when the muscles are stimulated electrically.

Finally, it is widely accepted that the increase of muscle size that accompanies regular strength training for many months is not proportionately as great as the increase in ability to produce force. A muscle such as the gastrocnemius in man can increase its strength greatly with training and yet change very little in size. Unless some undiscovered changes are occurring in the muscles, it appears that a portion of the strength gain with training is because of a nervous system adaptation. Assuming this to be true, it is unfortunate that nothing is yet known about the precise location within the nervous system where this adaptation occurs (that is, whether in the motor cortex, reticular formation, spinal cord, muscle spindles, tendon organs or some other part of the nervous system) or the physical or chemical changes responsible for the adaptation.

Only slightly more is known about the mechanism by which individual motor units exert more force after training. It seems apparent that a nerve stimulus causes the activation of more actin-myosin cross bridges with maximal efforts after training. Such a change could occur if there were more muscle fibers (hyperplasia) in the trained muscle or if individual fibers increased in size (hypertrophy) because of a greater number of actin and myosin filaments after training. Although there is some evidence in laboratory animals that chronic exercise may help animals *retain* muscle fibers that are normally lost with advancing age, there is little or no evidence that typical training programs increase the number of fibers in skeletal muscles (6, 7). On the contrary, nearly all studies of this problem have concluded that muscles get larger after training because individual fibers hypertrophy.

Research has demonstrated that heavy overload training somehow stimulates the production of greater amounts of actin, myosin, and other myofibrillar proteins, so that more cross bridges are available to produce force during a maximal strength effort (6, 10, 11). In contrast, endurance training tends to increase the production of enzymes involved in providing energy for aerobic metabolism, namely, the enzymes of the mitochondria (11). The increase in myofibrillar protein that is brought about as a result of heavy resistance exercise could conceivably be the result of an increased rate of buildup (synthesis) of proteins from amino acids delivered to the muscle, a decreased rate of breakdown (degradation) of proteins to amino acids, or to a combination of increased synthesis and decreased degradation of proteins. In studies of compensatory hypertrophy of rat muscles (soleus and plantaris) that were forced to do more work than normal after the tendon of an assistant muscle (gastrocnemius) was cut, it has been demonstrated that both increased synthesis and decreased degradation operate to cause rapid muscle growth (9). With more normal laboratory animal-training programs, such as treadmill running, however, it appears that enhanced synthesis of proteins is more important than diminished degradation (19).

Exactly what transpires between strenuous muscle contractions and greater protein synthesis is unknown. Although the effect of male sex hormone (testosterone) on strength seems apparent when observing strength differences between males and females, efforts to find consistently higher plasma levels of testosterone in trained subjects, or higher uptakes of testosterone into trained muscle where the hormone works to promote protein synthesis, have not been encouraging. Since hypertrophy, in response to the surgical elimination of assistant muscles, occurs in animals that are diabetic and in animals that have had their pituitaries removed, it seems unlikely that either insulin or growth hormone (secreted from the pancreas and pituitary, respectively) is required for the hypertrophy associated with strength training in man (9).

Although the uptake of amino acids from the blood into muscles is depressed *during* exercise, it is increased above resting values for some time *after* exercise (17, 26, 27). Perhaps there is some local change in the muscle membrane brought about by strenuous contractions that makes the membrane more permeable to amino acids, so that they may more readily diffuse from the tissue fluids into the muscle cells to serve as building blocks for protein synthesis. A mechanical change in the shape of molecules in the muscle membrane because of tension on the membrane during contraction could be the critical initiating factor in stimulating amino acid uptake into muscle fibers and incorporation into myofibrillar proteins. Such a mechanism is highly speculative, but has been suggested because of experimental results demonstrating that simply stretching muscle fibers results in enhanced protein synthesis in those fibers (3, 9, 16).

Regardless of the precise physiological mechanism involved, it is now widely accepted that the greater size of trained muscle fibers results in part from greater amounts of actin, myosin and other intracellular proteins. In addition, muscle connective tissue, tendons and ligaments are strengthened by heavy exercise (2). Adaptations such as these would seem to be important in making trained muscles less susceptible to injury. These adaptations are, consequently, good justification for rigorous strength training programs prior to the initiation of seasonal athletic activities such as snow skiing, water skiing, football and wrestling.

EFFECT OF IMPROVED STRENGTH ON ATHLETIC SKILLS

Common sense suggests that greater muscular strength is more important for some athletic events than others. Performance in those events which rely on power (force × distance/time) logically should be enhanced by strength training more than performance in events which are governed more by endurance, and available research bears out this rationale. Performance is especially improved in events that involve less complex movements of one or two limbs. For example, research literature supports the conclusion that strength training improves performance in vertical jump, standing long-jump, softball, basketball and medicine ball throws for distance, baseball throwing speed and speed of limited arm and leg movements, such as arm movement in a horizontal plane from the side of the body to the front (4, 22). Mixed results have been reported for the effectiveness of strength training on track and swimming sprints that involve more coordinated movements of all limbs, and insignificant effects of strength training are usually found for events such as distance running or swimming (4).

Let us consider the basis for improvements in athletic power, that is, the ability to move the body or some implement such as a shot or discus rapidly through space. Increased arm strength or leg strength would be of no use in improving power unless that strength somehow enabled the movement to be completed more rapidly. If movement speed with the same load were improved by training, it should be apparent on a graph of speed plotted against load (1). In Fig. 9.2, two plots of movement speed versus load are shown on the same set of axes; curve A is the pretraining curve, and curve B is the posttraining curve. It is obvious that strength training resulted in an improved speed of movement for all loads. The mechanism underlying this improved speed is not known, but it seems that a certain percentage of the potential cross bridges in a muscle can be activated quickly (5) so that if one increases the number of cross bridges in a muscle with strength training, he increases the number that can be activated rapidly.

As an example of this highly speculative explanation, consider the case of that famous shotputter, Klaus Carbuncle, who, prior to training, had exactly 1,000 potentially active cross bridges in his

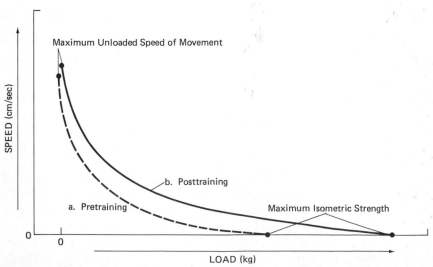

Figure 9.2. Approximate effects of strength training on muscle force-velocity curves.

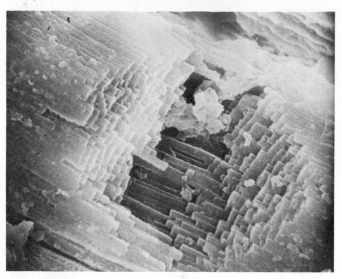

Figure 9.3. Stereo electron micrograph of a single muscle fiber. A section of the fiber has been removed to show internal arrangement of myofibrils. (Courtesy of R. E. Carrow, W. W. Heusner and W. D. Van Huss, Michigan State University, E. Lansing, Michigan.)

shotputting muscles. Of these 1,000 force-generating sites in his muscles, 40 per cent or 400 could be quickly activated, with the remainder more slowly entering into the contractile effort. After training, by lifting a hippopotamus every day from birth until it weighed 5,000 pounds, Klaus had increased the number of potentially active actin-myosin cross bridges in his muscles to 2,000 and the number of rapidly activated cross bridges to 800 (40 per cent of 2,000). Small wonder then that Mr. Carbuncle improved his putting speed (and, therefore, power) so that his shotput distance improved, according to legend, from 70 to 140 feet. It is not quite clear why other sons of hippopotamus trainers have not also become outstanding shotputters.

Whatever the actual explanation is for the improved speed of loaded movements that accompanies improved strength, it appears that, at least within a certain range of the force-velocity curve, speed must increase with greater strength. This increase in speed seems to be especially true for slower, more heavily loaded movements, perhaps because as the muscles are freed from loads, nerve coordination of progressively faster movements becomes relatively more important than muscle strength. This dominance of nerve coordination may account for the reported failure of strength-training programs to improve speed in more complex movements such as sprinting.

STRENGTH TRAINING AND MUSCULAR HYPERTROPHY

Two of the most common questions a physical educator or coach is faced with are: "How can I build up my muscles so I don't look so skinny?" and "How can I avoid getting big, ugly muscles when I start exercising?" The first question is usually asked by males, and the second, by females; the correct answers are not easy to give. The enhancement of muscular bulk or hypertrophy should accompany any type of overload training, but it is highly variable both in terms of which muscles increase in size and in terms of how great those size changes are. Three general principles pertaining to muscular hypertrophy can be gleaned from the research literature and from observing the effects of strength-training programs on various groups of people.

First, there are tremendous individual differences in the adaptation of muscles to training, with females usually demonstrating much less hypertrophy than males, probably due to differences in male sex hormones. Thus, most females need not worry about their muscles getting disproportionately large, and some males will gain very little muscle bulk, regardless of the type or amount of strength training they undergo. It is often helpful to point out to females that from the point of view of most males, a well-developed muscular symmetry in females is much more pleasing to the eye than the gaunt "prisoner of war" look and that enlargement of pectoral muscles is one of the few natural remedies for an obscure bustline. It is extremely difficult to predict which few females will adapt to training by developing knotty muscles, but experience suggests that girls and women who already are beginning to develop such muscles are probably the only females who should be concerned. Likewise, one who attempts to guess which males will fail to develop with training is likely to be incorrect many times, but usually it is the thin, ascetic type who will probably remain relatively thin and ascetic after training, and the mesomorphic, heavily muscled individual who will show dramatic increases in muscle growth.

Second, the greatest hypertrophy usually is shown by those muscles which in everyday life do the least work in relation to their genetic potential. Some of the fastest gains in muscle size have been reported in persons whose muscles have wasted away (atrophied) because of prolonged hospitalization. Accordingly, those whose lives have been relatively sheltered from physical work often show great increases in muscle bulk after a period of overload training. Also, larger muscles such as the pectoralis major and quadriceps femoris can usually be expected to show greater size changes than smaller muscles such as those of the forearm. However, well-defined appearance of muscular hypertrophy (often called "definition") can be obscured by subcutaneous fat tissue; consequently, this hypertrophic definition is also highly variable and dependent upon inherited patterns of localized fat deposition. This effect of fat on obscuring muscle definition probably also partly explains why females, who have more subcutaneous fat, are less apt than males to demonstrate enlarged muscles after training.

Third, the extent to which a muscle in any given individual gains in bulk depends not only on the severity of overload, but also on the total duration of the overload. Thus, most studies of the problem show that isometric training, which supposedly gives the maximal severity of overload, is not as effective in producing muscular hypertrophy as isotonic training. Isotonic training is usually less severe but has a longer total duration of contraction time. Even within the isotonic category of training, it appears that for most persons, sets of about 10 R.M. are better for developing bulk than are sets of 1–6 R. M. Again, however, it should be noted that individuals vary in their adaptations to these programs and that there are many exceptions to these principles. Although it is inefficient, the trial-and-error method of choosing a muscle bulking program is often useful. If the equipment is available, one might find that isokinetic exercise leads to greater muscular growth than isotonic training (22).

When designing a program to enhance body contours, it is important to include activities for all major muscle groups so that a pleasing body symmetry is achieved. The development of the male upper body to the exclusion of the legs, for example, is not uncommon among "Adonis" types, but it leads to a total appearance that suggests both physical and mental imbalance.

Finally, for those who wish to add pounds to a lanky frame, dietary advice is often essential. High calorie, high protein meals are usually recommended for those who would build muscle rapidly, even though there is little evidence that extra protein will be used for muscle growth. Young people should remember that bulk often comes with maturation, so that a little patience will be well rewarded. The majority of adults in Western countries are victims of too much body tissue, not too little. Slender individuals should perhaps be grateful for their appearance because they are given the best chance to avoid early death from obesity-related cardiovascular disease and other degenerative diseases. In any case, a high fat diet does not seem advisable for those on a muscle building program because of the apparent relationship between blood fat levels and the incidence of cardiovascular disease.

Review Questions

1. What is meant by "progressive overload" when applied to strength training?
2. List the advantages and disadvantages of isometric, isotonic, and isokinetic strength-training programs.
3. Why should strenuous isometric contractions be avoided by those afflicted with cardiovascular disease?
4. Explain why age and sex are important variables in determining responses to strength training.
5. What are the two general mechanisms underlying adaptations to strength training?
6. Describe some of the evidence that the nervous system is involved in adaptations to strength training.
7. Why should protein synthesis be related to strength improvement?
8. What types of athletic activities are most apt to be affected by improved muscular strength?
9. Explain why some persons do not exhibit substantial muscular hypertrophy as a result of strength training.

References

1. Asmussen, E. Growth in muscular strength and power. In G. L. Rarick (Ed.), *Physical Activity: Human Growth and Development.* New York: Academic Press, 1973, pp. 60–79.
2. Booth, F. W., and E. W. Gould. Effects of training and disuse on connective tissue. In J. H. Wilmore, and J. F. Keogh, *Exercise and Sport Sciences Reviews*, 1975, **3:**83–112.
3. Buresova, M., E. Gutmann, and M. Klicpera. Effect of tension upon the rate of incorporation of amino acids into proteins of cross–striated muscle. *Experientia*, 1969, **25:**144–145.
4. Clarke, D. H. Adaptations in strength and muscular endurance resulting from exercise. In J. H. Wilmore (Ed.), *Exercise and Sport Sciences Reviews*, 1973, **1:**73–102.
5. Davies, R. E. The dynamics of the energy-rich phosphates. In J. Keul (Ed.), *Limiting Factors of Physical Performance.* Stuttgart: Georg Thieme Publishers, 1973, pp. 56–62.
6. Edgerton, V. R. Exercise and the growth and development of muscle tissue. In G. L. Rarick (Ed.), *Physical Activity: Human Growth and Development.* New York: Academic Press, 1973, pp. 1–31.
7. Faulkner, J. A., L. C. Maxwell, D. A. Brook, and D. A. Lie-

berman. Adaptation of guinea pig plantaris muscle fibers to endurance training. *American Journal of Physiology*, 1971, **221**:291–297.

8. Gardner, G. W. Specificity of strength changes of the exercised and nonexercised limb following isometric training. *Research Quarterly*, 1963, **34**:98–101.

9. Goldberg, A. L., J. D. Etlinger, D. F. Goldspink, and C. Jablecki. Mechanism of work-induced hypertrophy of skeletal muscle. *Medicine and Science in Sports*, 1975, **7**:248–261.

10. Goldspink, G., and K. F. Howells. Work-induced hypertrophy in exercised normal muscles of different ages and the reversibility of hypertrophy after cessation of exercise. *Journal of Physiology (London)*, 1974, **239**:179–193.

11. Gordon, E. E., K. Kowalski, and M. Fritts. Adaptations of muscle to various exercises. *Journal of the American Medical Association*, 1967, **199**:103–108.

12. Hettinger, T. *Physiology of Strength*. Springfield, Ill.: Charles C Thomas, Publisher, 1961.

13. Ikai, M. and A. H. Steinhaus. Some factors modifying the expression of human strength, *Journal of Applied Physiology*, 1961, **16**:157–163.

14. Ikai, M. and K. Yabe. Training effect of muscular endurance by means of voluntary and electrical stimulation. *European Journal of Applied Physiology*, 1969, **28**:55–60.

15. Johnson, B. I., J. W. Adamczyk, K. O. Tennøe, and S. B. Strømme. A comparison of concentric and eccentric muscle training. *Medicine and Science in Sports*, 1976, **8**:35–38.

16. Mackova, E., and P. Hnik. Compensatory muscle hypertrophy induced by tenotomy of synergists is not true working hypertrophy. *Physiologia Bohemoslovaca*, 1973, **22**:43–44.

17. Makarova, A. F. Biochemical changes in animal muscles in experimental training of various kinds. *Ukrainian Biochemical Journal*, 1958, **30**:903–910.

18. Massey, B. H., R. C. Nelson, B. J. Sharkey, and T. Comden. Effects of high-frequency electrical stimulation on the size and strength of skeletal muscle. *Journal of Sports Medicine*, 1973, **5**:136–144.

19. McManus, B. M., D. R. Lamb, J. J. Judis, and J. Scala. Skeletal muscle leucine incorporation and testosterone uptake in exercised guinea pigs. *European Journal of Applied Physiology*, 1975, **34**:149–156.

20. Mitchell, J. H., and K. Wildenthal. Static (isometric) exercise and the heart: Physiological and clinical considerations. *Annual Review of Medicine*, 1974, **25**:369–381.

21. Morgan, W. P. Hypnosis and muscular performance. In W. P.

Morgan (Ed.), *Ergogenic Aids and Muscular Performance.* New York: Academic Press, 1972, pp. 193–233.

22. O'Shea, J. P. *Scientific Principles and Methods of Strength Fitness* (2nd ed.). Reading, Mass.: Addison-Wesley Publishing Co., 1976.

23. Pipes, T. V., and J. H. Wilmore. Isokinetic vs. isotonic strength training in adult men. *Medicine and Science in Sports*, 1975, **7:**262–274.

24. Schiaffino, S., and V. Hanzlikova. On the mechanism of compensatory hypertrophy in skeletal muscle. *Experientia*, 1970, **26:**152–153.

25. Stephens, J. A., and A. Taylor. Fatigue of maintained voluntary muscle contraction in man. *Journal of Physiology (London)*, 1972, **220:**1–18.

26. Yakovlev, N. N., A. F. Krasnova, and N. R. Chagovets. The influence of muscle activity on muscle proteins. In E. Gutmann and P. Hnik (Eds.), *The Effect of Use and Disuse on Neuromuscular Functions.* Prague: Publishing House of the Czechoslovak Academy of Sciences, 1963, pp. 461–473.

27. Zimmer, H.-G., and E. Gerlach. Protein synthesis in heart and skeletal muscle of rats during and subsequent to exercise. In J. Keul (Ed.), *Limiting Factors of Physical Performance.* Stuttgart: Georg Thieme, Publishers, 1973, pp. 102–109.

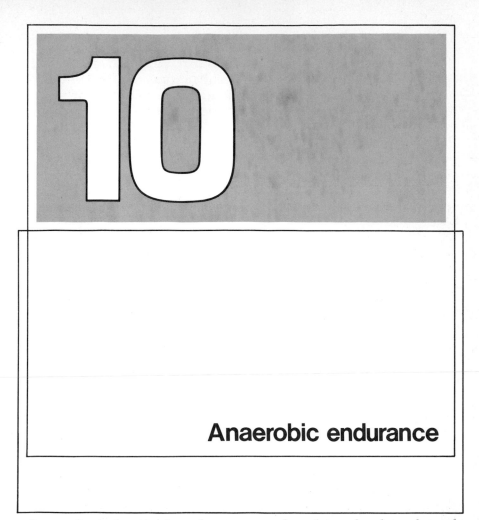

Anaerobic endurance

Some physical activities rely on strength and speed; others depend chiefly on the cardiovascular system to deliver oxygen. Between these two extremes are many types of exercise which are classified as *anaerobic endurance* activities.

These activities include the sprint events in track, in cycling and in swimming, vigorous wrestling competition, carrying heavy luggage or bags of groceries, vigorous shoveling of snow and the rapid manual sawing of wood. Anaerobic endurance activities may be dynamic, as in the case of sawing wood or sprinting, or static, as exemplified by carrying heavy loads, but all are characterized by strong muscular contractions that demand substantially greater rates of energy (ATP) production than can be provided by aerobic metabolism alone.

Let us define anaerobic endurance as *the ability to persist at the maintenance or repetition of strenuous muscular contractions that rely mainly upon anaerobic mechanisms of energy supply.* For most persons

155

this class of activities includes all those that, by reason of their high intensities, can be sustained for longer than 5 seconds but less than 1 or 2 minutes (2). Shorter duration activities are strength or power activities, whereas activities that can be sustained for longer than 1 or 2 minutes demand a substantial rate of oxygen delivery by the cardiovascular system and are designated aerobic endurance activities in this text. Accordingly, anaerobic endurance describes a type of physical fitness lying in the center of a continuum between strength fitness and aerobic (cardiovascular) endurance fitness. Remember that this sort of classification of the characteristics of physical fitness is arbitrary and that the boundaries separating the various categories are not precisely defined. For example, an activity that was originally classified in the anaerobic endurance category for an untrained indi-

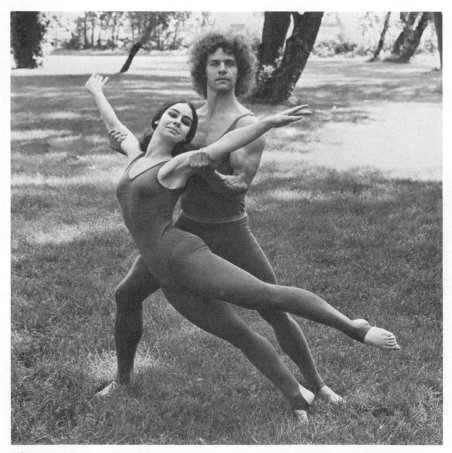

Figure 10.1.   Flexibility, strength and anaerobic endurance are essential to the dancer. (Courtesy of Office of Public Information, University of Toledo, Toledo, Ohio.)

vidual may be reclassified after a period of training as the person increases his ability to persist in the activity beyond the arbitrary 2-minute limit. These arbitrary classifications, although imprecise, serve a useful function by drawing our attention to the principal physiological mechanisms underlying various types of activities.

TESTS OF ANAEROBIC ENDURANCE

Static endurance of the elbow flexors could be measured as the time one can hold a 50-pound dumbbell at 90 degrees of elbow flexion. Common measures of dynamic endurance of various muscle groups would be the number of repeated knee extensions one could perform at a given rate with a given load, the distance during which one could maintain his maximal running speed, or the number of pushups, pullups, situps, or dips on the parallel bars one could perform at a given cadence. In the research laboratory, it is common to evaluate endurance as the time one can maintain a given force or the number of times one can produce a given force repetitively at a given cadence. Force in each instance is registered on a dynamometer, that is, a strain gauge or cable tensiometer. In the physical education setting, it is common to assess muscular endurance as the number of situps, squat-thrusts, pullups, pushups or dips one can perform at a given cadence. However, such measurements tend to favor lighter students because the greater muscular strength of heavier students does not compensate for their greater body weights (2). This is particularly true in the case of pullups. Therefore, if these activities are used to evaluate muscular endurance, normal values should be established for different body weight classifications.

Whenever endurance is to be measured, any instruments used should be calibrated, and the entire measurement procedure should be tested for its sensitivity and reproducibility as outlined for strength measurements in Chapter 9. Measurements of anaerobic muscular endurance are much less reproducible than strength measurements, probably because of variability in motivation for maintaining painful muscle contractions (3).

EVALUATION OF ANAEROBIC POTENTIAL

For the assessment of an athlete's potential to become an outstanding performer in a short-duration competitive athletic event, it would be helpful if there were some simple, reliable test of one's capacity to produce ATP anaerobically. Although it is possible to establish a profile of an athlete's anaerobic potential by analyzing muscle biopsy specimens for percentage of fast-twitch fibers, for ATP, creatine phosphate and glycogen stores, and for the activities of the enzymes in muscle which are used to catabolize those anaerobic energy stores, such tests are expensive and potentially hazardous. Consequently, several indirect measurements of anaerobic potential have been used.

Oxygen Debt Capacity as a Measure of Anaerobic Potential

As was indicated in Chapter 6, the oxygen debt is defined as the excess oxygen uptake during recovery from exercise, that is, the oxygen uptake above and beyond what would have occurred in the same time period had the subject remained at rest. *Oxygen debt capacity* is the greatest oxygen debt one can accumulate and is ordinarily achieved with exercise that can be sustained for 1–3 minutes (13). The reason that oxygen debt capacity has sometimes been used to estimate anaerobic potential is that some of the excess oxygen consumed after exercise is used by the mitochondria for replenishing the stores of ATP, creatine phosphate and glycogen that were depleted anaerobically during the exercise period. Thus, if there were a perfect relationship between oxygen debt capacity and anaerobic ATP production, oxygen debt capacity would obviously be a useful measure of anaerobic potential.

However, oxygen debt capacity is not solely related to the production of ATP anaerobically. It is thought, for example, that such factors as high adrenalin levels, elevated body temperature and increased oxygen uptake by the rapidly beating heart and by the respiratory muscles all contribute to the elevated rate of oxygen uptake during recovery from vigorous activity (13). Because of the above considerations, it is apparent that there is only a limited association between oxygen debt capacity and anaerobic potential. Nonetheless, oxygen debt capacities have been successfully used to distinguish between athletes and untrained persons by some (13), but not all, investigators (12). Athletes' oxygen debt capacities average about 10.5 liters (139 ml/kg) and 5.9 liters (95 ml/kg) for males and females, respectively, whereas corresponding values for untrained subjects are 5.0 liters (68 ml/kg) and 3.1 liters (50 ml/kg) (13). The variability of oxygen debt measurements for a given individual is quite substantial and has been reported to be associated with a coefficient of variation (Chapter 8) of 21 per cent (12). Also, in a group of subjects having similar physical characteristics, oxygen debt capacity cannot be used to accurately predict performance in short-duration activities (15).

Lactic Acid and Alactic Acid Components of Oxygen Debt. If oxygen debt and blood lactic acid levels are measured immediately after strenuous exercise lasting 5 seconds, 10 seconds, 20 seconds, 30 seconds and so on, it will be found that oxygen debts appear after even the shortest work period, and will increase in size until the oxygen debt capacity is reached after a work period lasting 1–3 minutes. However, lactic acid may not rise in the blood after the very short exercise periods. *Thus, there can be a small oxygen debt—the alactic acid oxygen debt—that is not associated with lactic acid production. In an exercise of more than a few seconds in duration, there will be a major portion of the oxygen debt—the lactic acid oxygen debt—that is associated with the production of lactic acid.*

The significance of the alactic acid component of the oxygen debt is that this portion of the extra oxygen consumed during recovery is thought to be used to provide energy for the resynthesis of ATP and creatine phosphate, and to replenish the oxygen stores of myoglobin and body fluids (7). The lactic acid component of the oxygen debt is used only to a slight extent to replenish glycogen supplies in liver and muscle because it takes about two days to replenish these stores. The remainder of this excess oxygen uptake during recovery is used in the ways that were described in the previous section. If one could easily partition that portion of the oxygen debt capacity that is alactic in nature from the lactic acid component, it would be possible to separate the anaerobic potential most useful in extremely brief types of exercise (sprints, static work and so on) from the anaerobic potential most needed in exercise of 1–2 minutes duration. Methods for accomplishing this objective are described in the following sections.

Alactic Acid Oxygen Debt Capacity. Because it has been shown that the alactic acid component of the oxygen debt occurs during the first 2 minutes of recovery from strenuous exercise (7), the alactic acid oxygen debt capacity is simply the measured oxygen debt during the first 2 minutes of recovery from maximal exercise lasting 1–3 minutes. This value can be further partitioned into the ATP-creatine phosphate O_2 debt by subtracting the oxygen used to refill myoglobin and tissue fluid stores of oxygen.

Accordingly, the ATP-creatine phosphate O_2 debt capacity has been estimated by the following equation:

$$\text{ATP-creatine phosphate oxygen debt capacity (cal/kg of body weight)}$$
$$= [(O_2 \text{ debt}_{2min}(ml) - 550) \times 0.6 \times 5]/\text{body weight (kg) (8)}$$

The first term of the equation is the oxygen debt measured during the first 2 minutes of recovery from maximal exercise of 1–3 minutes duration; 550 is the approximate amount of that 2-minute oxygen debt that can be attributed to refilling the oxygen stores of myoglobin and body fluids, 0.6 is the assumed efficiency of repayment of the alactic acid oxygen debt and 5 is the caloric equivalent of 1 ml of oxygen. (Note the use of calorie rather than kilocalorie.)

To illustrate the estimation of ATP-creatine phosphate oxygen debt capacity, suppose Hector Hawklips, famous track coach at Ballpoint University, wanted to determine the alactic potential of young Belding Fopswitch, a new candidate for the 400 meter dash. Belding ran as fast as possible for 3 minutes and then exhaled for 2 minutes of recovery into a large gas-collection bag. From this gas sample Mr. Hawklips determined the oxygen uptake for 2 minutes of recovery and subtracted from that figure the oxygen uptake that occurred during a pre-exercise 2-minute rest period. The 2-minute oxygen debt thus determined was 2.0 liters or 2000 milliliters. Belding's body weight was 40 kilograms because he subsisted on a diet of dandelions and lettuce. Thus, his ATP-creatine phosphate capacity was $[(2000-550) \times 0.6 \times 5]/40 = 108.75$ cal/kg. As this value was not particularly outstanding (8), the coach suggested that Belding take up distance swimming.

It should be noted that the equation for estimating ATP-creatine phosphate oxygen debt capacity assumes values that may be substantially incorrect for a given individual. As more data are published in studies of high-energy phosphate oxygen debt capacity, the validity of this equation can be better evaluated.

A typical value for ATP-creatine phosphate oxygen debt capacity is about 100 cal/kg or 1.5–2.0 liters of oxygen (6, 8). Fox (8) has shown that this capacity can be improved more readily with interval training regimens that rely on 30-second work intervals than with those that include 2-minute work periods.

Maximal Anaerobic Power. A person can maintain his greatest muscular force for only a few seconds. If this force is allowed to move a mass some distance, the maximal rate of performing work can be computed. Since the rate of performing work is defined as *power*, and since work at the maximal rate is performed at the expense of the anaerobic splitting of ATP and creatine phosphate, a measure of this maximal work rate is also a measure of maximal anaerobic power. If an athletic event or some industrial task can be completed in 5–10 seconds, a measure of maximal anaerobic power might prove valuable in the assessment of a candidate's ability to perform such a task. Short sprints and jumps are some of the athletic events that are obviously dependent upon maximal anaerobic power.

A rather simple test of anaerobic power consists of a fast run up a flight of stairs (9). The subject stands 6 meters in front of the stairs

Table 10.1. Classification of Anaerobic Power Scores[9]

Male Classification	Stair Climb (kg-m/sec) Age in Years		50 Yard Dash (sec) Age in Years	
	15–20	20–30	15–20	20–30
Poor	Under 113	Under 106	Over 7.1	Over 7.8
Fair	113–149	106–139	7.1–6.8	7.8–7.5
Average	150–187	140–175		
Good	188–224	176–210	6.7–6.5	7.4–7.1
Excellent	Over 224	Over 210	Under 6.5	Under 7.1
Female Classification	Age in Years		Age in Years	
	15–20	20–30	15–20	20–30
Poor	Under 92	Under 85	Over 9.1	Over 10.0
Fair	92–120	85–111	9.1–8.4	10.0–9.2
Average	121–151	112–140		
Good	152–182	141–168	8.3–7.9	9.1–8.7
Excellent	Over 182	Over 168	Under 7.9	Under 8.7

and runs up the stairs, three at a time, as fast as possible. On the third stair the subject steps on a switchmat that starts a timer, and on the ninth stair the subject stops the timer by stepping on a second switchmat. Time elapsed between the third and ninth stairs is recorded to the nearest hundredth of a second. Since power = (mass × distance)/time, one must know the weight (mass) of the subject in kilograms, the vertical height in meters between the third and ninth stairs, and the elapsed time between the third and ninth stairs in seconds to calculate power in kilogram-meters per second. For example, if the vertical distance between two steps is 16.9 cm., the total vertical distance between stairs three and nine is 6 × 16.9 = 101 cm. = 1.01 m. If the subject weighs 70 kg. and the elapsed time between the two switchmats is 0.50 sec., power (kgm/sec) = (70 × 1.01)/0.50 = 141.4 kgm/sec.

If a staircase or timing apparatus is unavailable, another estimate of anaerobic power can be obtained by timing a subject in a 50-yard dash with a 15-yard running start. Table 10.1 shows a classification scheme for maximal anaerobic power based on the staircase or 50-yard dash scores (9).

Maximal Capacity for Anaerobic Glycolysis. Because most of the oxygen debt that can be accumulated with strenuous exercise is used to catabolize lactic acid to carbon dioxide and water or to resynthesize glycogen from lactic acid (2, 13), an evaluation of the energy resulting from lactic acid production during such an exercise bout should give some meaningful information about the amounts of glycogen and glucose that were broken down anaerobically during activity. Although a measurement of the concentration of lactic acid in the blood would certainly indicate the extent of anaerobic glycolysis, a more accurate picture would be provided if the amount of lactic acid throughout the body fluids was calculated. The equation used to estimate the energy provided by anaerobic glycolysis is as follows: *Energy from anaerobic glycolysis (cal/kg of body weight) = net blood lactic acid (g/l) × 0.76 × 222 (8)*. Net blood lactic acid is the difference between lactic acid at rest and the greatest lactic acid level observed 4–5 minutes after exercise, the time of peak lactic acid in the blood (16). The value 0.76 is a constant used to correct blood lactic acid levels to levels throughout the body fluids, and 222 is the caloric equivalent of a gram of lactic acid production. A typical value in men of college age for maximal energy derived from anaerobic glycolysis is about 200 cal/kg (8).

Since a high school coach is not likely to have the expertise or equipment to determine blood lactic acid levels, he must rely on performance tests of 1–3 minutes duration to help him assess the glycolytic capacity of his athletes. Of course, performance time in an 800-meter run, for example, is affected by factors other than maximal glycolytic capacity. Motivation and pain tolerance are two of the most important of these other factors, but such factors as running technique and sense of pace will also have a bearing on performance.

FACTORS RELATED TO ANAEROBIC ENDURANCE

Any factor that speeds or retards the onset of fatigue during high intensity work is obviously related to anaerobic endurance. Therefore, as will be described in Chapter 11, a reduction in energy stores, the onset of ischemia, excessively high temperature, or elevated lactic acid levels may enhance the development of fatigue. There are, however, four other factors not discussed in Chapter 11 that should be noted. These factors are strength, age, sex and muscle fiber-type profile.

Anaerobic endurance for simple, submaximally loaded movements is directly related to maximal muscle strength. In other words, a person who has maximal elbow flexor strength of 100 pounds at a joint angle of 90 degrees could expect to hold a 25 pound dumbbell at 90 degrees for about twice as long as a person who has a maximal strength of only 50 pounds (5, 19). For submaximal, static contractions at less than 60–70 per cent of maximal strength, there are at least two reasons for this relationship. First, the stronger person can produce a force of 25 pounds with fewer motor units than the weaker person.

Consequently, more motor units can be resting at any one time in the muscles of the stronger individual so that it will take longer to fatigue all his motor units. Second, in the case of static contractions, blood-flow is reduced in proportion to the relative severity of the muscle contraction. If the stronger person is contracting at only 25 per cent of his maximal strength, blood flow to his elbow flexors will be much less restricted than that to the muscles of the weaker subject, who must produce 50 per cent of his maximal force.

For static contractions with loads greater than 60–70 per cent of maximal strength, blood flow is totally cut off (10). For such contractions, the relationship between maximal strength and endurance is solely because of differences in the number of motor units that must be recuited to maintain the contraction for weaker and stronger persons. With *maximal* contractions, both static and dynamic, presumably the same total number of motor units must be recruited for both weak and strong persons so that there is little relationship between absolute strength and endurance with maximal loads (5). In other words, the weaker person will be able to exert less force for about the same time that the strong person exerts a greater force.

For submaximal dynamic contractions, stronger persons have greater endurance because they need to recruit fewer motor units to exert the same force. The reason for this is that the individual muscle fibers within each motor unit of the stronger person have more actin-myosin cross bridges to produce tension.

Just as contractions of 100 per cent of maximal strength can be held by the weaker person for about as long as the stronger one, so, too, a weaker person can persist at any given percentage of his maximal strength, whether it be 10, 40 or 70 per cent, for about the same time as a stronger individual. Another way of stating this is that *there is not a direct relationship between maximal strength and the time one can persist at producing force equal to any standard percentage of that maximal strength.*

Because there is a direct relationship between strength and endurance at submaximal loads, and because strength increases with age until about 30, before beginning a gradual decline (Fig. 7.17), *both strength and anaerobic endurance are affected in a similar fashion by age.* Likewise, *because males have greater maximal strength than females, they also have greater anaerobic muscular endurance for submaximal loads.* The age range of 12–15 years seems to be optimal for improving anaerobic endurance in simple movements (1). The underlying physiological mechanism for this phenomenon is not clear, although it may be explained by the fact that motivational levels are often high in young adolescents.

Finally, *anaerobic endurance at submaximal loads is greater for muscles that have greater proportions of slow twitch fibers* (14). This is true because the slow twitch fibers are better adapted to endurance activity by virtue of their better blood supply; their greater supply of mitochondria and mitochondrial enzymes of aerobic energy metabolism; their lower actin-myosin ATPase activity, which makes the maintenance of tension more efficient; and their greater supply of the protein, myoglobin, which acts as a local store for oxygen somewhat as hemoglobin stores oxygen in the blood. All of these factors better enable slow twitch fibers to produce ATP aerobically so that less lactic acid will be produced as an end product of anaerobic glycolysis.

TRAINING FOR IMPROVED ANAEROBIC ENDURANCE

As was seen in Chapter 9 regarding strength training, an important factor in establishing a training routine is to try to develop exercises that will train the body in a highly specific manner, improving its response to the precise demands that will be placed upon it in competition, manual labor or daily life. In other words, *unless one wishes simply to develop a general sort of endurance, the exercises used to improve endurance should mimic the actual task performance that the trainee is attempting to improve.* If he wishes to have better endurance at swinging a heavy ax, he should train with movements similar to, if not identical to, that task; but if he wishes to improve his ability to engage in a highly isometric type of performance such as moving furniture, he should probably exercise isometrically for much of his training. By training in a specific manner, it is thought that the appropriate adaptations in the nervous system are more effectively brought about. Thus, if one is training to improve an isokinetic or isotonic type of performance, it is probably best to design a program that emphasizes isokinetic or isotonic exercises.

Anaerobic Endurance Training for Dynamic Activities

As was described in the introduction of this chapter, there is a wide range of physical activities that might be classified as anaerobic endurance exercises. Dynamic anaerobic endurance includes such activities as chopping wood at a fast rate; sprinting for up to 1–2 minutes in track, swimming or cycling; wrestling; and the prolonged sprinting phases of such sports as basketball, soccer, field hockey, canoe racing and football. Also, although running, swimming and cycling over long distances depend much more on the cardiovascular system's delivery of oxygen, champions in these activities also have the capacity to sustain anaerobic sprints at the finish of their events.

Consequently, distance performers must not overlook the anaerobic aspects of their training.

Because of the varied nature of these dynamic anaerobic endurance activities, it is impossible to give specific training programs for each of them. The physiological principles for the development of specific programs are, however, similar for all types of dynamic anaerobic endurance events. It is these principles, with some examples, that will be described in the following discussion.

The body adapts to repeated exercise sessions so that subsequent exercise of a similar nature is tolerated more easily. Therefore, *it is important in training sessions to produce as much high-quality work as is feasible.* This means that the type of movement, the strength of the muscle contractions, and the speed of movement must be similar to what one is striving to accomplish as a training goal. Accordingly, if a beginning high school runner is trying to achieve a time of 2 minutes in an 800 meter competition, most of his training should be at that pace or faster, that is, he should run repeat 100's in no less than 15 seconds, 200's in 30 seconds and 400's in 60 seconds or faster. Likewise, a wrestler whose goal is to wrestle intensely for three 3-minute periods should practice intensely for repeated bouts of less than 3 minutes in length and not for long durations at low intensity.

The use of repeated work periods interspersed with recovery periods to help adapt the body to stressful demands placed upon it is known as *interval training*. In interval training the exercise periods are commonly called *work intervals* and the rest periods, *recovery intervals*. Although it is true that some championship performers have achieved greatness by training only at a slow pace for long durations, it is likely that many who train at a slow pace become better equipped to perform at that slow pace. Since the accumulation of lactic acid in muscle is greater in interval than in continuous exercise (11), interval training is especially useful for stressing anaerobic energy systems.

Because very little work can be performed at a *fast pace* when a continuous long-duration type of training is used, it is important to use repeated work intervals of rather short duration for the bulk of the training sessions. (Remember, though, that such training is extremely exhausting and must occasionally be interrupted by other types of training for the sake of variety; any method, no matter how grand in theory, is useless if the exerciser drops out of the training program.)

Because energy for anaerobic endurance activities is mostly provided by anaerobic mechanisms, training programs should be designed to stress or overload the cellular machinery responsible for producing ATP anaerobically. This means that the exercise periods must be very intense to place the greatest possible demands on the enzymes involved in anaerobic energy production, namely, the enzymes used to break down creatine phosphate and muscle glycogen. *Accordingly, work intervals should last no longer than 1–2 minutes.* Work intervals longer than 1–2 minutes do not increase the load on anaerobic capacity, but rather begin to rely more on aerobic energy supply (11). Since only a few long-duration work intervals can be tolerated in any given training session, it is important to keep the exercise periods under 1–2 minutes to maximize the total amount of work at the greatest anaerobic loads.

Also, it has been demonstrated that work intervals shorter than about 20 seconds do not bring about the maximal amount of anaerobic energy production if interspersed with recovery intervals of similar length (2, 11). This may be due to the ability of oxygen stored in muscles to promote aerobic ATP replenishment during the recovery intervals (2). Oxygen is stored in the muscles by being bound to *myoglobin*, which may release its oxygen to the muscle cells during periods of great oxygen demand (2). With interval training that includes very short work intervals, it is thought that myoglobin-bound oxygen is used during the work intervals, but can be rapidly replenished during rest intervals of similar length, so that anaerobic energy reserves such as creatine phosphate and glycogen are conserved (2). Consequently, *if work intervals of less than 20 seconds are used, recovery intervals should be limited to about 10–15 seconds so that myoglobin cannot be fully recharged with oxygen during the recovery intervals.* After a few repeats of such intervals, a more complete recovery period (15–20 minutes, for example) is required before beginning another set of work intervals.

Recovery intervals to follow work intervals longer than 20 seconds must be long enough to allow substantial recovery of the muscles, so that an adequate number of high-quality work intervals can be completed during a training session, but not so long that subsequent work intervals are not somewhat more stressful than the preceding ones. *Therefore, recovery intervals following short work intervals (20–30 seconds) should be about 1–2 minutes long, and longer work intervals should be followed by more complete recovery periods of 2–15 minutes.* The longer recovery intervals for a given work interval are needed for younger athletes or those with poor anaerobic capacities. Since lactic acid is removed more rapidly when mild exercise is performed during recovery than with complete inactivity (11), slow jogging, swimming and so on during recovery are often prescribed.

The exercise performed during work intervals designed to improve dynamic anaerobic endurance must be at maximal or near–maximal intensities. A commonly used rule of thumb suggests that anaerobic capacity begins to be taxed at about 80 per cent of one's maximal effort for a given duration of exercise (2). To insure a near-maximal reliance on anaerobic capacity, therefore, it would be wise to exercise at no less than 90 per cent of maximal effort in longer duration activities (1–2 minutes), and to exercise maximally for shorter work intervals. Thus, if a runner's best time for a 400 meter run is 60 seconds (6.67 m/seconds), he could run 400 meter intervals in 66.7 seconds (400/(6.67 × 0.90)), or he could run 360 meters in 60 seconds (90 per cent of 400 = 360) to insure that he would stress his anaerobic capacity.

The number of training sessions per week needed to cause the greatest improvement in anaerobic capacity is not well established, but some evidence indicates that 3–4 training sessions per week may be optimal, at least with unconditioned college males (9).

Table 10.2 summarizes information on interval training for improving anaerobic endurance. The suggested scheme in Table 10.2 should be useful in devising appropriate training procedures for any type of activity, especially when the work is performed at maximal intensity. It should be noted that a training program could include more repetitions with shorter recovery intervals than are shown in Table 10.2, but the work done then would be of relatively poor quality.

There are many combinations of work and recovery intervals that could be used during any training session. One might wish to combine 10-second work intervals and 2-minute work intervals in the same session, by completing perhaps 12 repetitions of the suggested routine with 10-second work intervals; then one could finish the session with 4 or 5 repetitions of the 2-minute work and recovery intervals. It bears repeating that the suggestions presented in Table 10.2 are meant to serve only as rough guidelines for training. Younger or less capable performers may not be able to complete as many repetitions or recover adequately with the recovery intervals suggested, and better performers may not be adequately stressed with these routines.

Table 10.2. **Suggested Scheme of Interval Training for Improving Anaerobic Capacity and Dynamic Local Muscular Endurance.**

Length of Work Interval	Percent of Intensity of Effort	Length of Recovery Interval	Number of Work Intervals Per Session	Training Sessions Per Week
10 sec	100	10 sec	20–30	3–4
20 sec	100	15 sec	10–20	3–4
30 sec	100	1–2 min	8–18	3–4
1 min	95–100	3–5 min	5–15	3–4
2 min	90–100	5–15 min	4–10	3–4

Responses to Interval Training for Improved Anaerobic Capacity.
Do the interval-training programs described in this chapter actually
overload the biochemical mechanisms responsible for the anaerobic
replenishment of ATP in skeletal muscles? Evidence obtained from
analysis of blood and muscle tissue supports an affirmative answer to
this question (11,13, 17). In Fig. 10.2, there are illustrated the idea-
lized changes in the muscle stores of glycogen and creatine phos-

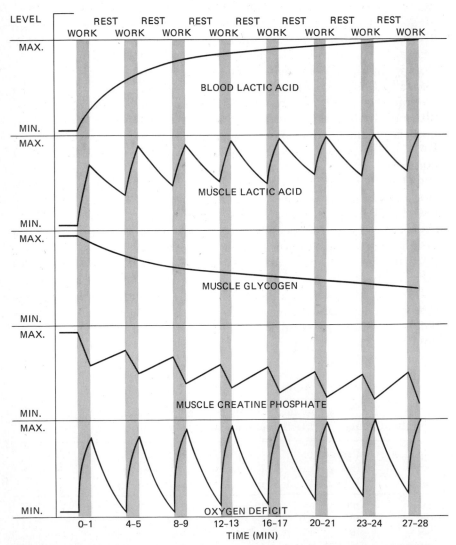

Figure 10.2. **Physiological changes occurring during interval training
session.**

phate, the accumulation of lactic acid in blood and muscle, and the repeated attainment of maximal capacity for oxygen deficit as the result of an interval-training session. As this illustration reveals, near-maximal or maximal oxygen deficit is reached during each of the eight work intervals. This shows indirectly that anaerobic mechanisms for supplying ATP are being heavily stressed. The other data shown in Fig. 10.2 give direct evidence that anaerobic events are occurring in the muscle: Creatine phosphate is gradually depleted during work and only partially replenished during each recovery period; glycogen is broken down; and extremely high levels of muscle and blood lactic acid progressively accumulate. Other evidence that interval training can be an effective means of stressing anaerobic capacity is that such training leads to adaptations in anaerobic enzymes and to improved oxygen debt capacity. This evidence will be discussed later in this chapter.

Maintenance of dynamic muscular endurance can be accomplished with one or two training sessions per week (9).

Improving Dynamic Anaerobic Endurance for Simple Movements. For dynamic endurance training of simple dynamic movements, such as repeated elbow flexions, most authorities conclude that repetition of movements is far more important than was true for strength training. Thus, *for dynamic endurance in simple movements, one should train with relatively light resistance and many repetitions.* However, it should be emphasized that strength improvement should probably be the most important secondary goal of any training program designed to enhance anaerobic endurance. Strength improvement in this context has such importance because of the strong relationship between strength and endurance. Accordingly, one should not stress repetitions over load until he has established a sound foundation of muscular strength (3). For most kinds of anaerobic endurance, training of a dynamic type (4–5 sets of 10–20 repetitions maximum) performed 3 or 4 days per week will approach the optimal general pattern of training. *Maintenance programs* for anaerobic endurance gained by training can be reduced to performance of the usual training routine once or twice per week.

Anaerobic Training for Static Activities

To improve static endurance one should perform many static contractions in each training session with a load greater than what will be faced in competition, on the job, or in daily life. One should start with intensive, short-duration contractions performed 10–20 times each session, 3–4 times per week. As strength improves, the program should be altered to include 5–10 long-duration contractions with loads just above those to be faced after training. In this way the organism can adapt to stress by improving not only strength, but also the ability of anaerobic metabolic systems to produce ATP under endurance conditions. Maintenance of static endurance can probably be achieved by repetition of the normal training session once per week.

As with strength and other types of fitness training, *it is important to vary the approach to anaerobic training so that boredom does not cause one to drop out of the training program.* An occasional training session of exercises that may not be ideal for improving endurance, but that are interesting to the trainee, are better than no training at all. One must not become too rigid in designing training programs lest no one be willing to become trained.

When designing training programs for the improvement of anaerobic endurance in physical education classes, many exercises can be accomplished in the form of sports activities or games, so that most students can better enjoy their fitness training. Rope climbs and "tugs of war" are good examples of activities that improve static endurance, whereas hopping races and relays in which participants must move on all four limbs can be used to improve dynamic muscular endurance. As was mentioned earlier in this chapter, excessive emphasis on pullups and rope climbs as tests of muscular endurance penalizes heavier students whose greater strengths do not compensate for their heavier body weights. Therefore, scoring on any such tests should be based on normative data for various weight classifications.

Duration of Training Effects on Anaerobic Endurance

As with gains in strength, improvements in anaerobic endurance for simple movements begin to be lost after about a month of inactivity. Much of the gains, up to 80 per cent in many cases, are retained for as long as 6 months, however (3). It seems likely that most of the retention of endurance gains for simple movements is because of the retention of strength improvements. The duration of training effects for activities such as swimming have not been adequately studied, but limited evidence suggests that a 2-month period of inactivity may completely obliterate any training effects (9).

PHYSIOLOGICAL MECHANISMS UNDERLYING IMPROVEMENTS IN ANAEROBIC ENDURANCE

In any attempt to assess the relative importance of possible mechanisms that could explain how a training program could enhance anaerobic endurance, one must consider the nature of the various types of anaerobic endurance, such as, the extent of static contractions, the degree of aerobic involvement and the relative intensity of the work, because it seems probable that different mechanisms may underlie gains in different types of endurance. With simple movements the only common factor that can help explain endurance improvements brought about by training is the gain in muscular strength associated with increased endurance of all types. However, strength gains cannot be the sole mechanism underlying endurance gains because strength rarely improves by as much as 100 per cent after a few months of training, whereas anaerobic muscular endurance may increase by more than 5,000 per cent for submaximal loads (2). Some of the other mechanisms that may be responsible for endurance improvements are described in the following paragraphs.

Intense Static Contractions

If one were to maintain a severe static contraction of the knee extensor muscles at a joint angle of 90 degrees for as long as possible, and then undergo an intensive training program concentrating on the improvement of the strength of the knee extensors, a posttraining test at the pretraining load would show a gain in holding time from a pretraining time of about 10 seconds to a posttraining time of perhaps 20–30 seconds. Because any static contraction at a load greater than 60–70 per cent of maximal strength causes complete compression of the arteries, so that no blood enters the muscles (10), the contraction must be maintained almost totally anaerobically, and improvements in circulation do not enter into the explanation of endurance gains. Also, muscle pain is not usually a major factor in limiting such brief contractions. Therefore, the mechanism responsible for these gains could involve two factors—a reduction in the number of motor units recruited to perform the task (because the trained muscle fibers in each motor unit can produce more force) and an increase in the capacity of the muscle to supply ATP anaerobically.

Regarding this latter possibility, some studies have shown increased muscle stores of ATP and creatine phosphate and a slight improvement in the capacity of the muscle to break down glycogen (11). However, most of the increased ATP content of the muscles after training is thought to reflect a greater storage of ATP in the mitochondria. This mitochondrial ATP is not useful for intensive static contractions. Accordingly, it appears that most, if not all, of the improvement in holding time for a very intense static contraction is because of the gains in strength that allow the muscle to rest some motor units that would have been recruited immediately to maintain the contraction prior to training. Since gains in holding time for such intense static contractions are rather modest, there is little reason to believe that factors other than strength improvements are involved in these endurance gains.

Moderate Static Contractions

For static contractions held at less than 60 per cent of maximal strength, substantial endurance training effects can be shown. Much of this gain in endurance is undoubtedly because of a greater strength of individual motor units, so that fewer need to be recruited at any one time after training, but other factors also probably play a role. These factors include a greater potential of the trained muscle to produce energy, an improved blood supply, a reduced production of lactic acid early in the work and perhaps a greater tolerance to the fatiguing effects of lactic acid later in the effort.

Little direct evidence is available, but it seems likely that muscles trained for anaerobic endurance have greater stores of glycogen and creatine phosphate which can be heavily used if the contraction is greater than about 20 per cent of the maximal strength (the level at which arterial blood flow begins to be reduced). Thus, trained muscles probably are better equipped to provide energy for sustained contractions than are untrained muscles.

For static workloads up to about 60 per cent of maximum strength, an improved circulation of blood to working muscles may contribute to enhanced endurance performance if the relative intensity of the contraction is less after training because of improved strength. In other words, prior to training, maintenance of a 15 kilogram load may have required 50 per cent of one's maximal strength, whereas after training the same load may demand only 30 per cent of a maximal contraction. Thus, a corresponding lesser restriction of blood flow to the working muscles would have been accomplished.

Assuming that endurance-trained muscles have a greater oxygen supply during heavy work, less demand is placed upon the anaerobic breakdown of muscle glycogen to lactic acid for energy supply. Consequently, the trained individual produces less lactic acid for a static contraction that produces a given force. If lactic acid limited performance prior to training (Chapter 11), it is then less apt to cause fatigue after training. With heavier static work that eventually does lead to a buildup of lactic acid, the trained person may not tire until he has a greater level of acid in his tissues than the untrained has. This may indicate a better ability to tolerate the lactic acid, or it may reflect a greater muscle glycogen store and improved capacity to break down glycogen to form lactic acid.

Dynamic Contractions

An enhanced anaerobic endurance for dynamic contractions after training is brought about by most of the mechanisms described for improvements in static endurance. Improved strength of individual motor units would allow the same force to be exerted by fewer motor units contracting at one time. Both a greater capacity to produce energy and a greater tolerance to lactic acid or greater capacity to produce lactic acid could contribute to improved endurance for both moderate and heavy dynamic contractions. There is evidence that training can increase both total (13) and alactic oxygen debt capacities (8). Enhancements have also been shown in the capacity to store glycogen (2, 21) and to catabolize it to lactic acid (19). These changes are sometimes associated with alterations in the activities of enzymes responsible for glycogen synthesis and degradation (11, 18, 20, 21).

In addition, better circulation is probably important in bringing more oxygen to, and removing more metabolic "waste" products from, muscles that are performing heavy (but not lighter) dynamic contractions. For lighter contractions a somewhat reduced blood supply after training has been reported; trained muscle apparently can make better use of a smaller oxygen supply to produce ATP by aerobic metabolism, so that less lactic acid has to be produced by anaerobic glycolysis (4).

For skilled movements that require a substantial amount of neuromuscular coordination, an additional mechanism is a major factor in improved endurance. That factor is the elimination of unnecessary contractions by muscles that are not required to perform the movement under the newly acquired pattern of skill. For example, a beginning swimmer uses many unnecessary muscles as he begins to develop skill. Those extraneous muscle contractions are gradually eliminated as the swimmer learns to use only the muscles actually required. As the swimmer's skill develops, he finds that his endurance improves, too. Part of that improved endurance can be attributed to the fact that: The muscle contractions he has been able to eliminate from his movements are no longer consuming oxygen and requiring high rates of blood flow that can be better used by the muscles whose contractions are essential to the task.

Review Questions

1. List five athletic events and three daily activities that rely heavily on anaerobic metabolism for energy supply.
2. Briefly describe the techniques which can be used in the laboratory and in the school setting to evaluate one's potential for performing anaerobic exercise.
3. What is the function of the alactic acid oxygen debt, that is, what is the excess oxygen used for?
4. Explain how interval training can be used to maintain the quality of work performed in a training session. What implications does this maintenance of quality have for any neural adaptations that may occur with training?
5. Explain why a stronger child has greater endurance in sawing wood than a weaker child.
6. List the principles of training for anaerobic endurance and explain each one.
7. Based on appropriate physiological principles, design an interval training program for an anaerobic activity of your choice. Design the program for one week in the middle of the training season.

References

1. Asmussen, E. Growth in muscular strength and power. In G. L. Rarick (Ed.), *Physical Activity—Human Growth and Development*. New York: Academic Press, 1973, pp. 60–79.
2. Astrand, P.-O., and K. Rodahl. *Textbook of Work Physiology*. New York: McGraw-Hill, 1970.
3. Clark, D. H. Adaptations in strength and muscular endurance resulting from exercise. In J. H. Wilmore (Ed.), *Exercise and Sport Sciences Reviews, Vol. 1*. New York: Academic Press, 1973, pp. 73–102.
4. Clausen, J. P. Muscle blood flow during exercise and its significance for maximal performance. In J. Keul (Ed.), *Limiting Factors of Maximal Performance*. Stuttgart: Georg Thieme, Publishers, 1973, pp. 253–266.
5. deVries, H. A. *Physiology of Exercise for Physical Education and Athletics*, 2nd Ed. Dubuque, Iowa: W. C. Brown, 1974.
6. di Prampero, P. E. The alactic oxygen debt: Its power, capacity, and efficiency. In B. Pernow and B. Saltin (Eds.), *Muscle Metabolism During Exercise*. New York: Plenum Press, 1971, pp. 371–382.

7. di Prampero, P. E., L. Peeters, and R. Margaria. Alactic O₂ debt and lactic acid production after exhausting exercise in man. *Journal of Applied Physiology*, 1973, **34**:628–632.
8. Fox, E. L. Differences in metabolic alterations with sprint versus endurance interval training programs. In H. Howald and J. R. Poortmans (Eds.), *Metabolic Adaptation to Prolonged Physical Exercise*. Basel: Birkhauser Verlag, 1975, pp. 119–126.
9. Fox, E. L., and D. K. Mathews. *Interval Training—Conditioning for Sports and General Fitness*. Philadelphia: W. B. Saunders, 1974.
10. Funderburk, C. F., S. G. Hipskind, R. C. Welton, and A. R. Lind. Development of, and recovery from, fatigue induced by static effort at various tensions. *Journal of Applied Physiology*, 1974, **37**:392–396.
11. Gollnick, P. D., and L. Hermansen. Biochemical adaptations to exercise: anaerobic metabolism. *Exercise and Sport Sciences Reviews*, 1973, **1**:1–43.
12. Graham, T. E., and G. M. Andrew. The variability of repeated measurements of oxygen debt in man following a maximal treadmill exercise. *Medicine and Science in Sports*, 1973, **5**:73–78.
13. Hermansen, L. Anaerobic energy release. *Medicine and Science in Sports*, 1969, **1**:32–38.
14. Hudlicka, O. Differences in development of fatigue in slow and fast muscles. In J. Keul (Ed.), *Limiting Factors of Physical Performance*. Stuttgart: Georg Thieme, Publishers, 1973, pp. 36–41.
15. Katch, V., and F. M. Henry. Prediction of running performance from maximal oxygen debt and intake. *Medicine and Science in Sports*, 1972, **4**:187–191.
16. Margaria, R., P. Cerretelli, P. E. di Prampero, C. Massari, and G. Torelli. Kinetics and mechanism of oxygen debt contraction in man. *Journal of Applied Physiology*, 1963, **18**:371–377.
17. Saltin, B., and B. Essen. Muscle glycogen, lactate, ATP, and CP in intermittent exercise. In B. Pernow and B. Saltin (Eds.), *Muscle Metabolism During Exercise*. New York: Plenum Press, 1971, pp. 419–424.
18. Saubert IV, C. W., R. B. Armstrong, R. E. Shepherd, and P. D. Gollnick. Anaerobic enzyme adaptations to sprint training in rats. *Pflugers Archives*, 1973, **341**:305–312.
19. Simonsen, E. (Ed.). *Physiology of Work Capacity and Fatigue*. Springfield, Ill.: Charles C Thomas, Publisher, 1971.
20. Staudte, H. W., G. U. Exner, and D. Pette. Effects of short-term, high intensity (*sprint*) training on some contractile and

metabolic characteristics of fast and slow muscle of the rat. *Pflugers Archives,* 1973, **344:**159–168.

21. Taylor, A. W. The effects of exercise and training on the activities of human skeletal-muscle, glycogen-cycle enzymes. In H. Howald and J. R. Poortmans (Eds.), *Metabolic Adaptation to Prolonged Physical Exercise.* Basel: Birkhauser Verlag, 1975, pp. 451–462.

11

Muscular fatigue and soreness

Muscular fatigue is the inability to maintain or repeat the production of a given force by muscular contraction. Fatigue of muscles during physical exercise has been experienced by everyone. Its rate of onset often determines who will be a champion athlete, who will be the most productive laborer, and who will become the most easily frustrated when attempting to become physically fit. Accordingly, an examination of some of the possible mechanisms of fatigue is warranted in a text on exercise physiology. Because muscular fatigue is often studied under relatively anaerobic conditions of exercise, it seems especially appropriate to consider fatigue in a chapter following the analysis of anaerobic endurance.

It should be noted that there are other kinds of "fatigue" that are beyond the scope of this text. We will not consider the fatigue that comes with boredom, mental activity, emotional exhaustion, or psychological depression.

177

ANATOMICAL SITE OF FATIGUE

The limitation on one's ability to maintain muscular contractions at a given level of force conceivably could lie *in the central nervous system* (that is, in the nerve cells of the motor cortex of the brain which initiate the impulses for voluntary contractions or in the connections (synapses) between neurons that lie in the pathway from the motor cortex to the final motor nerve of the spinal cord). The site of fatigue could also be *in the final motor nerve itself, in the neuromus-*

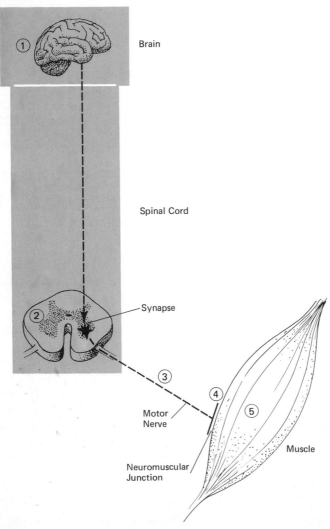

Figure 11.1. Possible sites of muscular fatigue.

cular junction (motor end-plate), or *in the muscle.* (See Fig. 11.1.) Unfortunately, about the only site that scientific experiments seem to have ruled out is the motor nerve that conducts the stimulus from the spinal cord to the muscle. It is exceedingly difficult to stimulate this nerve to the point where it fails to conduct an impulse; muscular fatigue always precedes nerve fatigue at these high rates of stimulation (24).

There is, however, some very persuasive evidence that under some conditions other cells or synapses in the central nervous system may stop transmitting impulses between nerve cells. For example, in some studies of human finger and thumb endurance, electrial stimulation of the nerve to the muscles caused strong contractions after voluntary efforts failed to produce contractions (24). These results suggest that neither the nerve-muscle junction nor the muscle itself is the site of fatigue, and that the failure must reside in the generation of impulses in the brain or in the synaptic transmission of those impulses in the central nervous system.

Other experiments show at least as persuasively that both the junction between nerve and muscle and the muscle itself may fail to perform adequately at the time of fatigue (25). In these experiments electromyographic (E.M.G.) recordings of the contractile stimuli (action potentials) showed that E.M.G. activity declined with the onset of fatigue, whether that fatigue was caused by maximal sustained voluntary contractions or by electrical stimulation of the nerve. This implicates the neuromuscular junction in the fatigue process because the impulses (E.M.G.) reaching the muscle should not have been diminished if the neuromuscular junction was still functioning properly. In these same experiments, however, a second phase of the fatigue process was shown where the continued decline in contractile force occurred more rapidly than the decrement in E.M.G. Accordingly, this phase of the fatigue process seems to rest in the muscle and not in the neuromuscular junction. Supposedly, higher threshold motor units consisting of fast-twitch muscle fibers are more susceptible to junctional fatigue, whereas lower threshold slow-twitch fibers eventually succumb to fatigue processes in the muscle fibers themselves. The neuromuscular junction failure is thought to be due to a diminished release of the chemical transmitter, acetylcholine, from the nerve ending. Possibilities for failure in the muscle itself are discussed in the following section.

In summary, after more than 50 years of scientific study, we are still uncertain about where to pin the anatomical blame for muscular fatigue. Perhaps it is logical to conclude that central nervous system, junctional and muscular failures all can occur with different types of exercise. If one were to speculate, it would seem reasonable that failure of the central nervous system would be most important in

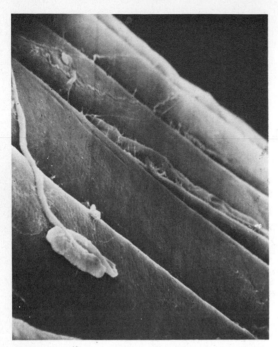

Figure 11.2. Stereo electron micrograph showing surfaces of four muscle fibers with white nerve fibril and large motor end-plate on lowest muscle fiber. (Courtesy of R. E. Carrow, W. W. Heusner and W. D. Van Huss, Michigan State University, E. Lansing, Michigan.)

long-duration activities characterized by repetitive movements that require a high degree of concentration. Factory workers who must sustain highly skilled movements for many hours may succumb to central nervous system fatigue. On the other hand, neuromuscular junction failure may be most important in sprint and power events that rely on fast twitch muscle fibers, and failure in the muscle itself may primarily affect performance in longer-duration events that are powered by slow-twitch motor units but require little cerebral concentration.

POSSIBLE CAUSES OF FATIGUE BECAUSE OF FAILURE OF MUSCLE CONTRACTION

If an exercise physiologist were asked to pick the most likely single site of fatigue, he would probably choose the contractile process in the muscle. One reason for this is that there are many experimental studies that demonstrate a rather straightforward relationship between the depletion of energy sources such as creatine phosphate and glycogen and the progression of fatigue (4, 14, 18, 19, 22). These relationships suggest, but do not prove, that fatigue is caused by a lack of energy stores to replenish the ATP needed for continued muscle contraction. It is also possible, of course, that the relationship between energy store depletion and fatigue is merely associative and not causative. Nevertheless, because this relationship is so consistent, and because there are so few other reproducibly demonstrated relationships with fatigue, the depletion of energy stores remains the most accepted explanation for fatigue. Let us take a closer look at the relationship between fatigue and energy stores.

Energy Depletion for Activities That Can Be Sustained Less Than 2–3 Minutes

For maximal or near-maximal contractions that can be sustained for between about 5 seconds and 2 minutes, oxygen delivery to the muscles is of limited importance. This is because the rate of energy expenditure is too high to be met aerobically or because in static contractions above about 60–70 per cent of maximal strength, blood flow is shut off by the strongly contracted muscles (9). What is important in these strenuous contractions is the rate at which ATP can be replenished by anaerobic metabolism, that is, by the anaerobic breakdown of creatine phosphate and muscle glycogen and glucose.

When energy stores in muscles are measured after contractions that can be maintained for less than 10 seconds, it is unusual to find a severe depletion of muscle glycogen, and only 20–50 per cent of the ATP and creatine phosphate stores may be depleted (3). Therefore, it seems likely that the *rate* of ATP utilization during severe muscle contractions is simply too great to be met by resupply from muscle stores of ATP and creatine phosphate (7). In other words, the making and breaking of actin-myosin cross bridges is happening too rapidly for the transfer of energy from stored ATP and creatine phosphate to keep pace. The work must slow down or stop so that ATP can move to the cross bridges from nearby storage sites.

For workloads that can be sustained for longer than 10 seconds, but less than about 2–3 minutes, a substantial drop in creatine phosphate stores (perhaps greater than 90 per cent, can be measured along with a 30–40 per cent decrease in ATP (3, 10, 18). Because much of the ATP seems to be stored in the mitochondria, the sarcoplasmic reticulum and in other compartments, a rather small fraction of the ATP is available for muscle contraction. Therefore, it appears that creatine phosphate depletion may limit the ability of the muscles to sustain contractions at these high loads. Glycogen breakdown does not seem to be able to provide the necessary ATP, because glycolysis is relatively slow, and because the lactic acid produced in glycolysis may depress the activities of some of the glycolytic enzymes, especially phosphofructokinase (Fig. 3.2, reaction C) (10).

Energy Depletion for Activities That Can Be Sustained More Than 3 Minutes

Any activity that can be sustained for longer than about 10 seconds is performed with some participation of aerobic energy metabolism, and beyond about 2 minutes, oxygen delivery to the muscles is progressively more important for meeting the energy demands of the muscle. This requirement for oxygen exists because anaerobic metabolism cannot continue to supply large quantities of ATP beyond about 60 seconds, perhaps because of progressively greater inhibition of glycolytic enzyme activity by lactic acid. Given that oxygen delivery to the muscles is important, it is still possible that depletion of fuel reserves may cause fatigue.

Physical exercise that can be sustained for 3–40 minutes does not seem to be limited by depletion of either ATP, creatine phosphate or glycogen. Although there is a large fall in creatine phosphate levels in the muscles, this reduction is similar for exercise that can be sustained for 6–7 minutes and for exercise lasting 20–25 minutes (18). (See Fig. 11.3.) Accordingly, if creatine phosphate depletion were the limiting factor for this type of exercise, it should be impossible to continue working beyond 6–7 minutes. However, since muscle glycogen falls by only 10–50 per cent in work of less than 40 minutes duration (22), and since it is widely agreed that neither fat nor blood

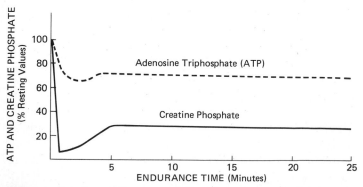

Figure 11.3. ATP and creatine phosphate depletion with exercise sustained for 1–25 minutes. Data primarily from reference 18.

glucose makes a significant contribution to activity that leads to exhaustion in less than 25 minutes, it seems that some factor other than depletion of energy reserves limits work of 3–40 minutes duration. Perhaps the lactic acid inhibition of glycolysis is that factor.

Glycogen depletion is associated with fatigue in heavy exercise that can be sustained for about 40–180 minutes (depending upon the condition of the exerciser) (22) (Fig. 11.4). Reductions in glycogen stores of about 60–90 per cent have been measured in muscle biopsy samples of humans in such diverse activities as cycling, skiing, running and soccer competition. It should again be noted that this is not necessarily a cause-and-effect relationship, but there is a logical and reproducible relationship between glycogen depletion and exhaustion at these heavy workloads. Additional evidence that supports a causal relationship is that when muscle glycogen stores are increased by dietary manipulation, endurance time also increases, whereas decreases in initial glycogen levels have the opposite effect. Therefore, it is now widely agreed that the depletion of glycogen is the most likely factor that leads to fatigue in activities lasting 40–180 minutes (22). In general, such activities require oxygen uptake from the blood at a rate of about 70–90 per cent of one's maximum capacity to consume oxygen.

When exercises of lower intensities are maintained for 4 hours or more, it is unlikely that exhaustion will be associated with an appreciable decline in muscle glycogen stores (Fig. 11.4), but there may be a fall in blood glucose levels that reflects a depletion of liver glycogen stores (15). Because the central nervous system is a high priority user

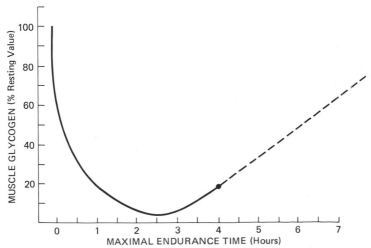

Figure 11.4. Glycogen values after exercise that can be sustained for various durations. Data principally from reference 22.

of blood glucose for energy, it seems possible that nervous system failure is a greater factor in fatigue for long-duration exercise than contractile fatigue in the muscle. This is logical because the glycogen and creatine phosphate stores left in the muscle at the time of fatigue should be able to continue providing energy if the nerve stimulus reaches the muscle unimpeded. Thus, we again have another case where depletion of energy reserves in the muscle does not adequately explain a failure of the muscle to sustain contraction. In the next section, other possible explanations of fatigue will be discussed.

Lactic Acid Accumulation in Muscles

The theory that lactic acid accumulation in the muscles limits muscular performance has been widely held since at least 1935 (24). There are several reasons why this idea has achieved such popularity. With most types of heavy work, fatigue is associated with high levels of lactic acid, and the rate of lactic and pyruvic acid accumulation in the working muscles is very closely related to the intensity of contractions (14). This relationship is shown in Fig. 11.5; it demonstrates that the time one can hold an isometric contraction decreases with increasing load and rate of acid accumulation in the muscle. Another piece of evidence taken to support the idea that the accumulation of acid or some other "toxic" substance leads to fatigue is that fatigued

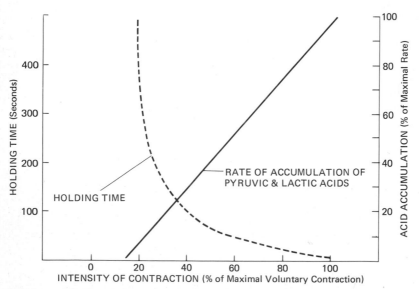

Figure 11.5.   Isometric contraction holding times and rates of accumulation of lactic and pyruvic acids at various intensities of muscular contraction. Data from reference 14.

muscles of laboratory animals can begin contracting anew if the muscles are perfused or washed out with a fresh salt solution after fatigue has developed (23). Since lactic acid is the most prevalent component of blood that differs between fatigued and rested muscles, it has usually been concluded that this washing out of the muscles removes excessive lactic acid.

The rationale that acid accumulation in muscles causes fatigue rests upon the effect of decreased pH (increased acid) on muscle contraction. There is some evidence that the formation of actin-myosin cross bridges may be inhibited by low pH (10). Also, several enzymes of energy metabolism may be inhibited by excess acid. Since muscle pH can fall from a resting value of about 7.0 to a maximal exercise value of about 6.5 or below, it is conceivable that phosphorylase or phosphofructokinase (Fig. 3.2), important regulating enzymes of glycolysis, or some other enzymes may be inhibited by lactic acid accumulation (10). In fact, muscle biopsy studies support the hypothesis that phosphofructokinase activity is inhibited with heavy exercise (4). It has also been shown that excess acidity can interfere with the transmission of the nerve stimulus across the neuromuscular junction (11). Therefore, the notion that lactic acid may be a causal agent of muscular fatigue has at least a theoretically sound basis. However, there are some other data that do not fit into the lactic acid scheme.

Evidence in Opposition to the Lactic Acid Accumulation Theory of Fatigue

As has been previously noted, the *rate* of lactic acid accumulation is related to the intensity of exercise (Fig. 11.5), and lactic acid levels are usually high at the time of exhaustion. But a closer look at the evidence reveals some contradictions to the theory that lactic acid accumulation causes fatigue. For instance, although the *rate* of acid accumulation is nicely correlated with the development of fatigue, *the total amount* of acid accumulated is not necessarily greatest at the time of fatigue (14). As can be seen in Fig 11.6, the greatest total accumulation of lactic acid does not come at 100 per cent of maximal voluntary contraction which can be held for 10 or 15 seconds, but at about 50 per cent of maximal voluntary contraction which can be held for 90–100 seconds. Of course, it is possible that somehow *the rate of change of pH* is more detrimental than the total accumulation of acid. But there are other types of physical activity that can be exhausting in the absence of high levels of lactic acid, so that doubt is cast upon the importance of the rate of accumulation of the acid. For example, if one runs at a constant speed on a treadmill for two exercise periods, one at a steeper treadmill slope than the other, the run up the steeper slope leads to exhaustion earlier but with a lower accu-

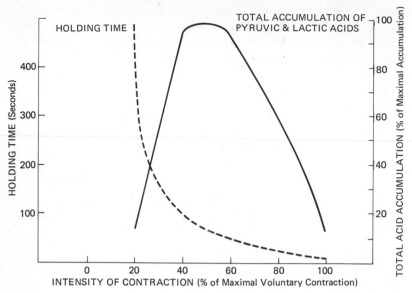

Figure 11.6. Isometric contraction holding times and total accumulation of lactic and pyruvic acids at various intensities of muscular contraction. Data from reference 14.

mulation of lactic acid (5). Also, lowering the muscle glycogen stores prior to an exercise test by consuming a low-carbohydrate diet or by prolonged exercising to exhaustion on a previous hour or day causes an *earlier* onset of fatigue with *lower* levels of lactic acid in the blood (15, 24). Therefore, there is abundant evidence that earlier fatigue is not necessarily associated with the greater accumulation of lactic acid that would be expected if lactic acid buildup were the sole cause of fatigue.

Another argument against the lactic acid accumulation theory of fatigue is that younger and older persons, who usually experience earlier fatigue in endurance activities than persons who are between 20 and 30 years of age, have lower lactic acid levels in their blood at exhaustion than those between 20 and 30 (Fig. 11.7). Although it is conceivable that there is some aging effect on muscular sensitivity to lactic acid, a simpler explanation is that lactic acid accumulation does not cause fatigue.

A final bit of information sometimes used to refute the lactic acid theory of fatigue is that training has often (but not always) been reported to increase one's capacity to produce lactic acid during maximal exercise (2, 19, 24). Because this greater production of lactic acid is associated with increased maximal work capacity and a delayed

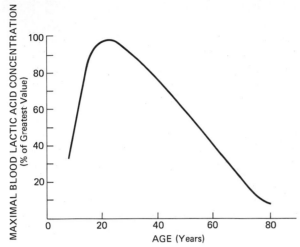

Figure 11.7. Maximal blood lactic acid concentration as a function of age. Data from reference 5.

onset of fatigue, it seems illogical to conclude that lactic acid causes fatigue. Proponents of the lactic acid theory might counter, however, with the idea that the untrained subjects in those studies that have shown a training effect on maximal lactic acid accumulation were inadequately motivated to continue working, and that the so-called training effect was simply due to an improved motivation to continue working in the face of increasing discomfort. Accordingly, there are two explanations of any training effect on maximal lactic acid accumulation. The first is that training improves motivation or improves tolerance to lactic acid, and the second is that more lactic acid is produced in the trained subject because he has greater stores of glycogen that can be called upon for anaerobic breakdown to lactic acid. The weight of evidence seems to support the latter explanation, and although it still has its vigorous supporters, the lactic acid accumulation theory of muscular fatigue is being confronted with more and more skepticism as research reveals greater numbers of possible explanations for fatigue.

Loss of Phosphate from the Muscle

As a muscle becomes fatigued, it loses progressively more phosphate into the tissue fluid and the blood surrounding the muscle (13). Since this phosphate is needed for the formation of ATP, it seems possible that a loss of phosphate might cause certain types of fatigue. In the laboratory, it can be shown that bathing a fatigued muscle in a phosphate solution tends to restore some of its contractility (13). As was discussed previously, though, a depletion of ATP and creatine phosphate can account for fatigue only in activities lasting less than a few minutes; exercise of longer durations can be continued with very little additional fall in these compounds. (See Fig. 11.3.)

Ischemia and Hypoxia

Ischemia is the condition of diminished blood supply to a tissue because of some obstruction of arterial blood flow, whereas *hypoxia* is a deficiency of oxygen that can be caused either by ischemia, by breathing air low in oxygen content or by other factors. Both ischemia and hypoxia can hasten the onset of fatigue, but their relative importance under normal exercise conditions is not fully established (3). Ischemia produced by the inflation of a blood pressure cuff around a limb decreases endurance time in all but very brief, near-maximal dynamic contractions and in all static contractions that require less than about 60–70 per cent of one's maximal strength to maintain. These exceptions are the types of contractions that are maintained without a major contribution of aerobic energy metabolism. Dynamic contractions lasting only a few seconds obtain energy at the expense of ATP and creatine phosphate, and static contractions held at greater than 60–70 per cent of one's maximal strength completely block the flow of blood to the muscles by compressing the arteries so that the blood pressure cuff has no additional effect (9).

Likewise, if persons breathe a gas mixture that has an abnormally low content of oxygen while performing exercise, endurance time will decrease except in anaerobic activities (17). Accordingly, because ischemia produces hypoxia, it is usually assumed that ischemia reduces endurance time by causing a state of hypoxia in the exercising muscles. However, some workers suggest that the adverse effect of ischemia on endurance is not because of hypoxia but, rather, to a disruption of afferent nerve impulses from the working muscles, or to a failure of the circulation to remove lactic acid and other "waste" products of metabolism. Experiments that have manipulated the amount of oxygen delivered to, or required by, the working muscles have, in fact, led some to the conclusion that hypoxia does not limit the endurance of muscles under normal exercise conditions where the exerciser breathes normal concentrations of oxygen (17). These experiments have mainly been concerned with *dynamic* work. In this type of work, hypoxia may not develop because blood flow is not drastically reduced as in intense static contractions. The bulk of the evidence points to ischemic hypoxia as a main cause of fatigue in strenuous *isometric* contractions.

Temperature

The temperature of working muscles has a somewhat variable effect on the onset of fatigue. Thus, warmup seems to prolong heavy exercise on a treadmill, probably because the increased body temperature is associated with increased blood flow to the muscles and because the enzymes of energy metabolism are somewhat more active at higher temperatures. But cooling of a muscle prolongs *static* exercise when blood flow is shut off by the sustained muscle contraction (24). The beneficial effect of cooling on holding time for a static contraction is thought to be due to a decreased activity of the myosin ATPase enzyme (21). This decreased enzyme activity leads to reduction in the disengagement and reattachment of actin-myosin cross bridges, so that once the cross bridges are established at the beginning of contraction, less ATP must be expended for making new cross bridges.

Another adverse effect of increased body temperature as far as the prolongation of exercise is concerned is that blood must be diverted from working muscles to the skin for purposes of cooling the body. Accordingly, after a muscle reaches about 38° or 39°C., additional heat is detrimental because it leads not only to greater demand for ATP in the myosin ATPase reaction but also to a greater shift of blood away from the working muscles to the skin (24). As the blood is diverted to skin, the working muscles are deprived of some of the oxygen needed for aerobic energy metabolism, and more lactic acid is produced as anaerobic glycolysis contributes increasingly to ATP replenishment. This lactic acid, in turn, may further accelerate the development of fatigue.

Pain and Motivation

Finally, sustained work can produce discomfort and sometimes pain that causes the exerciser to cease working before there is any evidence that the muscles themselves could no longer be stimulated to contract. The pain limitation to endurance is especially apparent in maintained static contractions. For example, when one attempts to hang from a horizontal bar for as long as possible, excruciating pain of the forearms and hands forces one to give up before there is any sign of muscle fatigue (8). It is as though the motor nerves to the active muscles are receiving intensive volleys of inhibiting stimuli from the pain-sensitive areas of the brain, so that no matter how greatly the subject wants to keep on hanging, he must ultimately drop from the bar. The exact cause of this type of pain is unknown.

There are, of course, great differences in the motivation levels of individuals, so that perseverance in an activity such as a "bar-hang" also varies greatly. Although there is no totally accurate method to test one's motivation to persevere in endurance exercise, physiologists sometimes check blood lactic acid levels after exertion to determine whether the subject persevered long enough to significantly elevate his lactic acid levels.

In summary, muscular fatigue may have many causes depending upon the type of physical activity in question and upon individual factors such as motivation. Because it seems logical to expect that a specific malfunction in the contractile process or in nerve transmission should be a common cause of fatigue in all types of exercise, many have attempted to pinpoint a unique cause of fatigue that is applicable to all forms of physical activity. As we have seen, such attempts have not met with great success. Therefore, until some research breakthrough is made, we are forced to the intellectually unsatisfying conclusion that muscular fatigue is a phenomenon that may be caused by several different factors, and that some of these factors may bring about fatigue only when they act in concert with each other.

MUSCLE SORENESS CAUSED BY EXERCISE

There are two factors that probably keep more people from exercising regularly than any others—the soreness that follows exercise, especially in the unfit, and the usual requirement to change into and out of athletic apparel and to bathe after exercise. Although it seems unlikely in a culture that exphasizes bodily cleanliness that the requirement to bathe after vigorous physical activity will ever be changed, it is certainly possible with the present state of knowledge to minimize muscle soreness. In addition, if research can pinpoint the exact cause of soreness, it is conceivable that soreness of many types could be eliminated.

Although certain kinds of strenuous efforts are associated with muscle pain during the exercise period, muscle soreness usually develops some hours or even days after exertion. The soreness that begins as fatigue approaches during heavy contractions, especially those that have a large static component, is thought to be caused by an inadequate blood flow to the working muscles that deprives the muscles of oxygen and fails to wash "pain substances" out of the muscles. There are several products of contraction that could build up in the muscles or tissue fluid surrounding the muscles and cause pain by stimulating nerve endings in the muscle or connective tissue within the muscle. Lactic acid and potassium, for example, can cause local pain when they are injected into a muscle. A lack of oxygen by itself does not cause muscular pain, but hypoxia does have an indirect effect by increasing the diffusion of substances out of capillaries into tissue fluid so that fluid accumulates in these tissues' spaces, leading to swelling and consequent stimulation of pain in nerve endings in the area of the swelling.

There are three common hypotheses given to explain the soreness that occurs usually a day or two after strenuous exercise—the lactic acid accumulation hypothesis, the muscle spasm hypothesis and the muscle tear hypothesis. Those who believe that the accumulation of lactic acid is responsible for muscle pain may be correct for the type of pain that occurs *during* exercise, but they are not able to satisfactorily explain how lactic acid produced during exercise causes pain 24–48 hours later, when there is no significant accumulation of lactic acid in the muscles longer than 15–30 minutes after exercise (12). In fact, since subjects who cannot produce lactic acid (because of an enzyme deficiency) have great pain upon muscular exertion, it even seems unlikely that lactic acid causes the immediate pain during severe exercise.

Those who believe in the muscle spasm hypothesis say: a) that strenuous contractions cause a reduction in blood flow (ischemia) to the working muscles, b) that this ischemia in turn triggers the release of pain substances out of the muscle fibers into the tissue fluid where the pain substances stimulate nerve endings, and c) that the pain receptors cause reflex spastic contractions of the painful muscle fibers to produce further ischemia and continued release of pain substances to renew the pain cycle (6). This hypothesis is supported by electromyographic evidence that under some circumstances fatigued muscles may indeed fail to relax completely after exercise, and that stretching of the muscles reduces the contractile activity and the associated pain. However, it seems very unlikely that postexercise spasms occur after all types of exercise that can result in pain. For example, in untrained persons even the mere act of stretching in limbering-up exercises can result in pain the next day. Therefore, the spasm-pain substance hypothesis is not a completely satisfactory explanation of all muscle pain caused by exercise.

Another hypothesis that seems somewhat more attractive is that pain nerve endings are stimulated by the swelling (edema) of muscle tissue after microscopic tears of a relatively few muscle fibers or their connective tissue attachments. Although techniques of ordinary light microscopy do not usually reveal any tissue damage after exercise, polarized light microscopy has revealed structural deformations, especially in untrained animals, that could conceivably lead to muscle pain (26). The fact that pain is usually proportional to the relative severity of the load for any given person also supports the muscle damage hypothesis, although it is perhaps equally supportive of the other two hypotheses.

But the fact that muscle soreness has been reported to be greater after eccentric contractions than after concentric contractions with the same load seems to support the muscle tear hypothesis (1). Although the total energy expenditure for the eccentric contractions is lower, there are fewer muscle fibers active in supporting the same load eccentrically so that each of those fibers contracts more strenuously and is more apt to tear or pull away from its connective tissue attachments. Because submaximal eccentric contractions are associated with less ischemia and less lactic acid accumulation than concentric contractions with the same load, these experiments seem to be sound support for the tissue damage hypothesis.

Minimizing Muscle Soreness

Whatever the exact mechanism underlying muscle soreness may be, there are enough facts about the genesis of soreness that are known to enable us to minimize its development. It is known that soreness is more apt to occur with relatively intense, phasic or jerking movements and that soreness is more common in those who are undertaking an exercise program after a long period of inactive living. Therefore, a rational approach to the initiation of a fitness program is: Begin with *extremely* light activity that does not require any lunging or thrusting movements, conduct the exercise periods for only 15–20 minutes during the first few sessions, and progressively and slowly increase both the intensity and duration of the exercise sessions. This will allow the muscle fibers and the connective tissue in the muscle to have a chance to become toughened as an adaptive response to the training. Older trainees, especially, should be made aware of those activities that increase the risk of becoming sore. Vigorous attempts to bob down and touch the toes, all-out efforts to perform as many situps as possible, and repetitions of deep knee bends with a barbell on the shoulders are all the kinds of activities that new trainees should avoid in the early course of a fitness program. Slow, easy movements should be the rule at this stage of fitness improvement.

MUSCLE CRAMPS AND PAIN IN THE SIDE

There are many different origins of muscle cramps. These origins range from a central nervous system imbalance to a hypersensitive muscle membrane. Most cramps associated with extreme athletic exertion are probably caused by salt imbalances in the fluids surrounding the muscle fibers. A disruption in the normal relationships between sodium, potassium and chloride concentrations inside and outside the muscle fiber can cause spastic contractions, as can a failure in the ability of the muscle to withdraw calcium from the myofibrils back into the sarcoplasmic reticulum so that the muscle can relax. Unfortunately, by the time one can begin to measure all these factors in the tissues, a cramp has usually passed away.

The same problem besets any research into the mechanism underlying the pain or stitch in the side that often is experienced during distance running. Because it is difficult to produce pain in the side with any reliability, it is almost impossible to measure any of the possible disruptions in function that may cause this pain. There seems to be no good reason to believe one of the commonly offered explanations of pain in the side over any of the others. Explanations that have been presented, often by word of mouth, from one generation of athletes to the next include: spasm of the diaphragm, spasm of the intercostal muscles of the ribcage, ischemic pain of abdominal organs because of reduced blood flow, swelling of the liver, stomach spasm, swelling of the spleen and jouncing of abdominal organs during activity. Jouncing supposedly causes tension on nerves in the connective tissue that maintains the position of the abdominal organs in the abdominal cavity. Because there is so little objective evidence to support any of these proposed causes of pain in the side, one should pick one cause that is most attractive to him or contribute another. In the author's view, the "jouncing" explanation has some merit solely because pain in the side seems to be more common in distance running and even in motorcross competition than in other activities that are of a less "jouncing" nature. Also, this pain is felt more often when exercising soon after eating with extra weight in the stomach and intestines to intensify the "jouncing" phenomenon. However, there is no experimental evidence to support this opinion.

Review Questions

1. Outline the possible sites of fatigue and describe the evidence that supports each of these possibilities.
2. Defend the statement that lactic acid accumulation is not the sole cause of fatigue in all types of exercise.
3. State your opinion about the cause of exercise-induced muscle soreness and support your opinion with evidence from the text, from your personal experiences and from other sources available to you.

4. Poll the member of your class to determine by recall, a) the nature of pain in the side they have experienced, b) whether there was "jouncing" associated with the pain or not, c) whether they probably had food in their stomachs during the activity, and d) whether they have discovered any way to relieve the pain. See if this information can lead the class to an alternate hypothesis about the cause of pain in the side.
5. Outline the possible mechanisms of fatigue described in this chapter.

References

1. Asmussen, E. Observations on experimental muscular soreness. *Acta Rheumatologica Scandinavica*, 1956, **2:** 109–116.
2. Astrand, P.-O., and K. Rodahl. *Textbook of Work Physiology.* New York: McGraw-Hill, 1970
3. Barclay, J. K. and W. N. Stainsby. The role of blood flow in limiting maximal metabolic rate in muscle. *Medicine and Science in Sports*, 1975, **7:**116–119.
4. Bergstrom, J., R. C. Harris, E. Hultman, and L.-O. Nordesjö. Energy-rich phosphagens in dynamic and static work. In B. Pernow and B. Saltin (Eds.), *Muscle Metabolism During Exercise.* New York: Plenum Press, 1971, pp. 341–355.
5. Ceretelli, P., and G. Ambrosoli. Limiting factors of anaerobic performance in man. In J. Keul (Ed.), *Limiting Factors of Physical Performance.* Stuttgart: Georg Thieme, Publishers, 1973, pp. 157–165.
6. deVries, H. A. *Physiology of Exercise for Physical Education and Athletics*, 2nd Ed. Dubuque, Iowa: W. C. Brown, 1974.
7. di Prampero, P. E. The alactic oxygen debt: Its power, capacity, and efficiency. In B. Pernow and B. Saltin (Eds.), *Muscle Metabolism During Exercise.* New York: Plenum Press, 1971, pp. 371–382.
8. Elkus, R., and J. V. Basmajian. Endurance in hanging by the hands. *American Journal of Physical Medicine*, 1973, **52:**124–127.
9. Funderburk, C. F., S. G. Hipskind, R. C. Welton, and A. R. Lind. Development of, and recovery from, fatigue induced by static effort at various tensions. *Journal of Applied Physiology*, 1974, **37:**392–396.
10. Gollnick, P. D., and L. Hermansen. Biochemical adaptations

to exercise: anaerobic metabolism. *Exercise and Sport Sciences Reviews*, 1973, **1**:1–43.

11. Haralambie, G. Importance of humoral changes to physical performance. In J. Keul (Ed.), *Limiting Factors of Physical Performance*. Stuttgart: Georg Thieme, Publishers, 1973, pp. 189–200.

12. Hermansen, L., Anaerobic energy release. *Medicine and Science in Sports*, 1969, **1**:32–38.

13. Hudlicka, O. Differences in development of fatigue in slow and fast muscles. In J. Keul (Ed.), *Limiting Factors of Physical Performance*. Stuttgart: Georg Thieme, Publishers, 1973, pp. 36–41.

14. Hultman, E., and J. Bergstrom. Local energy–supplying substrates as limiting factors in different types of leg muscle work in normal man. In J. Keul (Ed.), *Limiting Factors of Physical Performance*. Stuttgart: Georg Thieme, Publishers, 1973, pp. 113–125.

15. Hultman, E., and L. Nilsson. Liver glycogen as a glucose–supplying source during exercise. In J. Keul (Ed.), *Limiting Factors in Physical Performance*. Stuttgart: Georg Thieme, Publishers, 1973, pp. 179–189.

16. Ikai, M., and K. Yabe. Training effect of muscular endurance by means of voluntary and electrical stimulation. *European Journal of Applied Physiology*, 1969, **28**:55–60.

17. Kaijser, L. Oxygen supply as a limiting factor in physical performance. In J. Keul (Ed.), *Limiting Factors of Physical Performance*. Stuttgart: Georg Thieme, Publishers, 1973, pp. 145–156.

18. Karlsson, J. Muscle ATP, CP, and lactate in submaximal and maximal exercise. In B. Pernow and B. Saltin (Eds.), *Muscle Metabolism During Exercise*. New York: Plenum Press, 1971, pp. 383–395.

19. Karlsson, J., L.-O. Nordesjö, L. Jorfeldt, and B. Saltin. Muscle lactate, ATP, and CP levels during exercise after physical training in man. *Journal of Applied Physiology*, 1972, **33**:199–203.

20. Kurihara, T., and J. E. Brooks. The mechanism of neuromuscular fatigue. *Archives of Neurology*, 1975, **32**:168–174.

21. Ruegg, J. C. Mechanochemical energy coupling. In J. Keul (Eds.), *Limiting Factors of Physical Performance*. Stuttgart: Georg Thieme, Publishers, 1973, pp. 63–66.

22. Saltin, B., and J. Karlsson. Muscle glycogen utilization during work of different intensities. In B. Pernow and B. Saltin (Eds.), *Muscle Metabolism During Exercise*. New York: Plenum Press, 1971, pp. 289–299.

23. Schottelius, B. A., and D. D. Schottelius, *Textbook of Physiology*, 17th ed. St. Louis: C. V. Mosby, 1973, p. 99.

24. Simonsen, E. (Ed.), *Physiology of Work Capacity and Fatigue.* Springfield, Ill.: Charles C Thomas, Publisher, 1971.

25. Stephens, J. A., and A. Taylor. Fatigue of maintained voluntary muscle contraction in man. *Journal of Physiology (London)*, 1973, **220:**1–18.

26. Vail, S. S. Changes in the muscles of the limbs in overstraining, in trained and untrained animals. *Arkhiv Patologii*, 1967, **29:**45–49 (Russian).

12

The physiology of aerobic endurance

Endurance or staying power in some physical activities such as basketball, soccer, distance running, swimming, and cycling is limited not so much by muscle strength or the local endurance of a few muscle groups but, rather, by the capacity of the circulatory system (heart, blood vessels, and blood) and the respiratory system (lungs) to deliver oxygen to the working muscles and to carry chemical waste products away from them. Such activities are often classified as "cardiovascular," "cardiorespiratory," "generalized" endurance, or, as in this text, aerobic endurance activities.

The degree to which circulation and respiration limit one's performance depends on many factors, chief of which are the intensity of the exercise, the duration of the activity, and the amount of static muscle contraction involved. In general, the lesser the intensity, the longer the duration, and the lesser the amount of static contraction involved, the more that performance in the activity will be limited by the functioning of the heart, blood vessels, blood and lungs. Dis-

Table 12.1.   Aerobic and Anaerobic Energy Production in Various Activities*

Activity	% Anaerobic Energy	% Aerobic Energy	Activity Classification
25 m. Swim 50 m. Sprint	95	5	Speed, Strength
50 m. Swim 100 m. Sprint	85	15	Speed, Strength
100 m. Swim 200 m. Sprint	80	20	Speed, Strength, Anaerobic Endurance
200 m. Swim 400 m. Sprint	70	30	Anaerobic Endurance, Speed, Strength
400 m. Swim 800 m. Run	60	40	Anaerobic Endurance, Aerobic Endurance, Speed
800 m. Swim 1500 m. Run	40	60	Aerobic Endurance, Anaerobic Endurance
1600 m. Swim 3000 m. Run Basketball (Fast Break Style) Soccer Fullback	15	85	Aerobic Endurance, Anaerobic Endurance
Marathon (26 mi.)	<1	>99	Aerobic Endurance

* Exact percentages depend on the state of training of the individual, and upon natural endowment in such factors as muscle fiber types, speed, muscle size, and body weight.

tance running, for example, is a relatively low-intensity, long-duration activity consisting mostly of rhythmic, nonstatic, muscle contractions and is limited mainly by aerobic capacity. Weightlifting performance, on the other hand, is limited mostly by the strength and endurance of a few muscles that are contracting statically to a large extent. These static contractions tend to close off blood vessels and restrict blood flow to the working muscles, so that the muscles must work in the presence of very little oxygen. Therefore, weightlifting would be categorized as an activity requiring relatively little aerobic endurance.

Some events, such as running from 400 to 800 meters or swimming for 200 meters, fall in between weightlifting and distance running since middle distance running and swimming events are not limited so much by endurance of a few muscle groups or by oxygen transport to working muscles, but by a combination of oxygen transport capacity and capacity for anaerobic energy (ATP) production in *many* large muscle groups. Thus, all "endurance" activities have both aerobic and anaerobic components, the shorter events having a larger anaerobic component, and the longer events being more aerobic in nature. Table 12.1 shows one way of classifying some activities based on the degree to which the energy for these activities is derived from anaerobic sources, that is, glycogen within the working muscles, or from aerobic sources requiring the transport of oxygen to the muscles. Note that the classification of staying power for an activity as "anaerobic" or "aerobic" is somewhat arbitrary and depends only on the extent to which muscular endurance is limited by anaerobic or aerobic energy production.

CARDIAC FUNCTION

It is known that a period of aerobic endurance training is followed by an increased ability to tolerate long distance running or swimming, that is, the trained person can run or swim farther and faster. Many physiologists believe that this increased endurance can be explained almost entirely by the improved functioning of the trained heart, and that other functional changes in the circulatory, respiratory and muscular systems are of little significance. Because the heart is the pump responsible for maintaining circulation, and therefore all organic function, it is certainly understandable that many have used cardiac function as the single criterion for determining endurance capacity and training effectiveness. However, as described later in this and subsequent chapters, factors other than heart function are also important in circulorespiratory endurance performance and must not be overlooked.

Cardiac Output at Rest and During Exercise

At rest the heart pumps about five or six liters of blood into the arteries of a healthy college-age male each minute. This rate of pumping is known as the *cardiac output*. It may be increased about four times to approximately 22 liters per minute in normal young men, or as much as six times to 30 liters per minute or more in highly trained athletes during maximal endurance work (19). A resting cardiac output of five liters per minute may be achieved if the heart rate is 65 beats per minute and if the stroke value (amount pumped per beat) is 77 milliliters ($65 \times 77 = 5005$ milliliters $= 5.005$ liters). During vigorous exercise, the cardiac output may be increased to 30 liters per minute by a tripling of heart rate to 195 beats per minute and a doubling of stroke volume to 154 milliliters ($195 \times 154 = 30.030$ liters). Therefore, the increased cardiac output that accompanies exercise is due to increases in both heart rate and stroke volume (19, 20).

If one were to measure his heart rate at rest, just prior to, during, and for several minutes after a vigorous bout of running or swimming, he would discover an anticipatory rise in heart rate just prior to exercise, a gradual leveling off during exercise (if the work is not maximal) and a slow decline back toward resting values following exercise (Fig. 12.1).

Anticipatory Rise in Heart Rate. The pre-event anticipatory rise in heart rate is thought to be due to a stimulation of the cardiac accelerator nerve centers in the medulla at the base of the brain by nerve stimuli coming from the limbic systems of the brain (hypothalamus, limbic lobe of the cortex) where the pre-event anticipation has generated the initial nerve impulses. This anticipatory rise in heart rate may also be caused in part by increased circulating adrenaline and nor-adrenaline from the adrenal glands and sympathetic nerves that have been stimulated by the limbic system. As one would expect, the anticipatory rise in heart rate is much greater during a highly competitive situation than during, for example, a noncompetitive practice session.

Exercise Heart Rate. Even in the absence of an anticipatory rise in heart rate, experts have detected that the heart beats faster almost instantaneously when exercise starts (17). The first beat of the heart after exercise begins is faster than the preceding ones. The speed with

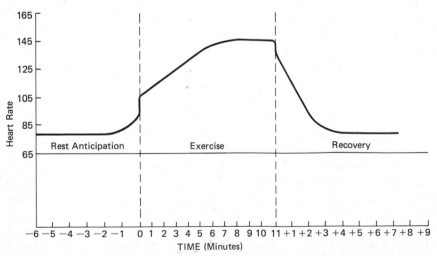

Figure 12.1. Heart rate response before, during, and after moderate exercise.

which this response occurs makes it apparent that it is caused by a nerve reflex, probably at least partly originating from receptors in the working muscles and/or joints (17). Both muscle spindles and receptors in joint capsules have been suggested as the receptors responsible for this instantaneous cardioacceleration as exercise begins. Thus, as muscles begin to contract and joints begin moving through a range of motion, impulses are generated in the spindles and joints receptors; these impulses then pass to the spinal cord and to the cardiac regulating center of the brain. There the vagus nerves are inhibited so that a rise in heart rate occurs. (The vagus nerves slow the heart when they fire.)

Other factors contribute to the tachycardia (high heart rate) associated with exercise. First, as the motor areas of the cortex of the brain become activated during voluntary movement, those areas send impulses not only to the working muscles but, also, to the cardiac regulatory centers of the medulla of the brain to excite the cardiac accelerator nerves and inhibit the vagus nerves. This effect is similar to that occurring when the limbic system is activated during the anticipatory rise in heart rate prior to exercise. Second, the heart is stimulated by adrenaline and nor-adrenaline. Third, as blood vessels serving nonworking muscles, kidneys, liver and other organs constrict, and as the working muscles "massage" the veins that run through them, more blood is returned to the right atrium than at rest. This increased filling of the right atrium causes the heart to beat faster to pump out the incoming blood. This effect, called the Bainbridge Reflex, operates through pressure-sensitive receptors in the walls of the right atrium and the great veins which enter it. These pressure receptors are activated as pressure increases. They send nerve impulses through sensory fibers of the vagus nerves to the medulla of the brain, where these impulses cause a slower rate of firing of the motor fibers of the vagus nerves that supply the heart. This inhibition of the vagus causes cardiac acceleration by reducing the slowing effect of the vagus nerves.

Fourth, during strenuous exercise the muscles produce lactic acid and lose potassium, both of which rapidly diffuse into the blood. As arterial blood pH is reduced from a normal 7.4 to about 7.0 because of the increased acid supplied by vigorously contracting muscles, this increased acid stimulates specialized nerve cells (chemoreceptors) located in the walls of the aorta and of the carotid arteries. These stimulated chemoreceptors then transmit nerve impulses to the medulla. At the medulla vagal output to the heart is inhibited and sympathetic output increased so that the heart speeds up. The potassium that leaks out of contracting muscles may also cause a reflex rise in the heart rate (9).

Finally, there seem to be factors in the heart itself that increase its rate during exercise. Such factors are called *intrinsic* mechanisms and are suggested by the fact that even when the nerves to the heart are blocked chemically or surgically, the heart still beats faster in response to exercise. Persons who have had their cardiac nerves blocked are not capable of working quite as hard as normal persons, but their heart rates can rise to 120 or so during treadmill running. One of the intrinsic factors is the increased rate of firing of the sinoatrial node in response to its being stretched as more blood returns to the right side of the heart during rhythmic exercise. Another intrinsic factor is the effect of temperature on the speed with which action potentials can be initiated in the heart. As the temperature of the heart rises during vigorous exercise, the heat causes a faster rate of development of the electrochemical impulses which stimulate the heart to beat. This effect can be observed also in the absence of exercise by drinking a hot drink and recording the gradual rise in one's heart rate as the heat passes through the body fluids from the warmed esophagus to the nearby heart.

Heart Rate After Exercise.   The heart slows rapidly when exercise stops. With a fall in accelerating influences from the limbic system and motor cortex, from muscle spindles and joint receptors, and from the Bainbridge reflex, it is easy to understand why the heart rate declines, but it is not so easy to understand why it doesn't return to normal even faster than it does. The accelerator effect of increased levels of hormones, such as adrenaline and nor-adrenaline, and of increased temperature of the heart may continue to operate until the body cools and the hormones are metabolized. Other unknown intrinsic mechanisms may also be operating. It also seems likely that some chemicals, such as lactic acid, potassium and carbon dioxide, which are produced by the working muscles, affect the cardioregulator centers of the medulla to maintain a high heart rate until the levels of these chemicals in the body fluids return to resting values. A summary of the probable factors involved in heart rate changes before, during, and after exercise is shown in Table 12.2.

Stroke Volume.   The amount of blood pumped into the aorta with each beat of the heart is known as the stroke volume, and the stroke volume increases up to twice that at rest when one exercises strenuously in an upright posture, for example, when running or cycling (10). This increased stroke volume is probably a result of increased stimulation of the heart muscle by adrenaline and nor-adrenaline from the sympathetic nervous system and the adrenal glands. These two hormones cause the heart to not only beat faster but to contract more forcefully and completely, thus ejecting more blood with each contraction. Also, the effect of increased amounts of blood returning

Table 12.2. Summary of Probable Factors Involved in Heart Rate Changes Before, During, and After Exercise

Factor	Heart Rate Changes		
	Anticipatory Rise	Exercise Rise	Postexercise Fall
Neural Activity Originating in the Brain			
1. Activity of the limbic system	Increase	Increase	Decrease
2. Activity of motor cortex		Increase	Decrease
Peripheral Nerve Reflexes			
1. Muscle/joint mechanoreceptor reflexes		Increase	Decrease
2. Muscle potassium receptor reflexes		Increase	Decrease
3. Bainbridge reflex		Increase	Decrease
4. Carotid/aortic chemoreceptor reflexes		Increase	Decrease
Circulating Hormones			
Adrenaline, noradrenaline	Increase	Increase	Decrease
Intrinsic Factors			
1. Stretch of sinoatrial node		Increase	Decrease
2. Temperature effect		Increase	Decrease

to the heart as a result of muscle action on veins may cause the fibers of the heart to be stretched. This results in a more forceful contraction of those fibers because of a more effective overlap of actin and myosin filaments. The effect (the Frank–Starling phenomenon) operates when nervous activity to the heart is blocked, but it is unclear whether the effect operates during normal exercise (18).

The increased stroke volume that occurs during exercise in an upright posture is not always seen when a person performs exercise while in a prone or supine position (20). For example, a swimmer would experience an increased cardiac output, but mostly because of a greater heart rate; stroke volume changes very little when going from resting prone or resting supine condition to exercising prone or exercising supine position. The explanation for this is that in a horizontal posture, the stroke volume is near maximal even at rest. The effect of upright exercise is simply to bring the stroke volume up to the value it would have achieved had the person been at rest in a prone or supine position.

Possible Heart Damage Because of Sudden Heavy Exercise —Value of Warm-up

The value of warm-up prior to strenuous physical activity has usually been attributed to the prevention of muscular or connective tissue injuries, or to a better circulation of oxygen and nutrients to the working muscles. However, a much more important value of warm-up may be the prevention of heart damage during the first few seconds of strenuous exercise. This has been suggested by the authors of a study which showed that most of the men who ran 9 mph up a steep grade on a treadmill, without a warm-up, exhibited electrocardiographic signs of decreased blood flow to the heart muscle and decreased blood pressure during diastole (relaxation phase) of the heart, the period when the heart receives the bulk of its blood supply (5). These signs that the hearts of the subjects were not obtaining a large enough blood supply were nearly all abolished when the strenuous run was preceded by a two–minute warm-up run on the treadmill. The warm-up precaution is advisable for everyone who engages in strenuous exercise and specially for older subjects who have a greater risk of heart damage.

CHANGES IN CIRCULATION DURING EXERCISE

During running, swimming, and other aerobic endurance activities, the working muscles may use oxygen at a rate ten to twenty times greater than when at rest. In order to supply the extra oxygen required, not only must cardiac output increase, but the circulation of blood through the working muscle must be dramatically increased. This increased cardiac output is delivered to working muscles by two changes in the vascular system—1) dilatation of blood vessels in the working muscles and 2) constriction of blood vessels in many tissues other than the working muscles.

Blood Flow in Working Muscles

In resting leg muscles, blood flows at a rate of about 5 milliliters of blood per 100 grams of muscle per minute. Thus, in a gastrocnemius muscle weighing 500 grams (a little over a pound) blood flows through at 25 milliliters (about 5 teaspoons) per minute. During heavy rhythmical exercise such as running, the blood flow in this muscle may increase by 15 times, up to 375 milliliters per minute (1). This enhancement of circulation is shown in Fig. 12.2, which also

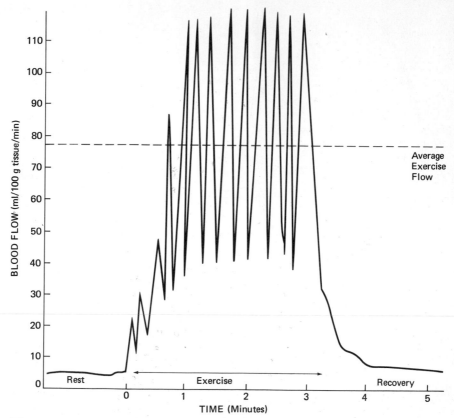

Figure 12.2. **Blood flow in working muscles.**

shows that blood flow falls sharply as the muscles contract and rises when they relax. This pattern of flow is caused by the rhythmical muscle contraction and relaxation, which alternately compresses the blood vessels to reduce blood flow and the allows dilatation of those vessels to increase flow.

The elevated blood flow in working muscle is caused by 1) the increased blood pressure that results from greater cardiac output, 2) the massaging action of the muscles on the veins, which helps pump blood through the muscles, and 3) a relaxation of the smooth muscle cells in the walls of arterioles and in the sphincters or valves that regulate the flow of blood to the capillaries as shown in Fig. 12.3. The greater blood pressure tends to drive more blood through the arterioles and capillaries of the muscle, and the massaging action of the muscle helps move blood out of the muscle and back to the heart muscle. But the chief factor that enhances blood flow to working muscles is the vessel dilatation caused by hypoxia and chemicals,

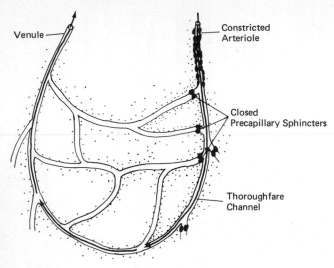

(a) Capillary network in rested muscle

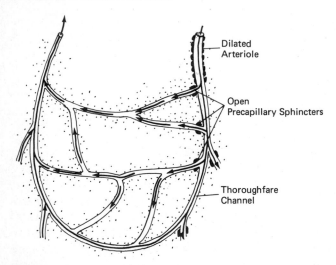

(b) Capillary network in exercising muscle

Figure 12.3. Local blood flow through skeletal muscle.

such as, potassium, lactic acid, and phosphate, that are produced by the contracting muscles (8). As muscles contract, they use up oxygen and release potassium, phosphate and other substances. This decreased oxygen, increased potassium, lactic acid, and phosphate and the leakage of other chemicals from muscle fibers into the tissue fluid (increased osmolarity of the tissue fluid)—all cause the smooth muscles of the arterioles and of the precapillary sphincters to relax

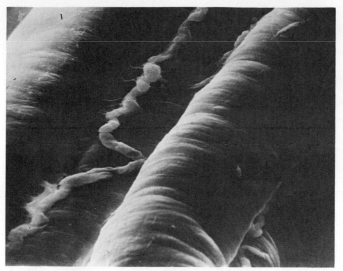

Figure 12.4. Stereo electron micrograph showing surfaces of three muscle fibers. A twisted white capillary is shown on surface of central muscle fiber. (Courtesy of R. E. Carrow, W. W. Heusner and W. D. Van Huss, Michigan State University, E. Lansing, Michigan.)

and thus widen the arterioles and open the capillaries so that more blood can flow closer to the active muscle fibers.

Another factor that accounts for some of the increased blood flow through active muscles is a relaxation of the normal intrinsic contractility of smooth muscle in arterial walls (8, 15). As skeletal muscles contract, they exert pressure on the outside of arteries, so that there is less need for arterial smooth muscles to contract to maintain the normal diameter of the arteries. Accordingly, during muscle contractions, the arterial smooth muscle relaxes so that vasodilatation occurs during subsequent relaxation of skeletal muscle fibers. This mechanism may be more important in prolonged exercise than in brief exercise (8).

Blood flow gradually returns to normal during recovery from exercise (Fig. 12.2) as the circulation carries away vasodilator substances and brings oxygen to the muscles. One reason for "tapering off," that is, slow jogging or swimming after an exercise bout, is to allow the circulation to remove substances such as lactic acid that may later contribute to muscle stiffness or soreness. A more important reason is to prevent the accumulation of blood in the legs that might cause inadequate venous return and inadequate cardiac output.

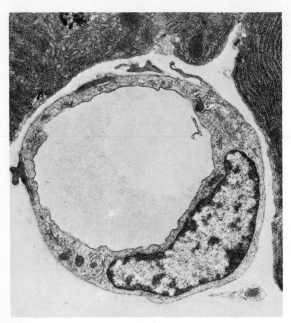

Figure 12.5. Electron micrograph of cross section of a capillary showing one large cell nucleus (magnification × 4,000). (Courtesy of G. Colin Budd, Physiology Department, Medical College of Ohio, Toledo, Ohio.)

It should be noted that the patterns of blood flow described in this chapter refer only to rhythmic work of an endurance nature. With static contractions blood flow is increased with light loads, but is increasingly occluded by the compression of the vessels caused by more severe muscle contraction. Thus, flow may be completely shut off above 60–70 per cent of one's maximal voluntary contraction strength (1).

Blood Flow in Nonworking Muscles

If all vessels of the circulatory system were dilated at the same time, there would be an insufficient amount of blood to fill them, venous return to the right side of the heart would fall, cardiac output would fall, and the organism would be in a state of circulatory shock and in danger of death. Thus, although there are about 6 quarts of blood in an adult, his potential circulatory capacity may be 15–20 quarts. Therefore, if blood vessels in working muscles are dilated, blood vessels elsewhere, that is, in resting muscles, visceral organs and skin, must constrict if cardiac output is to be maintained, to say nothing of increased. Resting muscles deliver a portion of their normal blood volume to the working muscles, principally because of an increase sympathetic nervous system outflow to vessels of the resting muscles. These impulses from the sympathetic nerves result in a contraction of smooth muscle in the walls of the blood vessels so that the flow of blood to the resting muscles is reduced.

It is thought that the sympathetic nervous system also sends constricting impulses to the blood vessels of working muscles but that the localized dilating effect of hypoxia, potassium, lactic acid, phosphate and other substances on the smooth muscle of the blood vessels is so great that the nervous stimuli have a negligible effect (6).

Blood Flow in the Viscera

Blood volume is also shifted to working muscles from liver, spleen, stomach, intestines and kidneys. Blood flow to these organs can be reduced by up to 80 per cent during severe exercise, probably as a result of the action of the sympathetic nervous system on the blood vessels serving these organs (20). One might wonder how an organ such as the liver can survive several hours of exercise with only 20 per cent of its normal blood flow. The answer is that although the liver and gut ordinarily receive about one fourth of the total cardiac output of 5 liters per minute, they remove only about 10 to 25 per cent of the available oxygen from the blood. Thus, these organs seem to be able to afford a drastic shutdown of their blood supply without any significant harmful effects; they simply extract a greater percentage of the smaller amount of available oxygen.

It should be pointed out that the degree of vessel contriction to these internal organs depends to a great extent on the relative severity of the exercise for a given individual (20). For example, an athlete capable of running a marathon race (26.2 miles) in three hours might experience an 80 per cent reduction in blood flow to his internal organs if he completed the marathon in three hours, but only a 30 per cent decrease in circulation if he ran the same distance in five hours. In other words, it is not necessarily true that all distance runners, or other endurance athletes, have a marked fall in blood flow to their internal organs when they compete. The extent of the circulation to the internal organs depends on the athlete's capacity and on how strenuously he competes.

It is not known how the body can precisely regulate blood flow to nonworking tissues depending on the relative severity of the workload for a given person. It seems that there must be a nerve reflex pathway originating in the working muscles, so that some receptor in these muscles is stimulated by a chemical such as lactic acid that is produced in greater quantities as the work becomes more strenuous (20). Unfortunately, such receptors have not been found.

Skin Blood Flow

After an initial small decline in skin blood flow as submaximal exercise begins, an endurance athlete ordinarily shifts some of his blood volume to his skin in order to carry away excess body heat; the extent of this shift may involve a skin blood flow during exercise of 4–7 times that at rest (1) (Fig. 12.6). However, with exhaustive, prolonged exercise, the working muscles apparently have first call on the blood, and some of the increased skin blood flow may be shifted back to the muscle (20). This phenomenon would occur in an athlete whose skin becomes more pale as he approaches an exhausted state. With heavy work lasting only a few minutes, skin vessels are constricted so that little or no increased flow to the skin occurs (20).

The shift of blood flow to the skin to remove heat is accomplished by the action of the hypothalamus, which is stimulated by the increasing temperature of the blood circulating through the hypothalamus during exercise, and by increasing skin temperature if work is performed in a hot environment. The hypothalamus, in turn, stimulates the nerves to the blood vessels of the skin by way of the medulla of the brain. These nerves cause relaxation of the smooth muscle around the vessels, and a resultant dilatation of those vessels

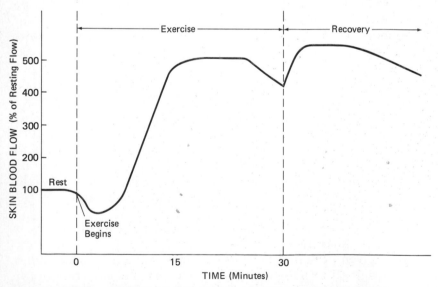

Figure 12.6. Skin blood flow during prolonged exhaustive work.

so that more blood can flow to the skin. At the beginning of exercise and at exhaustion, some unknown reflexes cause vasoconstriction of skin vessels.

Coronary Blood Flow

As the heart muscle works increasingly harder during exercise, its demand for more oxygen is met by an increase of blood flow through the coronary arteries up to five times the resting value (1). This increased flow is especially important for the heart because the heart normally removes 70–80 per cent of the oxygen from the blood of the coronary arteries. The coronary blood supply is enhanced by the action of adrenaline and nor-adrenaline, which are associated with a dilatation of the coronary arteries. Even more important are the dilating effects of a reduced amount of oxygen in the heart and the greater aortic blood pressure that forces more blood into the coronary arteries. (The coronaries originate in the aorta as it leaves the left ventricle.) This increased coronary flow occurs mostly during diastole (relaxation) of the ventricles because ventricular contraction (systole) collapses coronary vessels. Because physical training causes the heart to beat less frequently during submaximal exercise, the heart is resting more, so that greater coronary flow can be achieved.

Blood Flow of Lungs and Brain

Blood flow to the lungs is increased as the output of the right ventricle increases, but there is little evidence of changes in the overall supply of blood to the brain during exercise, although there are probably changes in flow within discrete regions of the brain itself (1).

Table 12.3.   **Summary of Regional Blood Flow Changes During Relatively Intense, Prolonged, Rhythmic Exercise**

Blood Flow To:	Exercise Blood Flow		
	Increased	No Change	Decreased
Working Muscles	X		
Nonworking Muscles			X
Skin	X		
Coronary Circulation	X		
Kidneys			X
Liver			X
Gastrointestinal Tract			X
Lungs	X		
Brain		X	

Intuitively, it seems reasonable that the blood flow to the brain should remain quite stable during exercise, so that neither fainting from a reduced blood supply nor the throbbing sensation and possible bursting of small vessels from an increased supply would occur.

In summary, blood flow during rhythmical exercise is increased to organs that must function at a rate greater than that occurring during rest, that is, to working skeletal muscles, heart, skin and lungs, but is decreased or remains stable to other organs such as resting muscles, visceral organs and brain (Table 12.3). These shifts in blood flow are accomplished both by mechanisms involving the hypothalamic, temperature-regulating nerve centers and the medulla of the brain and by local changes in the environment of the blood vessels, especially in the working muscle.

BLOOD PRESSURE DURING EXERCISE

Ordinarily arterial blood pressure changes are caused by alterations in cardiac output, blood vessel size, and blood volume. Increased cardiac output increases the flow of blood into arteries; this causes greater pressure within the vessels. Constriction of arterioles causes greater resistance to blood flow, so that the heart must pump more forcefully to drive blood through the narrowed arteries; this raises pressure. Vasodilation reduces arterial pressure. Greater blood volume increases, and lesser volume decreases, arterial pressure if other factors do not compensate for the volume changes.

During dynamic endurance exercise, such as running or cycling, the dilatation of thousands of blood vessels in the working muscles reduces the arterial resistance to blood flow more than the vasoconstriction in nonworking tissues increases resistance. Therefore, the net effect of changes in blood vessel size during exercise is to decrease blood pressure. Simultaneously, however, cardiac output is increasing during exercise, and that increased cardiac output causes a greater systolic blood pressure that more than counteracts the tendency toward reduced pressure caused by vasodilatation in the working muscles. Since only a slight fall in blood volume sometimes accompanies exercise, the *overwhelming effect of exercise on blood pressure is to increase systolic pressure, primarily because of the increased cardiac output.*

The effect of dynamic exercise, such as exhaustive cycling or distance running, on systolic and diastolic arterial blood pressure is shown in Fig. 12.7. As is shown, there is usually only a slight rise or no change in diastolic pressure during dynamic exercise. Diastolic pressure actually falls during sudden, strenuous, treadmill running (5). In static exercise both systolic and diastolic pressure can rise sharply,

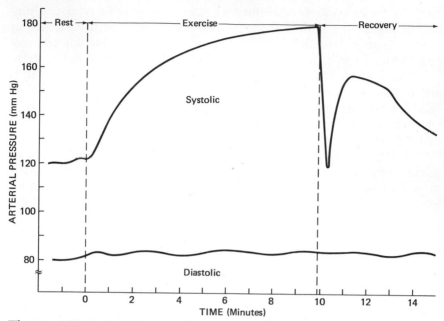

Figure 12.7. Systolic and diastolic blood pressure during dynamic exercise to exhaustion.

even when a finger or hand is contracting isometrically (3,4). The marked rise in blood pressure during static contractions seems designed to help drive more blood into the strongly contracting muscles, and is apparently caused by a nerve reflex arising in the working muscles (11). A greater than normal rise in blood pressure is also observed when one works dynamically with only small groups of muscles, for example, arms instead of legs, and especially, when one performs arm work with the arms above waist level (3). Such work is experienced by carpenters, painters and other tradesmen who must often work overhead. Because of the inordinately high blood pressures produced by static or overhead dynamic arm work, this type of work is contraindicated for those with cardiovascular disease (3).

Fig. 12.7 also shows a marked fall in systolic blood pressure immediately after completion of an exhaustive bout of dynamic exercise. Such a fall in pressure is not uncommon, especially if the exerciser is in an upright posture and stops all muscular activity immediately after completing the exercise. The fall in pressure can be explained by a pooling of blood in the still dilated blood vessels of the legs because of a cessation of the pumping action of the leg muscles on the veins of the legs. Since less blood returns to the heart, cardiac output may drop precipitously, and the exerciser may faint because of a lack of blood flow to the brain. This type of collapse can be observed after exhaustive work on a bicycle ergometer or after completion of a grueling endurance-type athletic event. The drastic fall in pressure can be avoided if the exerciser continues muscular activity at a reduced level for a few minutes after completion of the athletic event or work task, so that the vascular system has a chance to gradually adjust the flow of blood from working muscles and dilated skin vessels to the central circulation. If the exerciser is too exhausted to continue at a low level of work, he should be advised to lie down to avoid fainting.

The rise in blood pressure that accompanies exercise is related to the severity of the task so that heavier workloads are associated with higher blood pressures (4). Exercise blood pressure also tends to be higher in older subjects, who also usually have higher resting blood pressures (4).

BLOOD

The characteristics of the blood are very important for aerobic endurance exercise. Since hemoglobin in the red blood cells carries oxygen, it is obvious that the number of red blood cells and the amount of hemoglobin in those cells are important in determining how much oxygen can be transported to the working muscles. This fact has been amply demonstrated by the diminished endurance observed in subjects who have had some of their blood withdrawn (7). Blood is also vital for carrying away lactic acid, carbon dioxide, and other products of metabolism produced in the tissues during both rest and exercise.

The changes in the characteristics of the blood after a single bout of exercise or after physical training are not always easily predicted. There is a wide range of normal values for most of the constituents of blood at rest, and this range becomes even wider after exercise and training. The inconsistent effects of exercise and training on the makeup of the blood can be partly attributed to normal variation even at rest, partly to variations in exercise regimens and training programs, and partly to differences in methodology for blood analysis. At any rate, it is inaccurate to state that any tissue, and especially the blood, of all subjects responds in exactly the same manner to all types of exercise and training. When discussing "typical" responses of the blood to exercise, therefore, one must understand that there are many exceptions to those responses, usually only in terms of the magnitude of the response, but sometimes also in the direction of the response.

With the above qualifications in mind, let us examine Table 12.4, which describes some of the reported changes in the characteristics

Table 12.4.   Effects of Maximal Exercise and Physical Training on Characteristics of Blood in Young Adults*

Blood Characteristics	Untrained Male	Untrained Female	Trained Male	Trained Female
Total Blood Volume (liters)				
Rest	5.7	4.3	6.4	4.8
Maximal Exercise	5.5	4.2	6.1	4.7
Total Hemoglobin (grams/kilogram body weight)				
Rest	10.5	9.4	11.0	10.0
Maximal Exercise	No Change		No Change	
Red Blood Cell Count (millions of RBC/mm^3)				
Rest	5.4	4.6	No Change	
Maximal Exercise	5.7	4.8	No Change	
White Blood Cell Count (thousands of WBC/mm^3)				
Rest	7.0	7.0	No Change	
Maximal Exercise	15.0	15.0	No Change	
Total Red Blood Cells (trillions)				
Rest	30.8	19.8	34.6	22.1
Maximal Exercise	No Change		No Change	
Hemoglobin Concentration (grams/100 ml blood)				
Rest	16.0	14.0	No Change	
Maximal Exercise	17.6	15.4	No Change	
Hematocrit (%)				
Rest	47.0	42.0	No Change	
Maximal Exercise	50.0	45.0	No Change	
Arterial Oxygen Content (ml O_2/100 ml blood)				
Rest	19.5	16.8	No Change	
Maximal Exercise	No Change		No Change	
Arterial Oxygen Partial Pressure, $P_{a_{O_2}}$ (mm Hg)				
Rest	100	100	No Change	
Maximal Exercise	100	100	95–100	
Oxygen Content in Femoral Vein (ml O_2/100 ml blood)				
Rest	9.0	9.0	No Change	
Maximal Exercise	3.0	3.0	1.4	1.8
Oxygen Partial Pressure in Femoral Vein, $P_{v_{CO_2}}$ (mm Hg)				
Rest	30.0	30.0	No Change	
Maximal Exercise	13.0	14.0	10.0	11.0
Oxygen Content in Right Atrium (ml O_2/100 ml blood)				
Rest	13.0	11.0	No Change	
Maximal Exercise	5.5	5.7	4.0	4.0
Oxygen Partial Pressure in Right Atrium, $P_{\bar{v}_{O_2}}$ (mm Hg)				
Rest	40.0	40.0	No Change	
Maximal Exercise	18.0	19.0	15.0	16.0

(Continued)

Table 12.4. (continued)

Blood Characteristics	Untrained		Trained	
	Male	Female	Male	Female
Difference Between Arterial O_2 Content and Mixed Venous Blood (R. Atrium) O_2 Content, (A–$\overline{V}$ O_2 Difference), (ml O_2/100 ml blood)				
Rest	6.5	5.8	No Change	
Maximal Exercise	14.0	11.1	15.5	12.8
Arterial CO_2 Partial Pressure, $P_{a_{CO_2}}$, (mm Hg)				
Rest	40.0	40.0	No Change	
Maximal Exercise	38.0	38.0	No Change	
Femoral Vein CO_2 Partial Pressure, $P_{v_{CO_2}}$, (mm Hg)				
Rest	45.0	45.0	No Change	
Maximal Exercise	63.0	63.0	70.0	70.0
Right Atrium CO_2 Partial Pressure, $P_{\overline{v}_{CO_2}}$, (mm Hg)				
Rest	45.0	45.0	No Change	
Maximal Exercise	60.0	60.0	67.0	67.0
Lactic Acid in Arteries & Veins (mg/100 ml blood)				
Rest	12.0	12.0	No Change	
Submaximal Exercise (6 mph run)	50.0	50.0	18.0	18.0
Maximal Exercise	120	120	140	140
pH of Blood in Femoral Vein				
Rest	7.37	7.37	No Change	
Maximal Exercise	7.10	7.10	6.90	6.90
pH of Blood in Arteries				
Rest	7.40	7.40	No Change	
Maximal Exercise	7.20	7.20	7.0	7.0
Blood Temperature				
Rest	99.6°F, 37.6°C		No Change	
Maximal Exercise	104°F, 40.0°C		106°F, 41.2°C	

* There are wide individual and group differences for many of these blood characteristics. Values given should be considered as rough approximations only. Data from many sources, principally references 1, 4, 10, 12, 16, 19, and 21.

of the blood that occur with a single bout of maximal exercise and with endurance training. First of all, notice that a heavy bout of exercise often leads to a slightly reduced blood volume. This reduction in blood volume includes only plasma water and not any of the blood cells. Plasma water leaves the blood primarily because the high blood pressure in the capillaries of the working muscles forces water through the capillary wall into the interstitial spaces. The accumulation of water in the muscle tissues is partly responsible for the so-called "pumping-up" of the muscles that accompanies the repeated rapid lifting of dumbbells or barbells. Shortly after the exercise period, the excess water in tissues makes its way back into the blood-stream, so that blood volume returns to normal as does muscle size. The transfer of water from plasma to muscles results in *hemoconcentration*, or a thickening of the blood, due to a greater concentration of cells, especially red blood cells. Hemoconcentration is also partly attributed to a loss of plasma water because of increased sweating. Why males have higher red blood cell concentrations than females is not completely understood, but this phenomenon seems to be associated with the male sex hormone levels because the sex differences in blood develop at the time of puberty.

Physical training has often been reported to lead to a greater blood volume and hemoglobin volume because of an increase in both cells and plasma, but the exact mechanism responsible for this volume change is unknown (4). It is often suggested that the mechanism is the same as that invoked by high altitude living; that is, hypoxia in the tissues stimulates the production and release by the kidney of a hormone, erythropoietin, that stimulates red blood cell production by the bone marrow. Whether this is the case with exercise, where any hypoxia is of rather brief duration, is not clear.

The hemoconcentration that occurs with exercise explains the increases observed in red blood cell count, hemoglobin concentration, and hematocrit (Table 12.4), all of which reflect the greater concentration of red blood cells in a given volume of blood. On the other hand, the increased white blood cell count that often is seen after exercise is usually explained as an effect of the greater circulation during exercise "washing out" the white blood cells from their storage places in the lungs, bone marrow, liver and spleen (10). Such an explanation seems reasonable for the lungs and perhaps bone marrow, but blood flow in liver and spleen tends to decline with exercise. This white cell response is of no special benefit to the organism during exercise, and the white blood cell count resumes its normal value within a few hours after completing physical activity.

It is important to observe the lack of an appreciable exercise effect on arterial oxygen content and partial pressure. The lungs function so effectively that even under conditions of maximal exercise, most studies show little or no change in arterial oxygen levels. Likewise, physical training has no reproducible effect on arterial oxygen, and there is no good evidence to support the conclusion that regular exercise improves the ability of the lungs to deliver oxygen to the blood.

The reason that oxygen levels are lower in the femoral venous blood than in the arterial blood during leg exercise is that mitochondria of the leg muscles are using oxygen to carry away electrons and hydrogen ions in the electron transport system of aerobic metabolism. As the oxygen combines with hydrogen, water is formed so that the venous blood has less oxygen to deliver back to the heart and lungs. Oxygen in the right atrium of the heart is called *mixed venous oxygen* because venous blood from working muscles is mixed with venous blood from nonworking tissues. Accordingly, oxygen levels are higher in mixed venous blood than in venous blood from working muscles because there is a greater usage of oxygen in working muscles than in nonworking organs.

The difference between the oxygen content of arterial blood and mixed venous blood (A–$\overline{V}$ O_2 Difference) represents the amount of oxygen extracted from the blood and used by the tissues. Consequently, when the muscles are actively consuming oxygen during exercise, the arteriovenous oxygen difference increases. Training, especially in young adult males, sometimes is associated with increased arteriovenous oxygen differences after maximal exercise, probably because trained muscles have more mitochondria that can better utilize oxygen that is delivered to the muscles (20). These mitochondrial changes also explain the training-induced decreases in oxygen levels of femoral and mixed venous blood.

Carbon dioxide values are greater in venous blood than in arterial blood because the mitochondria of the tissues produce carbon dioxide as a product of aerobic energy metabolism. Training increases the output of carbon dioxide during maximal exercise because training causes an increased production of mitochondria that can, in turn, generate more carbon dioxide.

Lactic acid is a product of anaerobic glycolysis and is, therefore, found in greater amounts in the blood during exercise that is heavy enough to demand some anaerobic energy production. The trained person produces less lactic acid during submaximal work because he relies more upon aerobic metabolism as a result of increased effectiveness of skeletal muscle mitochondria. During *maximal* work, on the other hand, the trained individual can produce greater amounts of lactic acid because he has greater stores of muscle glycogen to break down to lactic acid, and/or because he can better tolerate increased levels of acid with improved motivation or some unknown physiological adaptations.

The acidity or pH of the blood during exercise is a direct reflection of the increased production of lactic acid. Accordingly, the lower pH (greater acid) in the blood of athletes during maximal exercise is because of the greater lactic acid generated in trained individuals.

Blood temperature increases during exercise because some of the chemical energy released by the breakdown of carbohydrates and fats in the muscle is lost as heat energy and because the process of muscle contraction itself produces heat. The trained person can generate more heat because he can work longer with heavier workloads than untrained individuals, and his muscles can, therefore, create more heat. The increased temperature and greater acidity of the blood circulating through the working muscles causes oxygen to be released somewhat more rapidly from the hemoglobin of the red blood cells. Thus, exercise changes in the muscles serve to increase oxygen delivery to those muscles. The increased carbon dioxide content of the blood does not have much effect on the release of oxygen from hemoglobin during prolonged exercise (21).

Blood Doping

The fact that physical performance is known to be poor after blood loss or withdrawal has led to experiments designed to discover whether *more* blood can enhance performance. In these studies subjects have a pint or more of their blood withdrawn, and after several weeks during which their bodies replace the lost blood, the previously withdrawn red blood cells are reinjected into the circulation (7,25). The rationale for this procedure, "blood doping," is that the extra red blood cells may be able to deliver more oxygen to the working muscles to improve their endurance. However, the results of such experiments are inconclusive with one (7) showing an improvement in maximal treadmill running time from 5.7 minutes before to 7.0 minutes after a month of training, and others (25) showing no improvement in performance. Whether the improved performance in the one experiment was because of the blood doping or the month of physical training cannot be answered definitely.

Regardless of the relative effectiveness of blood doping, it seems to be an artifical means of gaining a possible performance edge that should not become accepted practice. One can imagine the logical extension of such procedures to include surgical manipulations of the nerve supply to muscles in an attempt to form more slow twitch fibers or surgical alterations of tendon insertions to provide a more effective angle of pull. Such procedures are not in the best interests of individual athletes or of sport.

PULMONARY FUNCTION

During aerobic endurance activities, more oxygen must be delivered from the lungs to the working muscles, and excess carbon dioxide must be removed from the muscles. These processes require an accelerated exchange of oxygen and carbon dioxide between the lungs and the blood; they are accomplished by an increased flow of blood through the lung capillaries (increased pulmonary perfusion), by an increased rate and depth of breathing (ventilation), and by an increased rate of diffusion of oxygen from lungs into blood and of carbon dioxide from the blood to the air in the lungs.

Pulmonary Perfusion

The right ventricle pumps more blood to the lungs during exercise at the same time that the left ventricle delivers more blood to the working muscles and to the rest of the body. Even though there may be five times more blood pumped through the lungs during maximal exercise than at rest, there is only a slight rise in blood pressure within the lung capillaries (12). This rise in blood pressure means that there must be many more open capillaries in the lungs during exercise than at rest, and that the millions of tiny air sacs (alveoli) in the lungs must be much better perfused with blood. As a consequence of this increased perfusion or distribution of blood to the alveoli and of the increased rate of flow of blood through the lungs, more oxygen can diffuse into the pulmonary blood, and more carbon dioxide can diffuse out of the blood into the alveolar air.

Ventilation

At rest, the lungs are ventilated at approximately six liters per minute. This six liters is the result of breathing about 12 times per minute with the volume of each breath (*tidal volume*) being about one-half liter. During prolonged "steady state" endurance exercise, maximal ventilation is about 80–100 liters per minute. With short duration exercise, such as a 400 meter sprint, a ventilation rate of 140–160 liters per minute is not unusual (4).

The elevated rate of ventilation that occurs with dynamic exercise has been said to consist of two components, 1) a fast, *neurogenic* component and 2) a slow, *humoral* component (12). (See Fig. 12.8.) Within the first breath after exercise starts and stops, ventilation increases and decreases, respectively. This part of the exercise response occurs so rapidly that it is surely neurogenic (the result of a nerve reflex). After the initial neurogenic increase in ventilation, there is a slow rise in ventilation that seems to be humoral in nature, that is, caused by substances such as potassium (9), carbon dioxide (23) and lactic acid (13), which circulate in the blood. The neurogenic component is thought to result from impulses from blood vessels near the heart or the lungs (22, 24), to stimuli from receptors in the moving joints and contracting muscles (2), and to impulses from the limbic system of the brain and the motor cortex. All of these stimuli are transmitted to the respiratory control centers of the medulla of the brain (14). These neurogenic and humoral regulatory influences on ventilation are summarized schematically in Fig. 12.9.

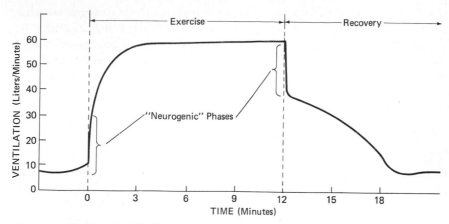

Figure 12.8.   Ventilation response to exercise.

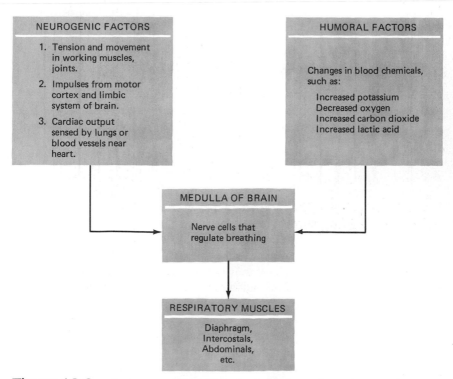

Figure 12.9.   Summary of neurogenic and humoral regulators of ventilation during exercise.

When one anticipates a competitive situation, it is not unusual for him to breathe more rapidly and deeply. This anticipatory response results from impulses radiating down to the medulla from the limbic system of the brain, and/or perhaps to the increased cardiac output that accompanies anticipation of exercise (22). As soon as the competitor begins moving his limbs, impulses from nerve endings and other receptors located in the working muscles and joints cause an immediate elevation in ventilation. Part of this rapid neurogenic phase of ventilation may also be the result of increased cardiac output that seems to be sensed somewhere between the pulmonary artery and the carotid arteries (22). A slower additional rise then occurs because of chemical factors such as lactic acid, potassium and carbon dioxide that are produced by the contracting muscles and released into the blood. These factors probably act on the neurons of the medulla that regulate respiration and/or upon chemoreceptors located in the carotid arteries (24). The neurons of the medulla that control ventilation apparently become more sensitive under exercise conditions, so that they have a greater response to normal or only slightly altered arterial oxygen, carbon dioxide and pH levels (2, 23).

Once the event has ended and there are no more nerve impulses from the muscles affecting ventilation, there is an immediate drop in ventilation, followed by a slower fall until the various chemicals that caused the humoral effect on ventilation are reduced to lower, ineffective levels in the blood.

It should be noted that with static exercise, there is no rapid neurogenic ventilation response (2). There must be movement of joints with dynamic activity if the neurogenic phase is to be observed.

Pulmonary Diffusing Capacity

The pulmonary (lung) diffusing capacity for a gas such as oxygen represents the rate of diffusion of the gas between the air sacs (alveoli) of the lungs and the blood of the lung capillaries. This capacity varies with many factors, including the thickness of the lung tissue, the thickness of the red blood cell membrane, the amount of plasma between the air sac and the red blood cell, and most important, the surface area of contact between alveoli and blood in the pulmonary capillary.

There is up to a 300 per cent increase in pulmonary diffusing capacity for oxygen during maximal exercise (12). This change is thought to be brought about almost entirely by the increased perfusion of blood around the air sacs of the lungs, as a result of a greater number of open capillaries in the lungs responding to a greater cardiac output during exercise. At rest in an upright posture, many of the pulmonary capillaries are closed, especially at the top of the lungs, because gravity tends to cause blood to pool in the lower parts of the lungs. Therefore, there is little or no diffusion of oxygen from many of the alveoli surrounded by the closed capillaries. However, as an elevated cardiac output during exercise forces more blood into the pulmonary artery, most of the pulmonary capillaries that were closed at rest become filled with blood. This creates a greater surface area for diffusion of oxygen from alveolar air to the pulmonary blood, and accounts for the increase in pulmonary diffusing capacity for oxygen during exercise.

Although the pulmonary diffusing capacity for carbon dioxide also increases during exercise as a result of a better perfusion of blood through the lungs, this phenomenon is of little consequence. The diffusion of carbon dioxide proceeds about 20 times faster than the diffusion of oxygen and would be rapid enough even if there was no exercise effect on the carbon dioxide diffusion capacity.

Pulmonary Function As a Possible Limiting Factor in Circulorespiratory Endurance

Most authorities believe that under normal circumstances in young persons, the lungs are perfectly capable of meeting the demands imposed by even the heaviest types of exercise stress (3, 12). The levels of oxygen and carbon dioxide in the arterial blood delivered from the left ventricle during maximal exercise are usually unchanged from resting values, ane one's maximal voluntary ventilation capacity of 160–180 liters per minute is not strained during long duration exercise where values of 80–100 liters per minute are commonly observed. Thus, the changes in lung perfusion, ventilation and diffusing capacity for oxygen during exercise are usually sufficient to keep arterial oxygen and carbon dioxide at values essentially unchanged from those at rest. However, as described in Chapter 14, elderly persons have lower maximal pulmonary ventilation rates, and their maximal oxygen uptakes may thus be limited by lung function.

SUMMARY

The physiological responses of the heart, lungs, and blood vessels are of primary importance in determining the ability of one to persist at prolonged physical activity. These responses are described in this chapter, and the mechanisms which bring about the responses are explained. A failure of any of these mechanisms to adequately provoke the appropriate responses may lead to diminished aerobic endurance performance, whereas improved responses can produce improved performance.

Exercise causes greater cardiac output by increasing both heart rate and stroke volume. A limited blood volume is effectively diverted to the working muscles by means of a widespread constriction of blood vessels supplying nonworking muscles and visceral organs, and a dilatation of blood vessels in the working muscles. A large increase in cardiac output overwhelms a small net decrease in peripheral resistance and is responsible for an elevated arterial blood pressure that provides the force to drive blood through the tissues during exercise. Pulmonary ventilation and diffusion of oxygen and carbon dioxide both increase so effectively during exercise that normal, young persons are not ordinarily limited in their aerobic endurance by an inadequacy of the lungs. Values of oxygen, carbon dioxide, lactic acid, and other chemicals in the blood during exercise reflect not only the changes in oxygen uptake and the production of carbon dioxide and lactic acid by the working muscles, but also a commonly observed hemoconcentration that occurs when high intracapillary pressures force fluid from the capillaries into the tissue spaces.

Review Questions

1. What is meant by the terms *neurogenic, humoral* and *intrinsic* in explanations of physiological changes?
2. List three factors that are probably involved in the immediate rise in heart rate at the start of exercise.
3. List two humoral stimuli that may cause a gradual rise in heart rate as exercise progresses.
4. Describe and explain the changes in stroke volume that accompany postural changes and exercise.
5. Explain why shifts in regional blood flow are required during exercise.
6. How is it possible for an organ such as the liver to sustain an 85 per cent decrease in blood flow during exercise and yet suffer no apparent damage?
7. Which is more important in determining arterial pressure during rhythmic exercise: changes in vascular resistance or changes in cardiac output? Explain your answer.
8. Examine Table 12.2 and explain each sex difference in blood characteristics and each exercise-induced and training-induced change in blood characteristics.
9. List three neurogenic factors and two humoral factors involved in the ventilation response to exercise.

10. Explain why pulmonary function in healthy subjects is ordinarily not considered a limiting factor in aerobic endurance performance.

References

1. Anderson, K. L. The cardiovascular system in exercise. In H. Falls (Ed.), *Exercise Physiology*. New York: Academic Press, 1968, pp. 79–128.
2. Asmussen, E. Ventilation at transition from rest to exercise. *Acta Physiologica Scandinavica*, 1973, **89**:68–78.
3. Astrand, I. ST depression, heart rate, and blood pressure during arm and leg work. *Scandinavian Journal of Clinical Laboratory Investigation*, 1972, **30**:411–414.
4. Astrand, P.-O., and K. Rodahl. *Textbook of Work Physiology*. New York: McGraw-Hill, 1970.
5. Barnard, R. J., G. W. Gardner, W. V. Diaco, R. N. MacAlpin, and A. A. Kattus. Cardiovascular responses to sudden strenuous exercise—heart rate, blood pressure, and ECG. *Journal of Applied Physiology*, 1973, **34**:833–837.
6. Costin, J. C., and N. S. Skinner, Jr. Competition between vasoconstrictor, and vasodilator mechanisms in skeletal muscle. *American Journal of Physiology*, 1971, **220**:462–466.
7. Ekblom, B., A. N. Goldbarg, and B. Gullbring. Response to exercise after blood loss and reinfusion. *Journal of Applied Physiology*, 1972, **33**:175–180.
8. Eklund, B. Influence of work duration on the regulation of muscle blood flow. *Acta Physiologica Scandinavia* (Supplementum 411), 1974.
9. Hnik, P., N. Kriz, F. Vyskocil, V. Smiesko, J. Mejsnar, E. Ujec, and M. IIolas. Work-induced potassium changes in muscle venous effluent blood measured by ion-specific electrodes. *Pflugers Archives* 1973, **338**:177–181.
10. Karpovich, P. V., and W. E. Sinning. *Physiology of Muscular Activity, 7th Ed.* Philadelphia: W. B. Saunders, 1971.
11. Lind, A. R., G. W. McNicol, and K. W. Donald. Circulatory adjustments to sustained (static) muscular activity. In K. Evang and K. L. Anderson (Eds.), *Physical Activity in Health and Disease*. Baltimore: William and Wilkins, 1966, pp. 38–63.
12. Margaria, R., and P. Cerretelli. The respiratory system and exercise. In H. Falls (Ed.), *Exercise Physiology*. New York: Academic Press, 1968, pp. 43–78.

13. Matell, G. Time-courses of changes in ventilation and arterial gas tensions in man induced by moderate exercise. *Acta Physiologica Scandinavica*, 1963, **58** (Supplementum 206): 1–53.

14. McCloskey, D. I., P. B. C. Matthews, and J. H. Mitchell. Absence of appreciable cardiovascular and respiratory responses to muscle vibration. *Journal of Applied Physiology*, 1972, **33**:623–626.

15. Mohrman, D. E., and H. V. Sparks. Myogenic hyperemia following brief tetanus of canine skeletal muscle. *American Journal of Physiology*, 1974, **227**:531–535.

16. Osnes, J.-B., and L. Hermansen. Acid-base balance after maximal exercise of short duration. *Journal of Applied Physiology*, 1972, **32**:59–63.

17. Petro, J. K., A. P. Hollandee, and L. N. Bouman. Instantaneous cardiac acceleration in man induced by a voluntary muscle contraction. *Journal of Applied Physiology*, 1970, **29**:794–798.

18. Roskamm, H. Myocardial contractility during exercise. In J. Keul (Ed.), *Limiting Factors of Physical Performance*. Stuttgart: Georg Thieme, Publishers, 1973, pp. 225–234.

19. Rowell, L. B. Circulation. *Medicine and Science in Sports*, 1969, **1**:15–22.

20. Rowell, L. B. Human cardiovascular adjustments to exercise and thermal stress. *Physiological Reviews*, 1974, **51**:75–159.

21. Thomson, J. M., J. A. Dempsey, L. W. Chosy, N. T. Shahidi, and W. G. Reddan. Oxygen transport and oxyhemoglobin dissociation during prolonged muscular work. *Journal of Applied Physiology*, 1974, **37**:658–664.

22. Wasserman, K., B. J. Whipp, and J. Castagna. Cardiodynamic hyperpnea: hyperpnea secondary to cardiac output increase. *Journal of Applied Physiology*, 1974, **36**:457–464.

23. Weil, J. V., E. Byrne–Quinn, I. E. Sodal, J. S. Kline, R. E. McCullough, and G. R. Filley. Augmentation of chemosensitivity during mild exercise in normal man. *Journal of Applied Physiology*, 1972, **33**:813–819.

24. Whipp, B. J. The hyperpnea of dynamic muscular exercise. *Exercise and Sport Sciences Reviews*, 1977, 5: In Press.

25. Williams, M. H., A. R. Goodwin, R. Perkins, and J. Bocrie. Effect of blood reinjection upon endurance capacity and heart rate. *Medicine and Science in Sports*, 1973, **5**:181–186.

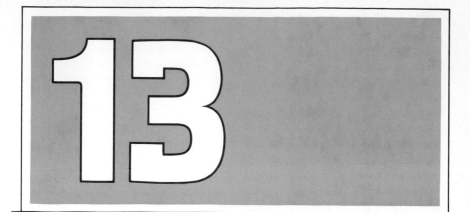

Evaluation of cardiovascular function and aerobic endurance performance

The principal limiting factor for most types of exercise that last longer than three or four minutes is the capacity of the heart, lungs and circulation to deliver oxygen to the working muscles. Therefore, if a physical educator, coach or physician wishes to evaluate one's circulorespiratory fitness or one's capacity for aerobic activity, he should try to estimate the maximal functional capacity of the heart, lungs and circulation of the student, athlete or patient. This maximal functional capacity of the circulorespiratory system is best evaluated with a test of the body's capacity to consume oxygen at a maximal rate, that is, with a maximal oxygen uptake test.

MAXIMAL OXYGEN UPTAKE

The rate of maximal oxygen uptake is abbreviated $\dot{V}_{O_2}$ max, where the V_{O_2} represents volume of oxygen consumed, usually in liters or milliliters, and the dot over the $\dot{V}$ is a notation that tells us that this volume is to be expressed per unit of time, usually per minute. Thus, the expression, $\dot{V}_{O_2}$ max $= 3$ l/min, means that a person can maximally consume oxygen at a rate of 3 liters per minute. The term *maximal oxygen uptake* is synonymous with the terms *maximal oxygen consumption, maximal oxygen intake* and *maximal aerobic power*, and represents the greatest difference between the rate at which inspired oxygen enters the lungs and the rate that expired oxygen leaves the lungs (Fig. 13.1). Therefore, in order to measure maximal oxygen uptake one must know the amount of oxygen inspired and the amount expired; the difference between these two values is the amount of oxygen that has been taken up and used by the electron transport system of the mitochondria to produce energy for the active tissues.

It is not unusual for oxygen uptake to increase about 10 or even 20 times when one passes from a condition of rest (about 0.25 l/min) to heavy endurance exercise (about 2.5 to 5.0 l/min). For young adult women maximal oxygen uptake is about 2.3 l/min, whereas men are apt to consume about 3.4 l/min under maximal exercise conditions (19). There is a fairly broad range of values for maximal oxygen uptake, depending on such factors as state of physical training, age, and sex. For example, the maximal oxygen uptake of typical college females may range from less than 1.7 to greater than 3.0 l/min, and

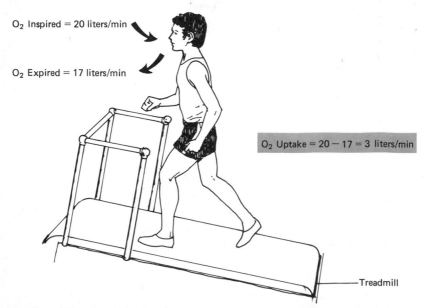

O_2 Inspired $= 20$ liters/min

O_2 Expired $= 17$ liters/min

O_2 Uptake $= 20 - 17 = 3$ liters/min

Treadmill

Figure 13.1   Schematic view of how oxygen uptake is measured.

for college males from less than 2.7 to greater than 4.0 l/min (19). Outstanding men and women cross country skiers in Scandinavia have had values reported as high as 6.0 and 4.0 l/min, respectively (4).

Because oxygen is used by all the body tissues, a larger individual has a greater oxygen uptake than a smaller one both at rest and during exercise. Accordingly, it is better for comparative purposes to record oxygen uptake values on the basis of body weight, ordinarily in terms of milliliters of oxygen per kilogram of body weight. Therefore, since a kilogram is equivalent to approximately 2.2 pounds, a man who weighs 154 pounds (70 kilograms) and has a maximal oxygen uptake of 2.8 l/min (2800 ml/min) can also be said to have a maximal oxygen uptake of 2800/70 = 40 ml/kg/min. When expressed in this fashion, typical maximal oxygen uptake values for college men and women might be about 48 and 40 ml/kg/min, respectively (19). Expressing the same data in terms of lean body mass or fat-free body weight is not usually advisable because such an expression unjustifiably penalizes those who are less fat (13).

Some Factors That Determine Maximal Oxygen Uptake

Let us review some of the physiological functions that are involved if one is to have a normal maximal oxygen uptake capacity. First, the heart, lungs, and blood vessels must be functioning adequately so that oxygen inhaled into the lungs is delivered to the blood. Second, the process of oxygen delivery to the tissues by the red blood cells must be normal; that is, there must be normal heart function, blood volume, red blood cell count and hemoglobin concentration, and the blood vessels must be able to shift blood from non-working tissues to the working muscles where the oxygen demand is greatest. Third, the tissues, especially the muscles, must have a normal capacity to use the oxygen that is delivered to them. In other words, they must have normal energy metabolism and mitochondrial function. As we have seen previously, the lungs of a healthy person do not limit his ability to consume oxygen (4). Also, a routine blood test can determine whether the characteristics of the blood are normal. Therefore, heart function, the ability to circulate blood to the active tissues, and the ability of the tissues to extract and utilize oxygen remain as factors to be evaluated by tests of maximal oxygen uptake in nonelderly persons who do not have pulmonary disease.

Heart function is reflected by cardiac output (CO). Both the ability of the circulatory system to transfer blood from inactive to active regions and the ability of the tissues to extract oxygen from the blood are reflected by the difference in the content of oxygen between arterial and venous blood (arteriovenous O_2 difference, A-$\overline{V}$ O_2 Diff.). A person who can shift most of his blood to working muscles during exercise will have a large arteriovenous oxygen difference because the active muscles will be able to extract more oxygen from the blood than would inactive tissues of the body. Likewise, one whose muscles have highly active mitochondria will be able to extract oxygen from the blood supply quite readily.

Assuming that the lungs and blood characteristics are normal, maximal oxygen uptake is a function of maximal cardiac output and maximal arteriovenous oxygen difference. This fact can be expressed in a simple equation as follows: $\dot{V}_{O_2}$ max = max CO $\times$ max A-$\overline{V}$ O$_2$ Diff. (22). Let us assume that a subject's maximal cardiac output is 25 liters per minute, that the oxygen content of the blood in his arteries is 20 milliliters of oxygen per 100 milliliters of blood, and that the oxygen content of his mixed venous blood sampled in the right atrium is 5 milliliters of oxygen per 100 milliliters of blood. The subject's max A-$\overline{V}$ O$_2$ Diff. is $20 - 5 = 15$ ml/100 ml or 0.15 liters of oxygen per liter of blood. Accordingly, this subject's maximal oxygen uptake is $25 \times 0.15 = 3.75$ liters per minute. Remember that the cardiac output represents the amount of blood potentially available for oxygen delivery to the active tissues each minute, and that the arteriovenous O$_2$ difference represents the degree to which the oxygen contained in the blood pumped out of the heart is used by the active tissues for aerobic energy metabolism.

$\dot{V}_{O_2}$ max and Endurance Performance

While it is true that a person's maximal oxygen uptake reflects the maximal functional capacity of his cardiovascular system, and the maximal functional capacity of the cardiovascular system is usually the most important determinant of one's performance in physical activity of an aerobic nature, it is not true that a person with a great maximal oxygen uptake is necessarily an outstanding endurance performer (4, 17, 19). Many other factors such as motivation and technique play a role in endurance performance. Thus, although an outstanding endurance athlete must have a relatively high maximal rate of oxygen uptake, it does not always follow that the best performer in a group of excellent performers has the greatest maximal oxygen uptake. A track coach who knows the maximal oxygen uptakes of all his freshman track candidates will be able to select those athletes who have the *physiological* potential to become good endurance performers, but he will not be able to predict very accurately from a test of oxygen uptake which of these potentially good performers may finally become champions. The *emotional, psychological* and *technical* characteristics of the athletes must also be considered.

$\dot{V}_{O_2}$ max and Cardiovascular Health

Although a test of maximal oxygen uptake can be useful to the physical educator or coach to determine those who are most fit for cardiorespiratory endurance activities, a much more important use of this test from the health standpoint is its use in the detection of cardiovascular disease, and in the assessment of one's capacity for exercise prior to the undertaking of an exercise program. The test is useful for normal fitness purposes as well as for the rehabilitation of patients who have suffered heart attacks or show clinical signs of cardiovascular disease. In recognition of the value of exercise testing, physicians, exercise physiologists and physical educators throughout the world are establishing testing and exercise centers where trained exercise technicians administer graded exercise tests, usually to those over 35 years of age. The results of these tests are used in the diagnosis of cardiovascular disease and in the prescription of exercise training programs that are conducted by skilled exercise leaders (2, 20).

Principles of Testing Maximal Oxygen Uptake

Routine testing of maximal oxygen uptake has been accomplished chiefly with three methods of exercise: treadmill exercise, bicycle ergometer exercise or bench stepping (6, 19). There are certain advantages to each of these procedures. For example, a stepping bench is inexpensive and portable; a bicycle ergometer can be used to measure the quantity of work performed very accurately; and in cycling, the upper body is relatively motionless for easy monitoring of electrocardiogram, blood pressure and other physiological measurements. Treadmill tests produce the highest values for maximal oxygen uptake and are subject to the least differences in skill and efficiency between subjects (19). One of the greatest problems inherent in the use of step tests is that at higher workloads for normal, active, and well-trained subjects, the height of the step and the rate of stepping become so great that it becomes increasingly difficult for the subject to maintain his balance and the appropriate stepping cadence (19). Both step tests and bicycle ergometry tend to place a great deal of stress on a relatively few leg muscles, so that performers often are forced to stop working because of muscle pain before maximal oxygen uptake has been achieved (19). Consequently, the treadmill test has achieved great popularity in the United States when precise measurements of maximal oxygen uptake are desired. That is not to say, however, that other procedures are not acceptable. The step test may be useful for testing patients with low capacities, and the bicycle ergometer is excellent as long as it is understood that it will probably underestimate maximal oxygen uptake by about 5–10 per cent, both because of the muscle pain factor and perhaps because of a smaller amount of muscle tissue involved in the bicycle work than in tread-mill exercise (19).

Criteria for Establishing That Maximal Oxygen Uptake Was Achieved. Probably the most important criterion for determining that one has achieved his maximal oxygen uptake for a given test pro-cedure is whether oxygen consumption reaches a plateau or perhaps declines slightly with increasing workloads (Fig. 13.2). Because it is known that oxygen uptake increases linearly with increasing work-loads up to the maximal rate of oxygen uptake, a plateau of oxygen uptake with an increasing workload is a sure sign that the subject has achieved his maximum. In the absence of such an observed plateau in oxygen uptake, one cannot be certain that the highest, or *peak*, ox-ygen uptake is indeed the subject's *maximal* oxygen uptake. Other evidence that may support the conclusion that a peak oxygen uptake is also the maximal uptake for a given subject might include a high level of blood lactic acid (above 70–80 mg/100 ml blood) and achieve-ment of near maximal heart rate (4, 15). Both of these factors usually are observed at the time of maximal oxygen uptake.

Additional factors to be considered in determining that maximal

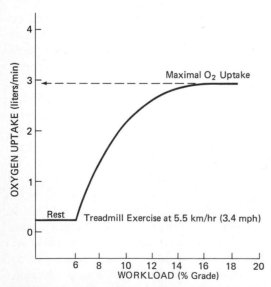

Figure 13.2. The plateau in oxygen up-take with increasing workload at maximal ox-ygen uptake.

oxygen uptake is measured for a particular test are exercise posture, muscle mass used in the exercise, exercise intensity, exercise duration, mechanical efficiency for the task, and the motivation of the subject (19, 22). Posture must be upright, either sitting or standing, because the highest oxygen uptakes observed in a horizontal posture while pedalling a bicycle ergometer or during swimming are almost always 5–29 per cent less than the highest uptakes for the same subjects on the treadmill (4, 18). World class swimmers, however, are capable of matching their bicycle maximal oxygen uptakes while swimming, but their swimming values are still 6–7 per cent lower than treadmill values, perhaps because swimming may require use of a smaller muscle mass than running (16).

Because the increased activity of skeletal muscles accounts for most of the increased oxygen uptake during exercise, it is obvious that large muscles must be used if maximal oxygen uptake is to be attained. In other words, one should not expect to get as great an oxygen uptake from arm work as from leg work, and arm work combined with leg work should give a somewhat greater oxygen uptake than either leg or arm work by itself (14, 23). About 50 per cent of the total muscle mass must be engaged in exercise before maximal oxygen uptake can be achieved (22).

Both exercise intensity and duration must be great enough to elicit a near-maximal response of the cardiovascular system if maximal oxygen uptake is to be attained. A minimum of about three or four minutes of running on the treadmill is required to achieve maximal oxygen uptake, whereas treadmill walking up progressively steeper grades may require 20 minutes or longer to elicit a maximal response (19). The intensity of the workload is increased progressively in tests of maximal oxygen uptake, so that eventually the intensity must reach a level sufficient to bring about a maximal response.

Finally, a good test of maximal oxygen uptake should not depend on the skill or motivational levels of the subject (22). It would be absurd to choose a hurdling task to measure oxygen uptake, for example, because of the high levels of skill and motivation required to perform such a task. Even in a simple task such as pedalling a bicycle ergometer, differences in efficiency among individuals can be about 6 per cent (4). Walking is a familiar task to most, and there are only negligible differences in walking efficiency among individuals (19). Some tasks, such as fast running on a treadmill, also suffer from the fact that many persons are either fearful of or are unwilling to persist in those activities. For both efficiency and motivational reasons treadmill walking up progressively greater inclines is a commonly used test of maximal oxygen uptake (5). Walking tests that are more prolonged in nature, that is, in which the intensity is only gradually increased, seem to be tolerated better than briefer walking tests, even though similar values in maximal oxygen uptake are achieved by both methods (10). For some subjects, however, shorter progressive treadmill running tests produce nearly 10 per cent greater oxygen uptakes than prolonged treadmill walking, perhaps because blood flow to the skin increases during prolonged exercise, and this may reduce blood and oxygen supply to the working muscles (12).

Predicting Maximal Oxygen Uptake from Physiological Responses to Submaximal Tests

During exercise of submaximal intensity, heart rate and ventilation rate increase approximately in proportion to increases in oxygen uptake. Consequently, numerous attempts have been made to predict maximal oxygen uptake from heart rate, ventilation rate and other variables during standardized submaximal exercise loads (11, 13, 19). In this way, an estimate of maximal cardiovascular function can be achieved without undue stress on subjects who may have unknown cardiovascular disease, without the need for the high levels of motivation required in tests that push subjects to near maximal levels, and without the need for complex, time-consuming direct determinations of oxygen uptake. Although these tests can usually provide a close approximation of maximal oxygen uptake, they are subject to a prediction error of around 10 per cent or greater (19). Thus, these tests often underestimate or overestimate maximal oxygen uptake by about 10 per cent for a given subject. Since the reproducibility of routine direct tests of maximal oxygen uptake is in the neighborhood of 2–4 percent, the prediction from submaximal test results is not entirely satisfactory. Some of the submaximal tests are terminated when the subject reaches a predetermined heart rate that represents a certain percentage (often 85 per cent) of predicted maximal heart rate for that subject. Unfortunately, there is a wide range of maximal heart rates for a given age group, so that prediction of maximal heart rate is often poor (6). This accounts for some of the poor predictions of maximal oxygen uptake obtained with submaximal tests.

Even though submaximal tests to predict maximal oxygen uptake are not satisfactory for research purposes, their use to assess maximal cardiovascular capacity is justified in situations where financial, personnel, subject safety, and time considerations prohibit direct determinations of maximal oxygen uptake. One of the simplest of these submaximal tests that has been validated for untrained college males is one where the subject pedals a bicycle ergometer at a speed of 60 revolutions per minute with a workload of 150 watts (900 kilopond meters per minute) for five minutes (11). Heart rate is measured during the fifth minute of the ride (HR_{150}), and maximal oxygen uptake is predicted from the following equation: $\dot{V}_{O_2}$ max (l/min) = 6.3 − .01926 HR$_{150}$. Accordingly, if a subject's heart rate during the fifth minute were 160 beats per minute, his predicted maximal oxygen uptake would be 6.3 − .01926 (160) = 3.218 l/min.

Other popular submaximal exercise tests include the Physical Working Capacity-170 test (24) and the Astrand-Rhyming test (3). These tests are more time consuming than the Fox test for predicting maximum aerobic power, but have been more widely used with various populations. Both use heart rate during submaximal exercise to predict maximal oxygen uptake.

Prediction of Maximal Oxygen Uptake from Running Performance

Because it is widely accepted that performance in distance running is dependent to a great extent upon cardiovascular function, several tests have been designed to estimate maximal oxygen uptake from running performance either on the treadmill or in the field. These performance measures include maximal running time on the treadmill (5, 7, 12), best time for running 600 yards, 1 or 1½ miles (1) or 2 miles (21), and maximal distance covered in 9 (1) or 12 minutes (1, 8). Performance on distance runs was initially reported to have a very strong relationship to maximal oxygen uptake (8), but later studies with more homogeneous populations (all subjects having similar ages, body weights, and physical condition characteristics) have showed rather poor predictions of maximal oxygen uptake from 12-minute-runs (13, 17, 19). One reason for this is that in addition to maximal cardiovascular function, factors such as motivation and pain tolerance are important in determining maximal run performance. It has also been demonstrated that maximal treadmill running time can be improved without any improvement in maximal oxygen uptake (12). Consequently, running performance does not seem to be an especially good predictor of maximal oxygen uptake and probably should not be used to estimate maximal cardiovascular function except as that function is involved in running performance. In other words, tests such as the Cooper test can only roughly assess cardiovascular function, but they are likely to give a very good indication of one's ability to persist at distance running.

In the physical education class or on the athletic field, however, the distance-run with all its drawbacks is undoubtedly the best practical indicator of cardiovascular function. Treadmill and bicycle work tests, whether maximal or submaximal, are simply too impractical to use with large numbers of students or athletes. Norms for performance on the Cooper test are provided in a popular format along with exercise programs designed to improve cardiorespiratory fitness (9).

EVALUATION OF AEROBIC ENDURANCE PERFORMANCE

The ability to perform well in aerobic endurance activities, such as distance running, cycling, and swimming, is best tested by having the subject engage in the actual activity for which he has been, or will be, trained. In other words, if one wished to know which of 100 boys were the best candidates for distance running training, he should have all the prospective trainees compete in a distance run, perhaps 1,500 or 3,000 meters (1 or 2 miles), and find out which candidates were the fastest finishers. This type of test measures not only cardiovascular function, but also motivation, pain tolerance, running efficiency, sense of pace, and race strategy—all of which contribute to performance in distance running. Likewise, cyclists should be tested by cycling, swimmers by swimming, and other performers by participation in their chosen event.

The physical educator or coach must be aware that such a test, if used to predict future performance, is biased in favor of those with greater experience. Therefore, if a mediocre finisher is obviously handicapped by a poor sense of pace, by poor mechanical skills, or by ineffective race strategy, the physical educator or coach should consider such handicaps carefully before deciding to expend most of his efforts on faster finishers who may have more nearly approached their maximal performance capacities. It would be unwise to conclude that performance on running tests could be used to predict accurately endurance performance in other types of activity. There are too many differences between performances in running and swimming, for example, to hope for an accurate prediction of one on the basis of knowledge about the other.

Review Questions

1. Describe the factors which determine maximal oxygen uptake.
2. Explain why maximal oxygen uptake can be used to evaluate maximal cardiovascular function in subjects who have no pulmonary disease. Write the equation that illustrates the relationship between maximal oxygen uptake and cardiovascular function.
3. Why is it not possible to predict aerobic endurance performance accurately from knowledge of a subject's maximal oxygen uptake?
4. List the principles of testing for maximal oxygen uptake and

the criteria used to determine whether one's maximal oxygen uptake has been achieved.
5. List several performance tests that have been used to predict maximal oxygen uptake. What are some advantages and disadvantages of such tests?

References

1. American Alliance for Health, Physical Education, and Recreation. *AAHPER Youth Fitness Test Manual*, Rev. Ed. Washington, D.C.: American Alliance for Health, Physical Education, and Recreation, 1975.
2. American College of Sports Medicine. *Guidelines for Graded Exercise Testing and Exercise Prescription*. Philadelphia: Lea & Febiger, 1975.
3. Astrand, I. Aerobic work capacity in men and women with special reference to age. *Acta Physiologica Scandinavica*, 1960, **49**:(Supplementum 169).
4. Astrand, P.-O., and K. Rodahl. *Textbook of Work Physiology*. New York: McGraw-Hill, 1970.
5. Balke, B., and R. Ware. An experimental study of physical fitness of Air Force personnel. *U.S. Air Force Medical Journal*, 1959, **10**:675–688.
6. Bruce, R. A. Methods of exercise testing. Step test, bicycle, treadmill, isometrics. *American Journal of Cardiology*, 1974, **33**:715–720.
7. Bruce, R. A., R. Kusumi, and D. Hosmer. Maximal oxygen intake and nomographic assessment of functional aerobic impairment in cardio vascular disease. *American Heart Journal*, 1973, **85**:546–562.
8. Cooper, K. H. A means of assessing maximal oxygen intake. Correlation between field and treadmill testing. *Journal of the American Medical Association*, 1968, **203**:201–204.
9. Cooper, K. H. *The New Aerobics*. New York: Bantam, 1970.
10. Falls, H. B., and L. D. Humphrey. A comparison of methods for eliciting maximum oxygen uptake from college women during treadmill walking. *Medicine and Science in Sports*, 1973, **5**:239–241.
11. Fox, E. L. A simple, accurate technique for predicting maximal aerobic power. *Journal of Applied Physiology*, 1973, **35**:914–916.
12. Froelicher, Jr., V. F., H. Brammell, G. Davis, I. Noguera, A.

Stewart, and M. G. Lancaster. A comparison of three maximal treadmill exercise protocols. *Journal of Applied Physiology*, 1974, **36**:720–725.

13. Gitin, E. L., J. E. Olerud, and H. W. Carroll. Maximal oxygen uptake based on lean body mass: A meaningful measure of physical fitness? *Journal of Applied Physiology*, 1974, **36**:757–760.

14. Gleser, M. A., D. H. Horstman, and R. P. Mello. The effect on $\dot{V}_{O_2}$ max of adding arm work to maximal leg work. *Medicine and Science in Sports*, 1974, **6**:104–107.

15. Graham, T. E., and G. M. Andrew. The variability of repeated measurements of oxygen debt in man following a maximal treadmill exercise. *Medicine and Science in Sports*, 1973, **5**:73–78.

16. Holmer, I., A. Lundin, and B. O. Eriksson. Maximum oxygen uptake during swimming and running by elite swimmers. *Journal of Applied Physiology*, 1974, **36**:711–714.

17. Jessup, G. T., H. Tolson, and J. W. Terry. Prediction of maximal oxygen intake from Astrand-Rhyming test, 12-minute run, and anthropometric variables using stepwise multiple regression. *American Journal of Physical Medicine*, 1974, **53**:200–207.

18. Magel, J. R., G. F. Foglia, W. D. McArdle, B. Gutin, G. S. Pechar, and F. I. Katch. Specificity of swim training on maximum oxygen uptake. *Journal of Applied Physiology*. 1975, **38**:151–155.

19. Nagle, F. J. Physiological assessment of maximal performance. In J. Wilmore (Ed.), *Exercise and Sport Sciences Reviews*. Vol. 1. New York: Academic Press, 1973, pp. 313–338.

20. Naughton, J. P., and H. K. Hellerstein (Eds.), *Exercise Testing and Exercise Training in Coronary Heart Disease*. New York: Academic Press, 1973.

21. Ribisl, P. M., and W. A. Kachadorian. Maximal oxygen intake prediction in young and middle-aged males. *Journal of Sports Medicine and Physical Fitness*, 1969, **9**:17–22.

22. Rowell, L. B. Human cardiovascular adjustments to exercise and thermal stress. *Physiological Reviews*, 1974, **54**:75–159.

23. Secher, N. H., N. Ruberg-Larsen, R. A. Binkhorst, and F. Bonde-Petersen. Maximal oxygen uptake during arm cranking and combined arm plus leg exercise. *Journal of Applied Physiology*, 1974, **36**:515–518.

24. Wahlund, H. Determination of the physical working capacity. *Acta Medica Scandinavica* (Supplementum 215), 1948.

14

Training for improved aerobic endurance

There are two principal reasons why an individual might with to improve his ability to persist in performing physical activities that demand an efficient heart and circulation. An endurance athlete is obviously interested in improving his aerobic endurance to enhance his athletic performance. But a more important consideration is the desire of many persons to improve their aerobic endurance in an effort to minimize their chances of becoming victims of heart disease early in their lives. Some of the evidence that suggests endurance exercise may offer some protection against the early onset of heart disease is presented in a later chapter. We will now describe some of the generally accepted principles of training for aerobic endurance improvement and explain some of the physiological adaptations that are commonly observed in trained individuals.

PRINCIPLES OF TRAINING FOR AEROBIC ENDURANCE

Before any strenuous training program is started, it is important to know if the trainee has any medical problems that might be aggravated by vigorous exercise or that might preclude a successful training outcome. Ideally, each trainee should undergo a complete physical examination, including an electrocardiogram taken during exercise, before engaging in the training program. Practically speaking, this ideal is rarely met because of financial costs and the lack of medical personnel and facilities for stress testing. However, those with known symptoms of cardiovascular disease, and all previously inactive individuals over the age of 35, should undergo a thorough physical examination (including exercise ECG) by their physicians to detect undisclosed cardiovascular disease (3). Young, healthy trainees should be carefully monitored during the first stages of a training program, so that any signs of inability to cope with the exercise stress can be detected before the stress becomes overwhelming. Extremely labored breathing, failure to keep up with one's peers, and any obvious symptoms of extreme physical discomfort should be taken as signs that a medical examination should be required and/or that the level of exercise for the individual should be reduced. Such signs of undue stress should, however, be rare occurrences if training programs are tailored to individual capacities as described in the next section.

Training Should Be Individualized and Should Progress Slowly. That there are great differences in aerobic endurance capacities among individuals should be recognized when undertaking or designing training programs. The program of world champion (at 77 km) Farely Fleetfoot is not appropriate for Pasquale Plumprump, whose most impressive distance performance is a train ride from Cucamonga to Kalamazoo. Training can be individualized in many ways, but two of the most commonly used procedures are to modify the exercise load according to a person's physiological response to exercise, such as ventilation or heart rate increase, or to base the target times for exercise on past performances. With these two procedures, trainees with lesser aerobic capacities than their peers will train at lower intensities than those with greater endurance. Trainees who work according to their capacities are not discouraged by their inabilities to meet unrealistic training goals. They are also less apt to experience minor medical ailments or, in the case of those with cardiovascular disorders, to precipitate a cardiovascular incident, such as a heart attack.

Another way to minimize the risk of cardiovascular incidents, muscle and joint injuries, and muscular soreness is to begin the training program at a very low level and to progress very slowly for the first 2–3 weeks of training. This precaution is especially important for those over 35 who have not been in training for two years or more, and for any person with cardiovascular disease symptoms. Even young participants are more likely to continue a training program if they can avoid severe muscular soreness at the start of the program. One simple criterion for minimizing the risk of exercising at too great an intensity is to work at levels that will allow one to carry on a normal conversation during the exercise.

Aerobic Training Should Impose Unaccustomed Demands Upon One's Potential for Aerobic ATP Replenishment. The ability to persist in prolonged rhythmic exercise depends largely on the potential of the cardiovascular system to deliver oxygen to the muscles and upon the potential of those muscles to utilize the delivered oxygen for ATP replenishment by aerobic metabolism. Just as confinement to a bed for several weeks reduces demands on the cardiovascular and muscular systems and diminishes aerobic endurance, increased demands imposed by vigorous exercise will stimulate adaptations in cardiovascular and muscular function which will enhance aerobic endurance (6, 8, 47). How can one determine that an exercise load is sufficient to bring about greater aerobic endurance? Any *regular* program of exercise that moderately elevates one's heart rate and breathing rate above resting values for at least 5–10 minutes will lead to some aerobic endurance benefits (18, 44). At low levels of training, these benefits may consist only of an enhanced ability to exercise without obvious physical discomfort. With more vigorous training programs, marked improvements in maximal oxygen uptake may occur. Those who are less fit may be satisfied with the endurance improvements brought on by a program of walking (18, 22), whereas endurance athletes will submit themselves to unbelievable rigorous training routines in efforts to compete successfully in aerobic endurance performances.

For those who are familiar with the strenuous training routines engaged in by endurance athletes, it is easy to be derisive about programs consisting of walking, mild calisthenics, and slow swimming or jogging. Although such moderate training routines cannot produce world-class endurance performers, they can improve the trainee's ability to exercise comfortably, and they may bring about measurable improvements in cardiovascular function and sometimes, even, in maximal oxygen uptake (44). Subjects in poor physical condition should be encouraged to do some type of endurance exercise. No matter how mild the program, it will undoubtedly be better than no program at all.

Intensity, Duration, and Frequency of Exercise Required to Improve $\dot{V}_{O_2}$ *max.* What is the minimal amount of exercise required to bring about measurable improvements in maximal oxygen uptake, the most commonly accepted measure of aerobic endurance fitness? Investigations of this matter have considered as little as 3 minutes of mild exercise per day to as much as an hour or more of heavy daily exercise (9, 10, 18, 22, 44, 50, 53). Subjects for most of the studies on exercise threshold for aerobic endurance enhancement have been adult males, and the training programs have usually emphasized continuous rather than interval exercise. A general conclusion that can be drawn from this research is that for most healthy, middle-aged men some improvement in maximal oxygen uptake can be expected if 1) the exercise intensity is at least that required to bring the heart rate above 130 beats per minute, 2) the duration of each exercise period at this intensity is at least 10 minutes, and 3) the frequency of training is at least three times per week. This minimum of 30 minutes per week does *not* include warm up time, does *not* include training for anything other than aerobic endurance fitness, and does *not* produce increases in maximal oxygen uptake for *every* trainee. It bears repeating, however, that a failure to produce changes in maximal oxygen uptake does not mean that a mild exercise program is totally useless. Other cardiovascular improvements may occur in the absence of changes in maximal oxygen uptake. For example, exercise at submaximal loads can be accomplished with lower heart rates, and more work can be accomplished without discomfort even though maximal oxygen uptake may not be enhanced.

Training Threshold for Improved $\dot{V}_{O_2}$ *max: Effects of Sex, Age and Fitness.* The minimal exercise program that can bring about increases in maximal oxygen uptakes for young adult women is similar to that for young adult men (27, 39). Accordingly, there does not seem to be a sex difference in adaptation to an aerobic endurance conditioning program. Age and pretraining physical condition are more important considerations, however. Research has shown that the maximal oxygen uptakes of youths and older adults are sometimes unresponsive to low-level training programs (9, 15, 41, 44). Other studies do show improvements in maximal oxygen uptakes for these extreme age groups, however (18, 23, 26, 44). Some of the discrepancies in results may be caused by differences in the total duration of the training programs or by differences in condition of the subjects before the training started.

Trainees who begin a conditioning program with a relatively high maximal oxygen uptake can expect either no changes or only minor improvements with mild to moderate training, whereas those who are in poor condition may experience increases of 30 per cent or more in maximal oxygen uptake (44, 46, 47). The usual improvement shown in maximal oxygen uptake for young and middle-aged subjects is about 15–20 per cent (44).

Suggested Ranges of Exercise Heart Rates for Aerobic Endurance Training. The practice of prescribing a single exercise heart rate, for example, 130 or 150 beats per minute, for aerobic training ignores the fact that such an exercise load might be too mild for a well-conditioned individual who wishes to achieve a *maximal* training effect but too severe for a trainee with cardiovascular disease. Even among normal untrained subjects there is a wide range of resting and maximal heart rates, depending upon age and heredity, so that exercise at a common heart rate will produce different relative intensities of work and different training effects (6, 52). Because of the age-related wide range of maximal heart rates, the practice of prescribing exercise solely as a percentage of maximal heart rate also will result in different relative exercise loads (17).

One way to facilitate exercise prescription is to estimate exercise intensity in relation to one's maximal oxygen uptake. Since at sub-maximal work loads, there is a linear relationship between heart rate and oxygen uptake (6), one can prescribe exercise at a heart rate that represents a given percentage of one's maximal oxygen uptake. Heart rates representing 40–75 per cent of maximal oxygen uptake have been suggested as target heart rates for aerobic training of nonathletic groups (17, 38, 45, 49, 51, 52). Unfortunately, it is not an easy matter to determine maximal oxygen uptakes for everyone who wishes to undertake an aerobic endurance training program. Consequently, an alternative method of prescribing target heart rates for training has been based on the difference between resting and predicted maximal heart rates and has found widespread acceptance (38). Karvonen (38) proposed that exercise heart rate should be at least the sum of the heart rate at rest plus 60 per cent of the difference between maximal and resting heart rates, that is,

$$HR_{Ex} = HR_{Rest} + 0.60 (HR_{Max} - HR_{Rest}).$$

Accordingly, if one's resting heart rate were 65 and his maximal heart rate were 205, the training heart rate should be greater than $65 + 0.60 (205 - 65) = 149$. The basis for this technique is that the difference between resting and maximal heart rates for a given person represents the reserve of his heart for increasing cardiac output. Exercise at a heart rate representing a high percentage of this reserve should then be adequate to bring about appropriate cardiovascular adaptations. The Karvonen technique is not without its detractors, however. It has been pointed out that the prediction of maximal heart rate, even when adjusted for age, is subject to error, especially when dealing with cardiac patients (34). For those in good health, however, the Karvonen technique seems to be a good compromise solution to the problem of exercise prescription.

In Table 14.1 are illustrated suggested ranges of exercise heart rates for aerobic endurance training of persons with various ages and resting heart rates. In each case, the low end of the range was determined by 1) substracting the resting heart rate from the predicted maximal heart rate for subjects of various ages (6, 52), 2) multiplying the difference so obtained by 0.5 (50 per cent of "cardiac reserve"), and 3) adding the value found in 2) to the resting heart rate to find the training heart rate. The high end of each range was calculated as 95 per cent of the trainee's predicted maximal heart rate. If a trainee were 15 years old with a resting heart rate of 80 beats per minute, his heart rate during exercise periods should be maintained above 142 (205 − 80 = 125; 0.5 × 125 = 62.5; 62.5 + 80 = 142.5). The exercise heart rate so determined should represent a minimal or threshold intensity of training for the individual to insure that the training will be strenuous enough to cause some adaptations of the heart and circulation and perhaps measurable improvements in maximal oxygen uptake (18, 19, 22, 34, 39, 44). For greater assurance of improvements in maximal oxygen uptake, one should exercise at greater than threshold levels. For the same 15-year-old trainee, the maximal

Table 14.1.   Suggested Ranges of Exercise Heart Rates for Aerobic Endurance Training. Training at low heart rates should improve endurance, but may not increase maximal oxygen uptake. Training at high heart rates will maximize rate of improvement in endurance and maximal oxygen uptake; it is recommended for athletes.

Age (years)	Estimated Max. H.R.	Heart Rate While Standing At Rest				
		50	60	70	80	90
5	205			138–195	142–195	148–195
10	210			140–200	145–200	150–200
15	205		132–198	138–195	142–195	148–195
20–25	200	125–190	130–190	135–190	140–190	145–190
30	195	122–185	128–185	132–185	138–185	142–185
35	190	120–180	125–180	130–180	135–180	140–180
40	185	118–176	122–176	128–176	132–176	138–176
45	180	115–171	120–171	125–171	130–171	135–171
50	175	112–166	118–166	122–166	128–166	132–166
55	170	110–162	115–162	120–162	125–162	130–162
60	165	108–157	112–157	118–157	122–157	128–157
65	160	105–152	110–152	115–152	120–152	125–152
70	155	102–147	108–147	112–147	118–147	122–147

training heart rate should be about 195 beats per minute (205 × 0.95 = 195). By exercising at 95 per cent of predicted maximal heart rate, the oxygen uptake during exercise should be maximal (6, 44). This high intensity of exercise is most often used in athletic training and is usually too high for ordinary conditioning programs.

If one exercises at an intensity greater than 95 per cent of maximal heart rate, maximal oxygen uptake will not increase further, but anaerobic metabolism will produce high levels of lactic acid, and less work will be accomplished during the training period. However, training at greater than 95 per cent of maximal heart rate is necessary for improving the anaerobic capacity of distance athletes, so that sprints at the start and finish of a race may be prolonged.

There are substantial individual differences in what constitutes the optimal exercise intensity for aerobic conditioning. The suggested ranges of exercise heart rates shown in Table 14.1 should encompass the optimal values for all trainees, with the possible exception of some patients with cardiovascular disease and some elderly persons who should perhaps exercise at lower heart rates (34). Exercise prescription has not been developed to the point where a simple measure can be used as the sole basis of a precise prescription for all individuals. It remains for the individual trainee, the exercise leader, the physician, the physical educator, and the coach to use judgement based on knowledge of the trainee to select the appropriate exercise heart rate within the ranges shown in Table 14.1 or to modify the ranges as necessary for unique individuals and circumstances.

Continuous and Interval Training. Both continuous exercise periods and interval training can produce similar improvements in aerobic potential, but it is generally agreed that more world–class athletes have achieved supremacy through interval training than through continuous training programs. Also, it seems that interval training can provoke endurance adaptations more rapidly than continuous training. It has been suggested that interval training may be superior in bringing about adaptations that result in a greater *rate* of aerobic and anaerobic energy replenishment, but that continuous training is preferred to increase one's capacity to work for prolonged periods *at a high percentage of maximal oxygen uptake* (6). The usual case is that athletes use both interval and continuous exercises in their training programs if for no other reason than to prevent boredom.

Nearly any form of rhythmic exercise, such as, running, cycling, swimming, handball, tennis, walking, and soccer, can be used in continuous or interval training with satisfactory results (44). Cooper (14) has produced a practical method of equating different types of exercise for their cardiovascular benefits, in which a variety of points are awarded for completion of various intensities and durations of activity. Both continuous and interval exercise should last a minimum of 10 minutes for each training period and should be repeated at least three times per week (29, 40, 44, 50). For athletic training, the usual weekly practice schedule includes 4–5 training sessions of 40–90 minutes each.

The optimal intensity of exercise programs has been discussed in the previous section and illustrated in Table 14.1. For high-level athletic conditioning with *continuous* exercise, heart rates of 160–175 during exercise are common for young adults. The high end of the ranges for exercise heart rates shown in Table 14.1 can be used to indicate training heart rates for interval training programs for athletes and others who desire high levels of aerobic fitness. When using *interval* training for the maximal improvement of aerobic potential, it is important to achieve maximal or near maximal oxygen uptakes during each exercise period, but not to exceed the exercise intensity that will provoke maximal oxygen uptake. The reason for this is that heavier loads must be met by progressively greater contributions of anaerobic metabolism, and exhaustion ensues more quickly to reduce the total work performed during the training session.

$\dot{V}_{O_2}$ Can Be Stressed Maximally by Working At Less Than Maximal Intensity. To place stress on the cardiovascular and muscular mechanisms that bring maximal improvements in maximal oxygen uptake, it is not necessary to work at maximal intensity. It has been demonstrated that maximal oxygen uptake is reached at about 95 per cent of maximal heart rate or at about 80 per cent of maximal performance speed for a given training distance (6, 44). Determining the appropriate speed for stressing maximal oxygen uptake at a given training distance becomes a simple matter if either maximal heart rate or fastest time for the distance is known. Thus, if Bjorn Blookerfeist has a maximal heart rate of 200 beats per minute and a best time of 120 seconds for the 800 meter run, he could run repeat 800's at a heart rate of $200 \times 0.95 = 190$ beats per minute. Since Bjorn's maximal speed for the 800 meters is $800/120 = 6.67$ m/sec, he could run repeat 800's at 80 per cent of that speed ($.80 \times 6.67 = 5.34$ m/sec). At this speed, Bjorn's training time for each 800 meter run would be $800/5.34 = 150$ seconds to insure that maximal oxygen uptake will be reached during most of the exercise periods (assuming short recovery intervals). As stated in previous paragraphs, it is not necessary to work at 95 per cent of maximal heart rate to bring about *some* improvement in maximal oxygen uptake. This type of high intensity work is needed only by those who want to get the greatest possible improvement in maximal oxygen uptake in the shortest possible time.

Suggested Lengths of Work and Recovery Intervals for Aerobic Interval Training. Convincing evidence that short work intervals produce lesser improvements in aerobic potential than longer intervals is not available. Although most trainees should be able to achieve maximal oxygen uptakes more consistently with 3–5 minute work periods (6), actual comparisons of adaptations in maximal oxygen uptake induced by short and long periods have produced discordant results (28, 40). The data of Knuttgen and his coworkers (40) suggested that 3-minute exercise periods interspersed with 3-minute recovery periods produced greater gains in maximal oxygen uptake than did a 15-second exercise and 15-second recovery regimen. On the other hand, Fox and his colleagues (28) found greater improvements in trainees who completed shorter work intervals (8–40 seconds) than in those who trained for longer durations (2½–5 minutes). Because of differences in subject populations, strict comparisons between the two studies are not possible. Therefore, it is suggested that both brief and longer periods be included in interval training programs to provide variety, to enhance anaerobic potential and to improve aerobic potential. However, the emphasis should be placed on equal work and recovery periods of 3–5 minutes duration to enable more trainees to maintain maximal oxygen uptake during more of the workout period (6). If shorter work intervals are used, the rest intervals should also be shortened to help maintain high oxygen uptakes throughout the training session (6).

Figure 14.1 illustrates the theoretical rise and fall of oxygen uptake and oxygen deficit during an aerobic interval training period.

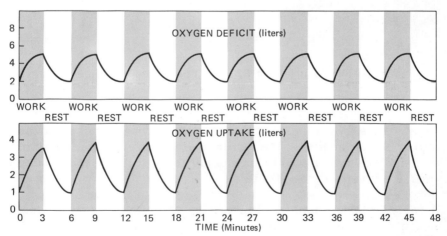

Figure 14.1 Hypothetical rise and fall of oxygen uptake and oxygen deficit during an interval training period designed to enhance aerobic endurance.

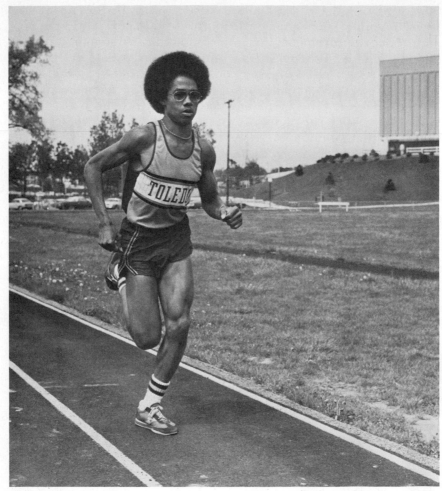

Figure 14.2. Work intervals must be of high intensity for optimal aerobic endurance training. (Courtesy of Office of Public Information, University of Toledo, Toledo, Ohio.)

Note that the trainee's maximal oxygen uptake of 4.0 liters is reached during all but the first of the 3-minute exercise periods, and that oxygen deficit is not allowed to accumulate to the subject's maximal oxygen deficit capacity of 6.0 liters.

Aerobic Training Should Be Progressive. As with any form of fitness training, aerobic conditioning programs are most effective when the exercise routines become progressively more difficult with increasing weeks and months of training. The reason for this is that the body adapts only to unaccustomed stress; as adaptations are made to one level of exercise training, that level no longer provides an unaccustomed stress, so what was once difficult becomes relatively easy. Therefore, the cardiovascular system and other organ systems that have adapted to one intensity of exercise must be overloaded by greater intensities of exercise if greater adaptations are desired.

There are two common methods used to ensure the progressive nature of an aerobic training program. One is to predict (guess) the appropriate times to increase the exercise load, duration and frequency on the basis of past experiences with similar trainees. This is the method used by some athletic coaches who plan a detailed training schedule for their athletes for the entire season without the slightest bit of evidence that those athletes have adapted to each step of the training routine. While it is true that those coaches with great experience may be very successful with this sort of program, it is also true that some individual trainees in such a program would be better suited to a more individualized approach, based on physiological evidence that adaptations to one level of training were achieved before subsequent levels were attempted.

A second method of ensuring the progressive nature of aerobic training is to base the training intensity upon a certain exercise heart rate, that is, 95 per cent of maximal heart rate, 50 per cent of maximal heart rate, heart rate of 130 beats per minute, 170 beats per minute, and so on. The principle underlying this training scheme is that as the body adapts to exercise, the resting heart rate and the heart rate for a given submaximal exercise load will be reduced (6). Therefore, as the individual becomes better trained, a greater exercise load will be required to elicit a given heart rate. For an untrained person, it takes very little activity to bring about a heart rate of 150; up to a point, a much greater work load is required to elicit a heart rate of 150 after a period of training. Likewise, 80 per cent of maximal heart rate can be achieved by a smaller intensity of exercise before training than after some weeks of training. This technique of basing exercise load on heart rate obviously requires that the trainee become accustomed to measuring his heart rate several times during each workout.

At that point in a training program, when one has increased his maximal oxygen uptake to its hereditary limit, a plateau will be reached at which there is no longer a reduction in heart rate for a given exercise load, no matter how long one trains at that load. At this point, a training program based solely upon exercising at a given heart rate (with the possible exception of extremely high rates such as 95 per cent of maximum) will no longer insure the attainment of progressive increases in exercise load and aerobic endurance capacity. When, after a few weeks of training at a given load, the trainee finds that he does not have to exercise at a faster rate or with a heavier load to attain the same exercise heart rate, he must conclude that he has reached a heart rate plateau. He must then work at a higher level that will elicit a faster heart rate if he is to continue improving his capacity to persist in exercise at a high percentage of his maximal oxygen uptake. (Even though one reaches a limit in $\dot{V}_{O_2}$ max improvement, he can continue to enhance his ability to work for longer times at greater percentages of that $\dot{V}_{O_2}$ max.)

LOSS OF AEROBIC FITNESS UPON CESSATION OF TRAINING

If one who has become conditioned to aerobic forms of exercise stops training, he can expect to lose most of the benefits of training within two weeks to three months (11, 21, 30, 42, 45). Values of maximal oxygen uptake, heart rate response to submaximal exercise, heart rate recovery after exercise, and resting heart rates usually revert to pretraining levels faster than the total capacity for submaximal work. Thus, part of the increased endurance to submaximal work tasks that is brought on by training must result from such "psychological" factors as increased tolerance to pain, greater motivation, or reduced anxiety, in addition to improvements in cardiovascular and muscular function (5, 30). The "psychological" improvements seem to persist longer than the cardiovascular changes. The fact that aerobic fitness is transient in nature illustrates the need for *regularity* in exercise training. It is not possible to retain a moderate level of aerobic fitness by playing golf once a week or even daily during the summer months alone. It does not make sense to plan for aerobic fitness during only four or five months of the year. On the other hand, training during the summer, providing it progresses slowly, is better than no training at all, and absence from a training program because of prolonged illness does not mean that prior training was necessarily wasted; but the evidence suggests that regularity in exercise programs should be the goal of all types of fitness conditioning.

MAINTENANCE OF PREVIOUSLY ACQUIRED AEROBIC FITNESS

A general principle of fitness programs is that it takes less activity to maintain an established level of fitness than to acquire it in the first place. This principle also is applicable to aerobic fitness. Several studies have reported that after vigorous conditioning programs, aerobic fitness (usually assessed by measures of maximal oxygen uptake) can be maintained by workouts 30–60 minutes long, 1–3 times weekly (11, 29, 45). These studies have included training and maintenance programs conducted for relatively short periods, and it is unknown whether low level maintenance programs can maintain fitness for a year or longer. From the data available, however, we conclude that a conservative recommendation for maintenance of aerobic fitness is a 30-minute training session three times weekly, with an exercise load similar to that used originally to acquire aerobic fitness. Although this recommendation may include more work than is absolutely essential, it seems advisable to risk such an error than to risk advising a program that may not be adequate to maintain fitness.

ADAPTATIONS TO AEROBIC ENDURANCE TRAINING

The physiological effects of physical training with continuous, rhythmic exercise have been frequently studied for many years. Although there are many contradictory reports that have resulted from these studies, there are, nevertheless, some generally accepted accounts of "typical" or expected adaptations to regular endurance training. As these adaptations are described, the reader should keep in mind that many factors can minimize or enhance the likelihood that any given adaptation will occur. Some of these factors are set forth below.

Cardiovascular Function During Maximal Work

It is widely recognized that aerobic endurance training can improve physical performance by causing substantial changes in cardiovascular function during maximal work. Because of the widespread interest in discovering means to prevent the early onset of degenerative heart disease, the role of exercise in improving cardiovascular function has come under increasing scrutiny. The most accepted measure of the effectiveness of exercise training in enhancing cardiovascular function is the nearly universal increase in maximal oxygen uptake that occurs with training.

Maximal Oxygen Uptake.   As described in the previous chapter, maximal oxygen uptake is, in those without lung pathology, a function of maximal cardiac output (the ability of the heart to deliver blood to the working muscles) and maximal arteriovenous oxygen difference (the ability of the circulation to shift blood from non-working regions of the body to working muscles, and the ability of those muscles to extract the oxygen from the blood so that ATP can be replenished aerobically). Therefore, maximal oxygen uptake can be viewed as a measure of maximal cardiovascular function, and improvements in maximal oxygen uptake after exercise training must be caused to some extent by improved maximal cardiovascular function.

Factors Influencing Improvement in Maximal Oxygen Uptake. Changes in maximal oxygen uptake as a result of aerobic training range from no improvement to increases as great as 43 per cent and more (44). The extent of any training effect depends on many factors, including physical condition prior to initiation of training, age, mode of exercise during assessment of maximal oxygen uptake, heredity, and type of training program. Both males and females respond to aerobic training with similar increments in maximal oxygen uptake, so *sex of the trainee is not an important factor in predicting improvements in maximal oxygen uptake* as long as other factors, especially the type of training, are equal (44). Whether or not training at a high altitude has a beneficial effect, compared with sea-level training, on maximal oxygen uptake is controversial. There seems to be no value in training at 2,300 meters as opposed to sea level (2), but this altitude may be below the threshold altitude (3,000 m.?), above which benefits have been observed in other studies (16, 20).

Physical Condition Prior to Training. Increases in maximal oxygen uptake in response to a training program are the least in those persons who are most fit, and the greatest in those who are least fit before the training program begins (6, 44, 47). Subjects who have been bedridden for several weeks or completely inactive for several years can expect to achieve a 30 per cent increase in maximal oxygen uptake (47), whereas fit endurance athletes may experience no further gains in maximal oxygen uptake with an additional training period (46). The underlying basis for this phenomenon is that each individual has a certain potential for optimal cardiac development, circulatory function, and muscular development, so that inactive persons have further to go to achieve their potentials than do habitually active persons. Most studies of changes in maximal oxygen uptake caused by aerobic endurance training in untrained men have shown improvements of 15–20 per cent (44, 47).

Age. Comparisons of improvements in maximal oxygen uptake for various age groups is somewhat difficult because of the scarcity of literature describing changes in very young and very old subjects, and because it is rare that very young or old subjects train at the high intensities often achieved by young and middle-aged adults. Thus, training programs are often not strictly comparable. From the evidence available, it appears that youths 10–15 years of age can achieve the same percentage increments in maximal oxygen uptake as older subjects (23, 41), but that elderly trainees can expect somewhat lesser improvements in aerobic power (44, 47). The apparent reason why elderly trainees do not experience as great a percentage improvement in maximal oxygen uptake is that they may be functioning closer to their maximal cardiovascular potential than younger persons. This is because age is associated with a reduction in maximal cardiac output as maximal heart rate falls from 200 in youth to about 160 at age 65 (6). Also, maximal pulmonary ventilation during exercise of short duration is lowered from 140–160 l/min at age 25, to 80 l/min or less in those 65 years of age and older (48). This reduction in maximal exercise ventilation is probably due to connective tissue changes in the joints of the rib cage that lead to stiffening of those joints and to gradual deterioration in lung and bronchial structure so that airway resistance is increased (48).

It should be emphasized once again that part of the lesser improvement in maximal oxygen uptake observed in elderly trainees is probably accounted for by the fact that exercise programs for the elderly tend to be very conservative with rather mild intensities of work prescribed. It may be that an older subject who engages in *heavy* training may experience just as great an improvement in aerobic power as his younger counterpart.

Mode of Exercise During Assessment of Maximal Oxygen Uptake. The magnitude of any effect of aerobic endurance training on maximal oxygen uptake depends to some extent on whether the exercise task used to evaluate oxygen uptake is similar to the exercise used in training. For example, if one trains by cycling but is tested for maximal oxygen uptake on a treadmill, smaller gains in aerobic power are apt to be observed than if the trainee were tested on a bicycle ergometer (43). Likewise, training by swimming increases maximal oxygen uptake when measured during tethered swimming, but not when measured with a treadmill test. The apparent reason for different maximal oxygen uptake adaptations when different types of exercise tests are used is that muscles specifically trained in one type of exercise, for example, arm muscles in swim training, do not have the same involvement in one form of exercise test as in another, such as, treadmill walking versus tethered swimming. Consequently, training–induced adaptations in the ability of muscles to extract oxygen from the blood or improvements in local circulation to the working muscles may not be evaluated properly with an exercise test that does not specifically stress those muscles.

A practical consequence of this phenomenon of exercise specificity in maximal oxygen uptake adaptations is that aerobic endurance training in one form of exercise is not necessarily of benefit when the trainee performs another type of physical activity requiring the use of untrained muscles. This is the common experience of many who, thinking themselves to be in "good shape" because they practiced basketball regularly, find that they become rapidly fatigued in a game of squash, in swimming, or in some other activity for which they have not specifically trained.

Heredity.   Not all trainees of the same environmental, social, economic, and educational background improve their maximal oxygen uptakes to the same extent with the same type of training. In other words, there seem to be some inborn factors that predispose certain individuals to have greater adaptations to training than others (44). Whether differences in populations of muscle fiber types, pain thresholds, emotions, enzyme systems, or some other differences in biological characteristics will eventually be shown to explain the variability in maximal oxygen uptake adaptations to training remains to be seen.

Type of Training.   Previously in this chapter, we learned that marked differences in the degree of change in maximal oxygen uptake are associated with differences in training programs. A program consisting of 5–10 minutes of walking twice per week will almost certainly produce no change in maximal oxygen uptake, whereas large increases in oxygen uptake can be produced as adaptations to more strenuous types of training (44).

Maximal Cardiac Output, Heart Rate and Stroke Volume.   In previously sedentary young adult males, about 50 per cent of the increase in maximal oxygen uptake that occurs with endurance training is associated with an increased maximal cardiac output, and 50 per cent, with an increased maximal arteriovenous oxygen difference, whereas in fit young males, in older males, and in females nearly all of the increase in maximal oxygen uptake has been attributed to a greater maximal cardiac output (6, 46, 47). Accordingly, it can be stated that the improvement in maximal cardiac output with aerobic training is at least as important as any other change in maximal cardiovascular function and may be the *only* significant change observed in some subjects (46).

The maximal cardiac output typically rises from untrained values of 22 or 16 *l*/min in young adult males and females, respectively, to 24 and 18 *l*/min after aerobic endurance training (6, 47). This training-induced rise in maximal cardiac output is not a function of a greater maximal heart rate after training because, if anything, the maximal heart rate declines slightly with training (6, 44, 47). Consequently, the greater maximal cardiac output after training must be the result of a greater stroke volume (6, 46, 47). Pretraining maximal stroke volumes of 110 and 80 ml for young adult males and females, respectively, typically increase to 122 and 96 ml after several months of aerobic training (6, 47).

The increased stroke volume observed as an adaptation to aerobic endurance training is often related to an increased heart volume, which also results from such training (6). Accordingly, a larger, stronger heart is able to deliver more blood to the arteries than an untrained heart. However, greater stroke volume is sometimes found in the absence of cardiac hypertrophy (8). This suggests that the greater stroke volume may be the result of greater cardiac contractility. In animal studies, exercise training has been associated with improvements in cardiac contractility, but whether or not a similar adaptation in humans is responsible for the greater stroke volume after training remains to be firmly established (8, 46).

Maximal Arteriovenous Oxygen Difference, Muscular Blood Flow and Oxygen Extraction. In untrained young men, maximal differences between oxygen in arterial and mixed venous blood average about 14.4 ml O_2 per 100 ml blood, whereas after training that value may be raised to 15.5 ml O_2 per 100 ml blood (47). This 8 per cent rise in maximal arteriovenous oxygen difference can account for half the observed increments in maximal oxygen uptake in many subjects. This greater arteriovenous oxygen difference could be produced by training if a greater fraction of the cardiac output were shifted to the working muscles, but this does not seem to happen (46). Although there may be a greater maximal blood flow to trained working muscles (a point of controversy (13)), there is also more blood delivered to nonworking regions (46). The problem of whether training increases maximal muscular blood flow remains unresolved because of technical difficulties in measuring this flow, but evidence is accumulating that maximal blood flow is *not* increased by training (36).

Accordingly, the increase in maximal arteriovenous oxygen difference caused by training must be the result of some factor(s) that increase the rate of oxygen extraction from the blood by the working muscles. The precise mechanism by which this increased oxygen extraction is accomplished is unknown. Three of the possibilities that have been suggested include: 1) an enhanced diffusion of oxygen from capillary to muscle because of greater stores of myoglobin in trained muscles, 2) a greater number of capillaries for each muscle fiber so that oxygen can diffuse more readily to the working fibers, and 3) a greater ability of skeletal muscle mitochondria to make use of delivered oxygen (46). There is evidence that aerobic training does result in greater myoglobin concentrations in trained muscles (36), but the role of myoglobin in promoting diffusion of oxygen during exercise is not proved. Although experiments with laboratory animals suggest that training produces more capillaries per unit area of muscle, these results are not necessarily representative of what happens in man (47).

Holloszy (36) has speculated that the greater maximal arteriovenous oxygen difference observed after training may be the result of an increased number and/or size of mitochondria, which can consume more oxygen. He illustrates this possibility by citing a hypothetical case wherein oxygen delivery to an *untrained* muscle working maximally would be adequate to allow the mitochondria of that muscle to consume 98 per cent of the oxygen that those mitochondria could potentially consume. If there is no greater maximal blood flow to the working muscle after a physical training program (47), the fact that more work is done with maximal exercise after training means that more oxygen must be consumed by the muscles, and that the level of oxygen in the muscle and muscle capillaries must be lower during maximal exercise after training. If during the training the number and/or size of mitochondria in the muscle cells increased 50 per cent, the oxygen level in the muscles during maximal exercise might fall to the point where the mitochondria could consume oxygen at a rate equal to only 75 per cent of their maximal potential. Assuming that the maximal oxygen-consuming capacity of the untrained mitochondria was 100, then oxygen consumption of these *untrained* mitochondria during maximal exercise was $0.98 \times 100 = 98$. *After training*, the maximal capacity of the mitochondria increased by 50 per cent to 150, so that when working at 75 per cent of capacity during maximal work, the oxygen consumption of the trained mitochondria was $0.75 \times 150 = 112.5$, an increase of 14.8 per cent in oxygen consumption over the 98 found in the untrained muscles. This 14.8 per cent hypothetical increase in maximal oxygen consumption was accomplished by a 50 per cent increase in mitochondrial mass, a very reasonable estimate (36). Thus, even though blood flow to the working muscles may ultimately limit maximal oxygen uptake (7, 25), it is possible that mitochondrial adaptations can allow greater extraction of the delivered oxygen in trained muscles to increase maximal oxygen uptake.

Blood Pressure During Maximal Exercise. There is no evidence that blood pressure during maximal exercise is changed with training. Of course, more work at the maximum level is done after training, so the trained person has a lower blood pressure per unit of work accomplished during maximal effort.

Blood Characteristics

Changes in the blood at rest and during maximal effort, as the result of aerobic training, are described in Chapter 12. Most of the changes, such as, lower venous oxygen content, higher venous carbon dioxide content, and greater venous and arterial lactic acid concentration, are secondary effects of the greater aerobic and anaerobic capacities of the trained skeletal muscles and the greater capacity of the heart to deliver oxygen to these muscles.

Aerobic Endurance Performance

Improvements in performance of such aerobic activites as running, swimming, and cycling cannot be entirely accounted for by improvements in maximal oxygen uptake. As Saltin (47) has pointed out, endurance athletes of recent years have maximal oxygen uptakes that are similar to endurance athletes of the 1930's. But contemporary competitive endurance performance records are substantially improved over the older records. Also, the improvement in maximal oxygen uptake with training is usually restricted to about 15–20 per cent in healthy persons, but performance times often can improve by 30 per cent or more in this same training period. Both of these observations support the contention that factors other than improved maximal cardiovascular function are involved in the improved performances that accompany aerobic endurance training. It seems likely that two of those additional factors are an improved anaerobic capacity and an enhanced tolerance to the physical and psychological discomfort experienced during heavy work. For work lasting longer than about 10 minutes, another important factor may be an improved ability to work at high percentages of one's maximal oxygen uptake with a lesser contribution of anaerobic metabolism. This possibility is discussed in more detail later in this chapter.

Cardiovascular Function During Submaximal Work

Except for athletes, a more important consideration than adaptations during maximal work are adaptations resulting from aerobic training that enable one to persist at higher levels of submaximal work with less disturbance of homeostasis. Such adaptations enable one to perform occupational labor more easily at higher rates, perform work around the home or garden with less distress, and engage in more demanding recreational pursuits for longer periods with more gratification.

Oxygen Cost of Submaximal Work (Mechanical Efficiency). For a given submaximal work load in a simple task such as walking at 2.5 miles per hour, it is generally conceded that the trained person requires the same amount of oxygen to perform the task as he did before training (6, 36). This means that training in a task such as walking produces no great change in *mechanical efficiency* (calories of work produced/calories of energy expended to produce the work). For fast running or for more complex tasks, such as, swimming, shoveling or lifting, small improvements in efficiency do result from training as the trainee gradually learns to use only the necessary musculature required to accomplish the task. In this way, oxygen consumption by extraneous motor units is eliminated.

It might also be expected that the reduced reliance on anaerobic energy production in trained persons would reduce total oxygen cost since the theoretical oxygen cost of removing lactic acid during recovery is twice as great as the oxygen equivalent of the energy released by the lactic acid production (35). However, actual measurements appear to show a 1 to 1 relationship between oxygen deficit and oxygen debt in steady state, short duration exercise (31). Thus, with heavy submaximal exercise where no skill learning is involved, oxygen uptake *during exercise* increases due to greater aerobic contributions to ATP replenishment, but oxygen uptake in *recovery* is reduced since less oxygen deficit is accumulated in the trained state. The *total* oxygen uptake is unchanged by training.

Cardiac Output, Heart Rate, and Stroke Volume During Submaximal Work. Most experiments show that there is no significant change in cardiac output during submaximal work as an effect of training, but some show a small reduction of cardiac output in the trained state (6, 47). Heart rate during the work is nearly always reduced and the stroke volume increased with training (6, 47). The increased stroke volume is probably the result of a greater heart volume and/or improved cardiac contractility (8). Accordingly, if a subject could run at 7 miles per hour with a cardiac output of 14 liters per minute, a heart rate of 165 beats per minute, and a stroke volume of 80 milliliters before training, he might be able to run at the same pace with the same cardiac output, but with a heart rate of 150 and stroke volume of 93 milliliters after several months of aerobic training.

Arteriovenous O_2 Difference, Muscle Blood Flow and O_2 Extraction During Submaximal Work. As discussed previously, oxygen cost is usually unchanged, and cardiac output during standard, submaximal work is unchanged or is slightly reduced with training. Therefore, arteriovenous oxygen difference must increase during the exercise to account for an increased contribution of aerobic energy production as a result of training (6). Contrary to popular opinion, blood flow to working muscles after training is somewhat reduced from the values found before training (13). Accordingly, the greater arteriovenous oxygen differences found in trained subjects exercising at a standard work load cannot be caused by a greater shift of blood volume to the working muscles, and must be the result of a greater extraction of oxygen by those muscles. This greater extraction of oxygen during submaximal work is simply the result of the increased diffusion gradient for oxygen from the blood to the muscle as the partial pressure of oxygen in the muscle cell and tissue fluid is reduced by mitochondrial activity. In other words, there is a reserve of blood flow to the working muscles that can be reduced by training with no adverse effects; the decreased flow is compensated for by more rapid diffusion of the decreased oxygen supply. During submaximal work, oxygen delivery is not limiting for muscular work.

Blood Pressure During Submaximal Exercise. Systemic arterial blood pressure during a standard submaximal work task has been found to be either decreased (12), unchanged (6) or slightly increased (4) as an effect of training. A decreased blood pressure could be the result of reduced peripheral resistance as more blood flows through nonworking regions (46). An increased pressure could be viewed as a means of providing greater force to drive blood into contracting muscles. After training, cardiac output is either unchanged or reduced with submaximal work, blood flow to nonworking regions of the body is increased (46), and the blood volume is only slightly greater (6). Therefore, it appears that any increased blood pressure must be caused by a decreased vasodilatation in the working muscles as evidenced by reported reductions in muscle blood flow during submaximal work (13).

Blood Characteristics During Submaximal Exercise

At light work loads, one would not expect to find any major effects of physical training on blood characteristics because there are so few other functional changes that are observed during such work. At higher work intensities, the major effect of training is a reduction in blood lactic acid and a concomitant rise in pH as a result of a decreased reliance on anaerobic glycolysis for energy. This decreased anaerobic contribution to ATP replenishment is brought about by a greater size and/or number of mitochondria as will be described.

Pulmonary Function During Submaximal Work

There is little or no effect of endurance training on pulmonary function during very light, submaximal work loads, with the possible exception that the breathing rate is reduced and the depth of breathing increased (6). At heavier work loads, where there is less anaerobic involvement after training than before, the ventilation rate is somewhat lower after training, and the ventilation volume per liter of oxygen consumed is reduced (6). This adaptation is achieved as a direct result of the decreased lactic acid in the blood of the trained person at a heavy, submaximal work load. With less lactic acid production, there is less acid to stimulate breathing by way of the arterial chemoreceptors.

Endurance to Submaximal Work Loads

A universal adaptation associated with training is that the completion of previously difficult tasks becomes easier, and progressively greater work loads can be accomplished without undue discomfort and fatigue. The mechanisms underlying this adaptation probably vary with work intensity. With mild work where there is no substantial accumulation of oxygen deficit or lactic acid, it seems likely that improvements in 1) mechanical efficiency (for complex skills only) and 2) psychological tolerance to the work are mostly responsible for an enhanced ability to persist at a given task. With heavier work that relies to a moderate extent on anaerobic glycolysis for ATP replenishment, that is, work that can be tolerated for 10 minutes to 1 hour or more, additional factors that contribute to increased endurance are 1) greater anaerobic capacity, 2) greater glycogen stores, 3) improved temperature regulation and 4) greater mitochondrial capacity for aerobic ATP replenishment. Improvements in anaerobic capacity and glycogen storage have been described in Chapter 10 and 5, respectively, and the faster sweating response to exercise in trained persons, which reduces the amount of blood that must be shifted away from muscles to the skin for cooling purposes, will be described in the following chapter. The enhanced mitochondrial capacity for aerobic energy production deserves further comment.

It has been conclusively shown in laboratory animals and in man that aerobic endurance training causes a substantial increase in the synthesis of mitochondrial membranes as reflected by greater numbers and/or sizes of mitochondria in trained muscles (36, 37). These structural changes are accompanied by greater capacities of the trained mitochondria to produce ATP as a result of greater activities of enzymes of the Krebs Cycle, the electron transport system, and other metabolic systems related to ATP production (36). These mitochondrial changes can explain how trained muscles produce less lactic acid for a submaximal work load than do untrained muscles. First, one must be aware that important enzymes of glycolysis are stimulated by a buildup of ADP in the sarcoplasm of the muscle; the greater the concentration of ADP, the faster the rate of glycolysis. Therefore, any factor that leads to a *reduced* level of ADP in the sarcoplasm can reduce the rate of glycolysis and lactic acid production. Second, it is known that the consumption of oxygen by mitochondria (and the associated production of ATP) is dependent upon the presence of ADP. Thus, for a given steady-state level of oxygen consumption by a single mitochondrion to occur, there must exist a certain mitochondrial concentration of ADP. This ADP diffuses into the mitochondria from the sarcoplasm. Accordingly, in a trained muscle with more mitochondria or a greater number of electron transport assemblies in larger mitochondria, each mitochondrion or electron transport assembly would have to consume proportionately less oxygen, at lower concentrations of ADP, to produce the same total oxygen consumption in the entire muscle. Since a lower concentration of ADP is thereby required, aerobic ATP replenishment can reach a steady state more rapidly with less oxygen deficit, less anaerobic glycolysis, and less lactic acid production (Fig. 14.3) (36).

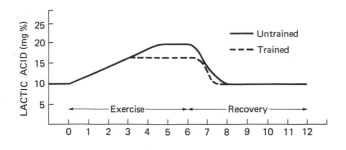

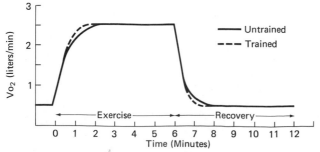

Figure 14.3. Effect of training on oxygen uptake and lactic acid accumulation during submaximal exercise.

As an illustration, assume that before training, a small muscle had 100 mitochondria, and that this muscle could perform a certain type of work with a total oxygen uptake of 1,000 atoms of oxygen per minute, that is, each mitochondrion consumed 10 atoms of oxygen per minute. Assume, further, that there had to be 5,000 ADP molecules in the sarcoplasm of the muscle to provide for diffusion of enough ADP into each mitochondrion to stimulate oxygen consumption at a rate of 10 atoms per minute. After training, assume that the muscle had twice as many (for example, 200) electron transport assemblies, either because of more mitochondria, more assemblies in larger mitochondria, or both. In this trained state, each mitochondrion of the muscle had to consume oxygen at only 5 atoms per minute to achieve the same total oxygen uptake of 1,000 atoms per minute for the submaximal work load. But since a lower concentration of ADP is required to stimulate an oxygen uptake of 5 atoms per minute rather than 10 by each electron transport assembly, perhaps only 2,500 ADP molecules were needed in the sarcoplasm of the muscle to provide adequate delivery of ADP to the mitochondria. Therefore, a steady state of oxygen uptake to balance ATP breakdown could be achieved faster at a lower concentration of ADP and with a reduced production of lactic acid.

An additional adaptation to aerobic training that is observed during submaximal exercise is a greater use of fat for energy (6, 36). Not only does training reduce respiratory exchange ratio (respiratory quotient) during exercise, but it also increases the rate of carbon dioxide production by muscles from radioactively labeled fatty acids (36). Both of these results support the belief that trained muscles oxidize relatively more fat than untrained muscles. The mechanism responsible for this change in energy metabolism is not entirely clear, but may involve a greater capacity of mitochondria in trained muscles to oxidize fatty acids (36). This adaptation in fat metabolism is important because the increased reliance on fat for energy allows muscle glycogen to be spared. Since muscle glycogen stores are directly related to endurance in moderately heavy work, a conservation of carbohydrates can extend performance time. Also, greater reliance on fat means that less energy is required from the anaerobic breakdown of glycogen to lactic acid.

Cardiovascular Function at Rest

It is generally agreed that resting rates of oxygen consumption in trained persons do not differ significantly from those in untrained persons (6). Also, resting cardiac output, regional blood flow, and arteriovenous oxygen difference are usually unchanged after training (6). Resting heart rate is almost invariably reduced 5–10 beats per minute with at least a few weeks of aerobic endurance training (6, 44). This training *bradycardia* is probably caused by increased activity of the parasympathetic nerves to the heart or by greater stores of acetylcholine in the heart itself, but some believe a decreased sensitivity to the sympathetic transmitters, adrenaline and noradrenaline, is also important (8). This bradycardia at rest and during submaximal exercise probably results in lower oxygen consumption by the heart, an adaptation that may help to explain the protective effect of exercise in minimizing the risk of early death from coronary heart disease (8).

If a normal resting cardiac output is to be maintained with a decreased heart rate, it is obvious that stroke volume must be greater at rest in trained individuals. This increased stroke volume, for example, from about 70 ml. before training to perhaps 81 ml. after training, may be due to greater heart size or to improved cardiac contractility (8).

Resting Blood Pressure.   Any reduction in resting arterial blood pressure in trainees who begin training with blood pressures in the normal range is minimal and unpredictable (12, 44). Exercise programs seem to have the greatest value in lowering blood pressure in older patients and in hypertensive patients (12, 44).

Pulmonary Function at Rest

In normal subjects little or no change in pulmonary function at rest is usually observed as a result of training. If subjects specifically improve the strength of their breathing musculature, they may experience some increase in vital capacity (especially in swimmers), and in maximal breathing capacity. Otherwise, only slight decreases in the breathing rate at rest and slight increases in tidal volume (depth of breathing) are sometimes reported (6, 47).

Other health-related adaptations to aerobic endurance training will be described in Chapter 18.

Review Questions

1. Describe four principles of aerobic training.
2. What is the minimal exercise program that one could expect to cause an improvement in maximal oxygen uptake in young adults?
3. What are some ways of prescribing appropriate intensities of exercise on an individual basis?
4. How large a percentage increase in maximal oxygen uptake

could one expect to result from an endurance training program? What are some of the factors that contribute to differences in the magnitude of this adaptation?

5. Outline an interval training program designed to improve aerobic potential in a high school student who has a maximal heart rate of 200 beats per minute and a best time of 5 minutes for the mile run. Begin by listing the general principles that should underlie any such program. The program should encompass a 10-week period.

6. Describe and explain the cardiovascular adaptations to endurance training. Include in your discussion the possible role of altered mitochondrial function in contributing to a greater maximal arteriovenous oxygen difference.

7. What accounts for the improved tolerance to submaximal exercise observed in trained persons? What is the likely role of the skeletal muscle mitochondria in this adaptation?

References

1. Adams, G. M., and H. A. deVries. Physiological effects of an exercise training regimen upon women aged 52–79. *Journal of Gerontology*, 1973, **28:**50–55.

2. Adams, W. C., E. M. Bernauer, D. B. Dill, and J. B. Bomar, Jr. Effects of equivalent sea-level and altitude training on $\dot{V}_{O_2}$ max and running performance. *Journal of Applied Physiology*, 1975, **39:**262–266.

3. American College of Sports Medicine. *Guidelines for Graded Exercise Testing and Exercise Prescription.* Philadelphia: Lea & Febiger, 1975.

4. Andersen, K. L. The cardiovascular system in exercise. In H. B. Falls (Ed.), *Exercise Physiology.* New York: Academic Press, 1968, pp. 79–128.

5. Applegate, V. W., and G. A. Stull. The effects of varied rest periods on cardiovascular endurance retention by college women. *American Corrective Therapy Journal*, 1969, **23:**3–6.

6. Astrand, P.-O., and K. Rodahl. *Textbook of Work Physiology.* New York: McGraw-Hill, 1970.

7. Barclay, J. K., and W. N. Stainsby. The role of blood flow in limiting maximal metabolic rate in muscle. *Medicine and Science in Sports*, 1975, **7:**116–119.

8. Barnard, R. J. Long-term effects of exercise on cardiac function. *Exercise and Sports Sciences Reviews*, 1975, **3:**113–133.

9. Bar-Or, O., and L. D. Zwiren. Physiological effects of increased frequency of physical education classes and of endurance conditioning on 9–10 year-old girls and boys. In O. Bar-Or (Ed.), *Pediatric Work Physiology–Proceedings of the Fourth International Symposium.* Wingate Post, Israel: Wingate Institute, 1972, pp. 183–198.

10. Bouchard, C., W. Hollmann, H. Venrath, G. Herkenrath, and H. Schlussel. Minimal amount of physical training for the prevention of cardiovascular diseases. *Proceedings of the 16th World Congress for Sports Medicine, Hannover, Germany,* 1966, pp. 91–97.

11. Brynteson, and W. E. Sinning. The effects of training frequencies on the retention of cardiovascular fitness. *Medicine and Science in Sports,* 1973, **5:**29–33.

12. Choquette, G., and R. J. Ferguson. Blood pressure reduction in "borderline" hypertensives following physical training. *Canadian Medical Association Journal,* 1973, **108:**699–703.

13. Clausen, J. P. Muscle blood flow during exercise and its significance for maximal performance. In J. Keul (Ed.), *Limiting Factors of Physical Performance.* Stuttgart: Georg Thieme, Publishers, 1973, pp. 253–266.

14. Cooper, K. H. *The New Aerobics.* New York: Bantam Books, 1970.

15. Daniels, J., and N. Oldridge. Changes in oxygen consumption of young boys during growth and running training. *Medicine and Science in Sports,* 1971, **3:**161–165.

16. Daniels, J. and N. Oldridge. The effects of alternate exposure to altitude and sea level on world-class, middle-distance runners. *Medicine and Science in Sports,* 1970, **2:**107–112.

17. Davis, J. A., and V. A. Convertino. A comparison of heart rate methods for predicting endurance training intensity. *Medicine and Science in Sports,* 1975, **7:**295–298.

18. deVries, H. A. Exercise intensity threshold for improvement of cardiovascular–respiratory function in older men. *Geriatrics,* 1971, **26:**94–101.

19. deVries, H. A. Physiological effects of an exercise training regimen upon men aged 52 to 88. *Journal of Gerontology,* 1970, **25:**325–336.

20. Dill, D. B., and W. C. Adams. Maximal oxygen uptake at sea level and at 3,090-m altitude in high school champion runners. *Journal of Applied Physiology,* 1971, **30:**854–859.

21. Drinkwater, B. L., and S. M. Horvath. Detraining effects on young women. *Medicine and Science in Sports,* 1972, **4:**91–95.

22. Durnin, J. V. G. A., J. M. Brockway, and H. W. Whitcher, Ef-

fect of a short period of training of varying severity on some measurements of physical fitness. *Journal of Applied Physiology*, 1960, **15**:161–165.

23. Eisenman, P. A., and L. A. Golding. Comparison of effects of training on $\dot{V}_{O_2}$ max in girls and young women. *Medicine and Science in Sports*, 1975, **7**:136–138.

24. Ekblom, B. Effect of physical training in adolescent boys. *Journal of Applied Physiology*, 1969, **27**:350–355.

25. Ekblom, B., R. Huot, E. M. Stein, and A. T. Thorstensson. Effect of changes in arterial oxygen content on circulation and physical performance. *Journal of Applied Physiology*, 1975, **39**:71–75.

26. Eriksson, B. O., and K. Gunter. Effect of physical training on hemodynamic response during submaximal and maximal exercise in 11–13 year old boys. *Acta Physiologica Scandinavica*, 1973, **87**:27–39.

27. Flint, M. M., B. L. Drinkwater, and S. M. Horvath. Effects of training on women's response to submaximal exercise. *Medicine and Science in Sports*, 1974, **6**:89–94.

28. Fox, E. L., R. L. Bartels, C. E. Billings, D. K. Mathews, R. Bason, and W. M. Webb. Intensity and distance of interval training programs and changes in aerobic power. *Medicine and Science in Sports*, 1973, **5**:18–22.

29. Fox, E. L., and D. K. Mathews. *Interval Training: Conditioning for Sports and General Fitness*. Philadelphia: W. B. Saunders, 1974.

30. Fringer, M. N., and G. A. Stull. Changes in cardiorespiratory paramenters during periods of training and detraining in young adult females. *Medicine and Science in Sports*. 1974, **6**:20–25.

31. Girandola, R. N., and F. I. Katch. Effects of physical conditioning on changes in exercise and recovery O_2 uptake and efficiency during constant-load ergometer exercise. *Medicine and Science in Sports*. 1973, **5**:242–247.

32. Gollnick, P. D. Cellular adaptations to exercise. In R. J. Shephard (Ed.), *Frontiers of Fitness*. Springfield, Ill.: Charles C Thomas, 1971, pp. 112–126.

33. Hanson, J. S., and W. H. Nedde. Long-term physical training effect on sedentary females. *Journal of Applied Physiology*, 1974, **37**:112–116.

34. Hellerstein, H. K., E. Z. Hirsch, R. Ader, N. Greenblott, and M. Siegel. Principles of exercise prescription for normals and cardiac subjects. In J. Naughton and H. K. Hellerstein (Eds.), *Exercise Testing and Exercise Training in Coronary Heart Disease*. New York: Academic Press, 1973, pp. 129–167.

35. Hermansen, L. Anaerobic energy release. *Medicine and Science in Sports*, 1969, **1**:32–38.
36. Holloszy, J. O. Biochemical adaptations to exercise: Aerobic metabolism. *Exercise and Sport Science Reviews*, 1973, **1**:45–71.
37. Hoppeler, H., P. Luthi, H. Claassen, E. R. Weibel, and H. Howald. The ultrastructure of the normal human skeletal muscle. *Pflugers Archives*, 1973, **344**:217–232.
38. Karvonen, M. J., E. Kentala, and O. Mustala. The effects of training on heart rate. A longitudinal study. *Annales Medicinae Experimentalis et Biologiae Fenniae*, 1957,**35**:305–315.
39. Kilbom, A. Physical training in women. *Scandinavian Journal of Clinical and Laboratory Investigation*, 1971, **28 (Suppl. 119)**:1–34.
40. Knuttgen, H. G., L.-O. Nordesjo, B. Ollander, and B. Saltin. Physical conditioning through interval training with young male adults. *Medicine and Science in Sports*, 1973, **5**:220–226.
41. Massicotte, D. R., and R. B. J. Macnab. Cardiorespiratory adaptations to training at specified intensities in children. *Medicine and Science in Sports*, 1974, **6**:242–246.
42. Michael, E., J. Evert, and K. Jeffers. Physiological changes of teenage girls during five months of detraining. *Medicine and Science in Sports*, 1972, **4**:214–218.
43. Pechar, G. S., W. D. McArdle, F. I. Katch, J. R. Magel, and J. DeLuca. Specificity of cardiorespiratory adaptation to bicycle and treadmill training. *Journal of Applied Physiology* 1974, **36**:753–756.
44. Pollock, M. L. The quantification of endurance training programs. *Exercise and Sport Sciences Reviews*, 1973, **1**:155–188.
45. Roskamm. E. Optimum patterns of exercise for healthy adults. *Canadian Medical Association Journal*, 1967, **96**:895–899.
46. Rowell, L. B. Human cardiovascular adjustments to exercise and thermal stress. *Physiological Reviews*, 1975, **54**:75–159.
47. Saltin, B. Physiological effects of physical conditioning. *Medicine and Science in Sports*, 1969, **1**:50–56.
48. Shephard, R. J. *Alive Man! The Physiology of Physical Activity*. Springfield, Ill.: Charles C Thomas, 1972.
49. Shephard, R. J. Intensity, duration, and frequency of exercise as determinants of the response to a training regimen. *International Zeitschrift fur Angewandte Physiologie*, 1968, **26**:272–278.
50. Stoedefalke, K. G. Physical fitness programs for adults. *American Journal of Cardiology*, 1974, **33**:787–790.

51. Wilmore, J. H. Individual exercise prescription. *American Journal of Cardiology*, 1974, **33:**757–759.

52. Wilmore, J. H., and W. L. Haskell. Use of the heart rate—energy expenditure relationship in the individualized prescription of exercise. *The American Journal of Clinical Nutrition*, 1971, **24:**1,186–1,192.

53. Wilmore, J. H., J. Royce, R. N. Girandola, F. I. Katch, and V. L. Katch. Physiological alterations resulting from a 10-week program of jogging. *Medicine and Science in Sports*, 1970, **1:**7–14.

15

Temperature regulation

Man is able to maintain his body temperature within a very narrow range under normal, resting conditions. However, under extreme environmental conditions, with fever, and with prolonged vigorous exercise, the organism may be unable to regulate its temperature satisfactorily, and illness, or even death, can ensue. When the body cools to below 96°F (35.4°C), enzymes in the cells especially those of the brain, become less active and cellular metabolism can eventually become depressed so that vital functions such as respiration slow up and even stop. As the cells are cooled to the freezing point and below, intracellular crystals of ice that can irreversibly damage cell membranes form. On the other hand, increases of body temperature can elevate enzyme activities so greatly that important cellular functions, again especially in the brain, are accelerated too greatly, and integration of the cells' activities is disrupted. Above temperatures of 109°F (42.8°C) enzyme proteins begin to break down, and tissues are slowly cooked (Fig. 15.1). Consequently, temperature regulation is an

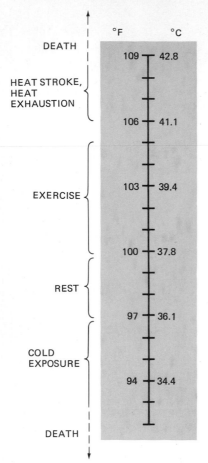

Figure 15.1. Range of oral body temperature.

important consideration in human physiology, particularly during conditions of prolonged exercise where the body can exceed temperatures of 105°F (40.6°C).

MECHANISMS OF HEAT TRANSFER

The human body is constantly exchanging heat energy with its environment. Whether the body gains or loses heat depends upon the operation of four different mechanisms of heat transfer: radiation, conduction, convection, and evaporation. *Radiation* is the transfer of heat energy in the form of electromagnectic waves (similar to light rays) through space from one object to another. All objects radiate heat to other objects in their environment; a person is warmed by radiation if objects in his environment (especially the sun) radiate more heat energy to him than he does to his surroundings. Conversely, if the surface of the body is warmer than one's surroundings, as for example, on a cold winter day, the body loses heat by radiation to its enviornment. Note that radiation does not require the presence of matter between objects that are exchanging heat energy by radiation. This is how the sun can radiate so much heat energy to us through outer space.

Conduction is the process whereby heat energy is transferred from a warmer to a cooler object with which it has direct physical contact, such as the transfer of heat from hot water in a bathtub to a body immersed in the water.

Convection is the transfer of heat between the surface of the body and the air (or water, if one is swimming) because of the circulation of air or water molecules next to the skin. For example, if cool air around a person is completely still and the person is immobile, heat is transmitted by conduction to a thin shell of air molecules that make contact with the skin, but if a breeze blows, the warm air molecules are displaced by cooler molecules that can, then, pick up more heat energy by conduction. The greater the difference in temperature between the skin and the neighboring air or water molecules, the greater the heat transfer.

Evaporation is the transfer of heat from the body surface through the change of liquid water on the skin to a gaseous water vapor in the environment. Just as one must impart heat energy to a kettle of water to make it turn into steam, body water must absorb heat from the body surface if it is to evaporate as water vapor. For every liter of sweat that is evaporated from the surface of the body, about 580 kilocalories of heat energy are removed from the body. Evaporation is vitally important to temperature regulation in a hot environment where heat is *gained* from the environment by radiation, convection and conduction, leaving evaporation as the only avenue for heat loss. Because evaporation is the diffusion of water molecules from the skin to the air, no evaporation can occur if the air is saturated with water vapor. Accordingly, when the relative humidity is high on a hot day, temperature regulation may not be possible if one is producing heat at a high rate while exercising. It is under conditions of high heat and humidity that most cases of heat illness occur.

PHYSIOLOGICAL CONTROL OF HEAT TRANSFER

There are two principal mechanisms by which the body can control the transfer of heat by radiation, convection, conduction, and evaporation between the surface of the body and the environment. First, the body can alter the temperature of its surface by changing blood flow to the skin. If skin blood vessels are open, warm blood from the core of the body is brought to the surface where the heat is then more easily lost by radiation, conduction, convection and evaporation. (Warmed perspiration evaporates more readily than cool perspiration.) On the other hand, if the blood vessels to the skin are constricted, heat will be conserved within the inner regions of the body, and less heat will be lost by radiation, convection, conduction and evaporation.

The second mechanism by which the body can control heat transfer between its surface and the environment is the control of sweat secretion by the sweat glands. Obviously, if more sweat is secreted, there will tend to be a greater loss of heat by evaporation.

Blood flow to the skin and sweat secretion are both governed by the activity of the hypothalamus at the base of the brain. The hypothalamus is responsive to changes in skin temperature, changes in the temperature of the blood and perhaps to temperature changes in other parts of the body. When the skin and/or blood are warmed, the hypothalamus generates nerve impulses which lead to the dilatation of cutaneous (skin) blood vessels and the secretion of more sweat. Under cool conditions of the skin and blood, the hypothalamus brings about cutaneous vasoconstriction and diminished sweating. The temperature of the face is especially important in determining the subjective sensation of a hot or cold environment and determining sweat rate (8). The thermal receptors in the skin of the face seem to be much more sensitive to temperature changes than those in other parts of the body. This accounts for the fact that a cool fan blowing on the face on a hot day is so pleasant, and for the common experience among distance runners that they would often rather pour water over their heads than drink it.

TEMPERATURE REGULATION IN A COOL DRY ENVIRONMENT

Heat production in a resting person is about 75 kilocalories per hour. Exercise may increase caloric expenditure by 20-fold, that is, to 1,500 kilocalories per hour for short durations. Obviously, most of this extra heat must be dissipated, or body temperature will rapidly rise above 43°C (109°F). Some of this heat is not removed during exercise, however. The body stores some heat and simply carries on its functions at a higher temperature during work and for 30 minutes (18) up to 11 hours (10) after the exercise is completed. It seems that the body must be somewhat more efficient during work at a tempera-

ture of 39°C rather than 37.5°C, perhaps because of more optimal enzyme activity at the higher temperature. It is as though the body's
hypothalamic "thermostat" were reset at a higher level to make exercise more efficient. This resetting of the hypothalamic thermostat
may be caused by increased sodium or decreased calcium ion concentration in the extracellular fluid bathing the hypothalamus (17).

In a cool, dry environment, for example, 70°F (21.1°C) and 50 per
cent relative humidity, the body can increase cutaneous blood flow
and increase sweating rate to help rid itself of excess heat during exercise. During movement, the hypothalamus responds not only to the
temperature of the warmed blood but also to reflex impulses originating in working muscles and/or joints (18). This is shown by the fact
that sweating begins within a few seconds of the start of movement,
long before any temperature rise of the blood or even muscles could
be detected (9, 18)). The increased sweating during exercise is useless,
of course, if evaporation is impeded because of high humidity, or because the individual wears clothing that does not allow the sweat to
evaporate. Sweating is especially blocked by plastic or rubberized
sweat suits, and the use of such clothing is dangerous if it causes the
body temperature to rise to critical levels.

In some persons, if the increased evaporative cooling caused by
sweating is sufficient to maintain body temperature below 39°C,
there may be no increased blood flow to the skin to increase heat loss
by radiation and convection (19). In fact, some of the blood flow to the
skin at rest may be shifted to the working muscles during exercise
(19). However, for work loads above about 1 liter of oxygen consumption per minute, there is usually an increased cutaneous blood flow as
the work progresses. Probably about 70 per cent of the heat lost
during exercise in a cool, dry environment is due to evaporation of
sweat, whereas about 15 per cent is lost as a result of radiation, and
15 per cent by convection (3). Because of the cooling effect of the
evaporation of sweat from the skin, skin temperature actually decreases during exercise except under hot, humid conditions (18).

EXERCISE IN THE COLD

Because of the potential 20-fold increase in heat production
during vigorous exercise, body temperature can be easily maintained, even in subzero conditions, as long as one continues to exercise. There is little danger of frostbite to fingers, toes and ears as long
as gloves, warm footwear and a head covering are worn. (A tremendous loss of heat can occur from an uncovered head because of a
poor vasoconstriction response of the blood vessels in the skin of the
head.) The ability of the exercising person to produce heat is, of

course, what makes skiing on a cold day enjoyable with only light-weight clothing for protection from the environment. This capacity to produce heat also enables swimmers to swim twenty miles or more in frigid water without freezing to death.

Thus, as long as one dresses warmly before and after exercise in the cold, there is little risk that the body will fail to maintain a near normal temperature. As a matter of fact, individuals who dress too warmly for exercise in the cold may find that they become intolerably warm. This is especially true if the clothing is such that evaporation of perspiration is hindered too greatly. A handy rule for dressing for exercise in the cold is to wear several layers of light clothing that can be removed or replaced separately as body heat rises and falls during work and rest periods.

Although there is little risk of failure in body temperature regulation during exercise in the cold, there is the possibility of discomfort from parched mouth and throat, and chapped lips because of the extremely low humidity present in cold air. Consequently, it is not uncommon for all-weather exercisers to wear protective scarves over their faces to retain some of the moisture in exhaled air near the sensitive membranes. There is no substantial evidence that lung tissues can be frostbitten during exercise in the cold.

EXERCISE IN HOT, HUMID CONDITIONS

Even under conditions of rest, prolonged exposures to hot and humid environments can lead to profound disruptions in the body's ability to maintain a stable internal environment for its cells and tissues. Exercise, especially endurance exercise, can accelerate the appearance of these harmful effects of heat exposure, not only because working muscles produce heat and thereby add to the heat load of the organism, but also because changes in the circulation that are associated with heavy exercise tend to decrease the body's ability to rid itself of excess heat. Certain types of athletic performance are not apt to be hindered by heat and, indeed, are probably aided by an elevated body temperature. For example, a single 100-meter sprint, a put of the shot or a single lift in weightlifting competition would not be adversely affected by heat. However, the *repetition* of these activities many times during a prolonged training session in hot, humid conditions could easily lead to a failure of the temperature regulating ability of the athlete. In fact, many of the most severe effects of prolonged exposure to heat are observed in football players during early season practice sessions, a time when the players rarely exert themselves strenuously for more than forty yards or a few seconds at a time. Unfortunately, the effects of heat on football players are aggravated by the helmets, heavy padding, and clothing they must wear to prevent injury. Such clothing obviously hinders heat loss.

Work Tolerance in the Heat

It is common knowledge that conditions of high heat and humidity can adversely affect performance in many athletic events. Some of this detrimental effect of heat on performance is undoubtedly due to motivational factors; that is, some persons are psychologically less tolerant of heat than others, and fail to maintain high levels of performance even when there is little evidence of physiological impairment (19). More often, however, the adverse effect of heat on performance is the result of the competing demands of the circulation to the working muscles and the circulation to the skin (13). Since the capacity of the heart to pump blood is less than the maximal rate of blood flow to working muscles plus skin, and since the total blood volume is less than the maximal volume capacity of the muscles and skin, either the muscles must be short-changed in their blood supply so that the muscles become fatigued or the skin receives less than the optimal amount of blood needed to cool the organism. Excess body heat will then cause discomfort and, perhaps, neurological malfunction. In either case, performance suffers. It should again be emphasized, however, that environmental heat and humidity have little effect on performance that is of short duration, perhaps less than 15 minutes. It is only in events lasting more than 15 minutes or in situations of repeated short work-bouts over a prolonged period that one must be concerned about performance detriments of physiological origin (19).

Females generally have somewhat less tolerance to work in the heat than men, probably because estrogen, the female sex hormone, inhibits sweating to some extent. Also, obese persons of either sex suffer more physiological strain while performing a standard task in the heat than lean persons do (12). Perhaps the most logical explanation of this effect of obesity is: Obese persons must work at a greater percentage of their maximal oxygen uptakes to accomplish a standard task, and this produces a greater strain on the circulation and on temperature regulation (12).

Maximal Oxygen Uptake in the Heat

If athletic performance suffers in hot, humid environments, it might be supposed that maximal oxygen uptake must also suffer. This relationship does not necessarily hold true. Some persons perform less well in the heat even though maximal oxygen uptake remains the same as that observed in a cool environment (7, 19). Another way to state this is that maximal oxygen uptake is a good indicator of maximal cardiovascular function, but not necessarily of *aerobic performance*. There are too many other factors, such as motivation, that are important in enabling one to express his functional capacity. Also, if one is inefficient in temperature regulation, for example, one has a poor sweating response to heat, more of the capacity for oxygen transport to working muscles must be used to deliver blood to the skin for cooling purposes than is the case for a similar subject with a good sweating response. It is known, for instance, that marathoners as a group have very high maximal oxygen uptakes, but *among* marathoners there is *no* linear relationship between maximal oxygen uptake and marathon time (6). It is apparent, therefore, that although a high maximal oxygen uptake is necessary if one is to compete successfully in a marathon, it is not sufficient; other factors such as high levels of motivation and efficient temperature regulation are also important.

Ordinarily, maximal oxygen uptake does not fall with short-duration exercise unless body temperature rises considerably, perhaps to 30°C (19). This condition can occur if persons are exposed to high temperature and humidity for some time before the maximal oxygen uptake test begins or if body temperature is elevated by prolonged submaximal work before the test. Although the fall of maximal oxygen uptake under circumstances of prior temperature elevation may be due to shifts of blood from working muscle to skin, it could also be the result of insufficient motivation to carry out the work task (19). Accordingly, the maximal oxygen uptake test under conditions of prior heating may not give a "true" maximal oxygen uptake. A third possibility is that cardiac output may be reduced under such conditions because of a reduction in stroke volume (19).

There are no conclusive studies to tell us which of these possibilities or combinations thereof explain the decline in maximal oxygen uptake that is observed in subjects preheated before short-duration, maximal exercise. Because of the subjective discomfort most persons experience in the heat, it seems very likely that at least some of this decrement in maximal oxygen uptake is due to motivational factors. This is probably especially true in those whose performance is of mediocre caliber.

A more consistent decline of 3–8 per cent in maximal oxygen uptake is observed after prolonged exercise, for example, an hour or longer, in the heat. This reduction may be because of a fall in cardiac output as venous return to the heart is reduced by a pooling of blood in dilated skin vessels. The fall in maximal oxygen uptake after prolonged exercise could also be the result of a decreased arterio-venous difference in oxygen content of the blood as blood is shifted from working muscles to the skin, where less oxygen uptake occurs.

Cardiovascular Function

For both short-duration (less than 15 min.) and long-duration, mild exercise in the heat, cardiac output often rises above that observed with the same work load in a cool environment. This increase in cardiac output is accomplished by an increase in heart rate because stroke volume often is diminished in the heat.

The extra cardiac output with submaximal work is directed to the skin so that more heat can be lost by radiation, convection and evaporation. (A warm skin increases the vaporization of sweat). Blood pressure during mild work in the heat is not noticeably different from that observed in cool conditions because the dilatation of skin vessels (which tends to lower blood pressure) is balanced by vasoconstriction in liver, kidney and nonworking muscles (19).

Cardiac output at more strenuous work loads in the heat is maintained throughout the exercise if it is a single, short–duration bout, but the output may fall toward the end of prolonged, vigorous exercise or after many repeated bouts of short–duration activity (19). Repeated windsprints in football practice could produce such falls in cardiac output. At the beginning of these strenuous exercise periods, cardiac output is maintained even with a reduced stroke volume by increases in heart rate, but as heart rate is increased to maximal levels, maximal cardiac output and maximal oxygen uptake must fall as a result of the decreased stroke volume (19). With the fall in cardiac output and increased vasodilatation in the skin, blood pressure also falls, sometimes by as much as 40 mm Hg. It is at this point of reduced cardiac output and lowered blood pressure that the danger of severe circulatory collapse and heat exhaustion occurs.

Body Fluids

Those who exercise for prolonged periods in the heat can lose more than 2 liters of body fluids (sweat) per hour and experience a total weight loss of 7 or 8 per cent of body weight in the course of an endurance event such as a marathon race (6). The body contains a total of only about 40 liters of fluid, including intracellular and extracellular compartments, and of that total, only about 5 liters are in the form of blood (3 liters of plasma and 2 liters of blood cells.) Therefore, if a major portion of the fluid lost during prolonged exercise in the heat were derived from the blood, it is obvious that blood volume, cardiac output and blood pressure would all fall precipitously. Fortunately, with severe dehydration (greater than 2.5 liters of water loss), much of the fluid lost in sweat seems to come from inside the body's cells, with less than a 20 per cent fall in plasma volume, that is, less than 600 ml., occurring during such exercise (3, 6, 11, 14, 20). There is a great variability in the effect on plasma volume of exercise in the heat, with some reports showing no change in plasma volume even with sweat losses greater than 2.5 liters (7), and others showing relatively greater losses of plasma volume by females than males (20). A fall in plasma volume contributes to the reduction in stroke volume, cardiac output and blood pressure seen with prolonged, vigorous exercise in the heat, and opposes the demands of the skin for more blood flow for cooling purposes.

A loss of body fluid during exercise is accompanied by a rise in body temperature partly because sweating is sometimes (14), but not always (7), less in a dehydrated state (2–3 liters of water loss). Therefore, it is important that body fluids be replenished to aid sweating and to help maintain body temperature at a lower level than would be the case in one who is badly dehydrated.

It is interesting that the thirst mechanism is inadequate to stimulate complete rehydration after heavy fluid losses due to exercise (7). This means that those who exercise in the heat will not voluntarily drink enough water to replenish body fluid stores after exercise, and body fluids are only gradually reestablished over a period of one or two days. Thus, an endurance athlete should learn to drink fluids even before he feels thirsty in order to delay dehydration as long as possible. If distance runners and football players would learn to drink a quart of water before competition and a cup of water every 10–15 minutes when they are exercising in hot, humid conditions, many problems of heat stress could be avoided (6, 7). As a check on fluid replacement, athletes should be weighed before and after practice to see that most of the sweat loss is replaced during the practice period. Coaches and physical educators should make certain that water is available at all times and should insist on regular water breaks in the heat.

During early season conditioning, a substantial amount of sodium chloride may be lost in the sweat, and if not replenished by extra salt in the diet or perhaps a daily salt tablet, this loss of body salt can result in "heat cramps," that is, muscle cramps resulting from disturbed concentrations of sodium, potassium, and chloride on either side of the muscle fiber membrane. Another adverse feature of this salt loss in the sweat is that as the water in the sweat evaporates, it leaves a coating of salt on the skin that increases the salt content of subsequent sweat secretions on the skin surface. As the salt concentration of sweat increases, it is more difficult to evaporate the sweat. (The heat required for vaporization of the sweat increases with increased salt concentration.) Therefore, it is probably beneficial to have some sweat drip off the body to carry excess salt with it and make evaporation more efficient. Although sweat that drips off the skin without evaporating does not directly contribute to cooling of the body, it indirectly helps by washing off salt that accumulates on the skin so that subsequent perspiration can evaporate more readily.

As training progresses, the sweat that is secreted has less salt than normal body fluids so that loss of fluid by sweating tends to increase the concentration of salt in body fluids, and a large intake of salt before or after exercise is neither helpful or desirable. Although consumption of several salt tablets per day is found to be beneficial for miners and others who labor in the heat for 6–10 hours daily, most authorities recommend that athletes should simply sprinkle a total of 2–4 teaspoons more salt on their food each day than they normally would or drink several glasses of water, each with a half teaspoon of dissolved salt (7, 15). Excess ingestion of salt is not mandatory during prolonged exercise in trained individuals and can be more harmful than no salt at all.

If too much salt in the form of tablets or a salt solution is taken into the stomach, body fluids will be drawn by osmosis into the stomach. This will increase the state of dehydration of the cells and make the athlete uncomfortably aware of a stomach filled with fluid (7).

Weight Loss in Wrestlers. It is common practice for wrestlers to attempt to gain advantages of leverage and maturity over their opponents by wrestling in a weight class lower than their normal body weights. Since wrestlers are very lean even before the training season (2, 21), much of the weight loss required to gain entrance to a lower weight classification tends to occur by voluntary dehydration a few days or hours before the weigh-in for certification. This rapid dehydration has both performance and health implications for the wrestler. There is conflicting evidence about the effects of dehydration on performance of the type seen in wrestling. Tolerance to prolonged exercise is definitely reduced, but the mechanism underlying that decreased tolerance and the effects of dehydration on muscular strength and anaerobic endurance are controversial (2, 7). Likewise, although dehydration may bring about severe changes in fluid volume, electrolyte balance, renal blood flow, and temperature regulation (2), there seems to be little conclusive evidence that these changes necessarily lead to heat illness, circulatory collapse or diminished growth and development. However, it is important that the wrestler and the coach understand the harmful potential of repeated episodes of rapid weight loss by dehydration for both wrestling performance and for health. It is the position of the American College of Sports Medicine (2) that wrestlers whose fat content is less than 5 per cent of their certified body weights (as assessed several weeks in advance of the competitive season [21]) should receive medical clearance before they are allowed to compete. Also, wrestlers should be discouraged from consuming less food than required to meet their minimal needs (1,200–2,400 kilocalories per day) and should not be allowed to attempt weight loss through the use of rubber or plastic suits, steam rooms, saunas, laxatives or diuretics (substances taken to cause greater fluid loss through the kidneys) (2).

MEASUREMENT OF HEAT STRESS

It has been seen that prolonged or repeated short bouts of exercise in the heat are associated with a potential hazard to cardiovascular function and temperature regulation. Since the body receives and gives up heat by radiation, convection and evaporation, a single measure of environmental temperature is not an effective means for evaluating heat stress on the organism. A better index of heat load would be one that combined estimates of heat stress because of radiation from the sun or environmental surroundings, heat stress because of humidity that impairs cooling by evaporation, and heat stress resulting from convection of warm air molecules next to the skin. Such an index, the Wet Globe Temperature, has been devised. It is measured with a Wet Globe Thermometer, an instrument available commercially from the Howard Engineering Co., P.O. Box 3164, Bethlehem, Pa. 18017. This instrument consists essentially of a thermometer enclosed in a copper sphere that is cover with wetted black cloth. The instrument is suspended in the air where radiant energy, convective heat transfer and evaporative heat loss all influence the temperature inside the copper sphere. Fig. 15.2 shows the estimated maximum Wet Globe Temperates that allow prolonged activity at various rates of energy expenditure. It should be emphasized that this chart assumes that an exerciser is wearing only light clothing, so that evaporative heat loss is able to occur at near maximal rates. Football players, rugby players and others who must have their bodies covered should exercise with extreme caution, that is, with many rest-and-water-breaks at Wet Globe Temperatures above 50°F (10°C). There have been football players who died at about 52°F (11°C) Wet Globe Temperature (15).

Distance runners are especially susceptible to heat stress, and most good marathons are run at dry bulb temperatures of about 40°F (4°C). Any time a marathon is run at dry bulb temperatures above 65°F (18°C), with more than 50 per cent relative humidity, many participants will be forced to stop because of heat stress (6). Distance runs on hot days should be conducted before 9:00 A.M. or after 4:00 P.M.

Since many will not have a wet globe thermometer available, a chart (Fig. 15.3) has been constructed using dry-bulb temperature

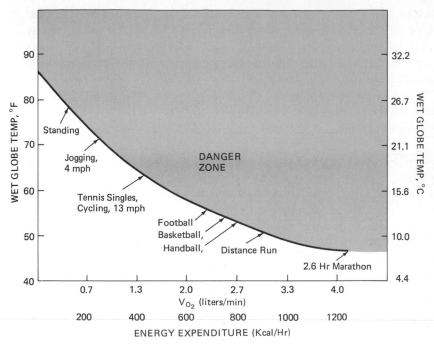

Figure 15.2. Wet-globe temperature danger readings for different rates of energy expenditure. (Data are extrapolated from reference 5.)

and relative humidity to suggest various combinations of temperature and humidity that could lead to heat illness in athletes. Note that this chart does not include any correction for direct exposure to the sun or for clothing or protective pads which may impose an additional heat burden upon the athlete. Therefore, this chart should be

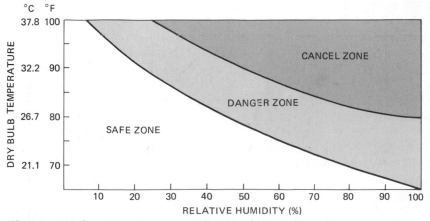

Figure 15.3. Exercise temperature and humidity guide.

conservatively interpreted under unusual conditions. When temperature and relative humidity intersect in the "Danger" zone of Fig. 15.3, athletes should take frequent rest- and water-breaks during prolonged exercise. Intersections of temperature and humidity in the "Cancel" zone should cause the cancellation of any prolonged activity or any athletic event such as a distance run or a football game that might lead to heat illness or even death.

ADAPTATION TO EXERCISE IN THE HEAT

After as little as 4–14 days of training in the heat, the human body is capable of exercising in hot, humid conditions with much less stress to the organism than prior to training (19, 22). The principal adaptation that is made is that the exerciser begins to sweat much more rapidly and profusely, and his sweat glands produce a more diluted and, therefore, more readily evaporated sweat (1, 19). The sweating adaptation is brought about by both an exercise effect and a heat effect (16). The physical training somehow makes the sweat glands more sensitive to signals from the brain, whereas the heat acclimatization causes the brain to begin sending those signals to the sweat glands more rapidly, that is, at lower body temperatures (16).

The reduced salt loss in sweat after acclimatization accounts for the less frequent "stinging" sensation in the eyes as training in the heat progresses. Because of this sweating adaptation, one who has been trained in the heat begins evaporative cooling of his body much faster, and continues this cooling at a faster rate than an untrained person; consequently, one can perform a standard, submaximal work task at a lower skin temperature, a lower rectal temperature and a lower heart rate than the untrained person (1, 19). The reduction in heart rate seems to be a reflex response to decreased skin and/or core temperature. Neither oxygen consumption nor cardiac output at submaximal loads commonly changes with heat acclimatization. Since cardiac output is unchanged and heart rate declines, it follows that stroke volume must rise in the acclimatized person. The increased stroke volume in acclimatized persons during exercise is still less than that seen in the same subjects working in a cool environment (19). The exact reason for this rise in stroke volume is not known, but it may be a simple adjustment to lowered heart rate. There does not seem to be enough of a rise in venous return to the right side of the heart to account for the increased stroke volume (19). Blood pressure during exercise is more stable after training in the heat, and there is a greater blood flow during mild work to the liver, kidneys and other nonworking regions, with the exception of the skin (19). The increased blood flow to the liver and kidneys is provided by a reduction in blood flow to the skin. Skin blood flow is less important for heat loss in the acclimatized person, who loses more heat by evaporation of sweat than the nonacclimatized person.

Finally, there is some evidence that body fluids are slightly increased with acclimatization to the heat. This change is exemplified by an increase of plasma volume by about 5 per cent (19). Such an increase in plasma volume could be of some importance in minimizing the fall in stroke volume and blood pressure that occurs with prolonged exercise, and other body fluid increases may contribute to the greater sweating response of acclimatized persons.

HEAT ILLNESS AND ITS TREATMENT

Some individuals tolerate heat poorly and experience a discomfort characterized by extreme fatigue, mental errors, and poor performance. These persons are suffering from *mild heat fatigue* and should rest in a cool place. A dramatic improvement in exercise performance has been observed when cold air is blown over a subject who seems to be approaching exhaustion from the heat. Heart rate falls dramatically, and the performer can continue a task that moments before had seemed too difficut. Indoors, or outdoors, if electrical outlets are available on the playing field, a large fan would give welcome relief to athletes on a rest-break or water-break.

Simple heat exhaustion (*heat syncope*) results from diminished cardiac output as a consequence of increased blood flow to muscles and skin, and may result in a feeling of dizziness or actual fainting (syncope) accompanied by a rapid pulse and often cool skin. Syncope is most apt to occur in those who must stand in an upright posture in the heat for prolonged periods (such as, Buckingham Palace Guards) or in persons who discontinue exercising in the heat and stand at rest. Because muscle contractions cease propelling blood back to the heart from the legs after exercise, the sudden reduction in venous return leads to a reduced cardiac output, a diminished flow of blood to the brain and sometimes fainting. Such victims should be placed in a comfortable reclining position in a cool location and given fluids to replenish body fluids lost through sweating.

Heat cramps may occur in those who lose excessive amounts of fluids and salts during prolonged exercise. This condition is rapidly alleviated by giving the victim salt tablets with plenty of water or several glasses of water, each containing a half teaspoon of dissolved table salt.

Heat stroke happens only rarely but is the most severe of the heat illnesses; victims of heat stroke often die. The symptoms of heat stroke include a high temperature (106°F, 41°C), absence of sweating (dry skin), and sometimes delirium, convulsions or loss of consciousness. These symptoms arise because the temperature regulating nerve cells of the brain succumb to the high body temperature and fail to regulate the sweating response (sweat gland fatigue). The body temperature must be immediately lowered with any means available, and a physician's assistance should be sought. Early warning signs that heat illness is impending include a sensation of chilling, nausea, a throbbing head, weakness and a dry skin.

It should be emphasized at this point that there should be no need to *treat* heat illness if proper precautions, as described in this chapter, are taken to *prevent* heat illness. If the athlete, coach and physical educator will insist on frequent rest- and water-breaks under conditions of moderately high heat and humidity, and will not participate in or allow prolonged endurance activities or football contests to continue under severe weather conditions, there should be little danger of severe heat illness occurring. There is no excuse for the loss of several lives each year on high school and college football fields because of heat illness. It is the responsibility of every coach to ensure that appropriate precautions, including the purchase of lightweight protective equipment for football, are taken to put a stop to such deaths.

Review Questions

1. Explain the various ways by which the body can conserve or rid itself of heat energy.
2. Describe the evidence that supports the idea that sweating is partly controlled by reflexes originating in working muscles and joints during exercise.
3. Why does skin temperature sometimes decline during exercise in the heat?
4. Describe the precautions one should take when exercising in the cold.
5. Explain why there is much greater risk of heat illness in humid weather rather than dry weather.
6. Describe the changes in cardiovascular function that occur in the heat under exercise conditions.
7. Describe the responses of body fluids when one exercises for prolonged periods in hot, humid conditions. What precautions should be taken with respect to fluid- and salt-replenishment before, during and after prolonged exercise in the heat?

8. Why is repeated rapid weight loss by dehydration in wrestlers frowned upon by medical authorities?
9. Describe the adaptations to exercise in the heat which occur with repeated exposures to exercise and thermal stress.
10. Describe the common forms of heat illness and their treatment.

References

1. Adams, W. C., R. H. Fox, A. J. Fry, and I. C. MacDonald. Thermoregulation during marathon running in cool, moderate, and hot environments. *Journal of Applied Physiology*, 1975, **39**:1,030–1,037.
2. American College of Sports Medicine. Position stand on weight loss in wrestlers. *Medicine and Science in Sports*, 1976, **8**:xi–xiii.
3. Astrand, P.-O., and K. Rodahl. *Textbook of Work Physiology*. New York: McGraw-Hill, 1970.
4. Benzinger, T. H. Heat regulation: Homeostasis of central temperature in man. *Physiological Reviews*, 1969, **49**:671–759.
5. Botsford, J. H. A wet globe thermometer for environmental heat measurement. *American Industrial Hygiene Association Journal*, 1971, **32**:1–10.
6. Costill, D. L. Physiology of marathon running. *Journal of the American Medical Association*, 1972, **221**:1,024–1,029.
7. Costill, D. L. Water and electrolytes. In W. P. Morgan (Ed.), *Ergogenic Aids and Muscular Performance*. New York: Academic Press, 1972, pp. 293–320.
8. Crawshaw, L. I., E. R. Nadel, J. A. J. Stolwijk, and B. A. Stamford. Effect of local cooling on sweating rate and cold sensation. *Pflugers Archives*, 1975, **354**:19–27.
9. Gisolfi, C., and S. Robinson. Central and peripheral stimuli regulating sweating during intermittent work in men. *Journal of Applied Physiology*, 1970, **29**:761–768.
10. Haight, J. S. J., and W. R. Keatinge. Elevation in set point for body temperature regulation after prolonged exercise. *Journal of Physiology* (London), 1973, **229**:77–85.
11. Harrison, M. H., R. J. Edwards, and D. R. Leitch. Effect of exercise and thermal stress on plasma volume. *Journal of Applied Physiology*, 1975, **39**:925–931.
12. Haymes, E. M., R. J. McCormick, and E. R. Buskirk. Heat tolerance of exercising lean and obese prepubertal boys. *Journal of Applied Physiology*, 1975, **39**:457–461.

13. Johnson, J. M., and L. B. Rowell. Forearm skin and muscle vascular responses to prolonged leg exercise in man. *Journal of Applied Physiology*, 1975, **39**:920–924.
14. Ladell, W. S. S. Terrestrial animals in humid heat: man. In D. B. Dill (Ed.), *Handbook of Physiology: Adaptation to the Environment*. Washington, D.C.: American Physiological Society, 1964, pp. 625–659.
15. Mathews, D. K., and E. L. Fox. *The Physiological Basis of Physical Education and Athletics* (2nd ed.). Philadelphia: W. B. Saunders, 1976.
16. Nadel, E. R., K. B. Pandolf, M. F. Roberts, and J. A. J. Stolwijk. Mechanisms of thermal acclimation to exercise and heat. *Journal of Applied Physiology*, 1974, **37**:515–520.
17. Nielsen, B. Effect of changes in plasma Na^+ and Ca^+ ion concentration on body temperature during exercise. *Acta Physiologica Scandinavica*, 1974, **91**:123–129.
18. Robinson, S. Physiology of muscular exercise. In V. B. Mountcastle (Ed.), *Medical Physiology* (13th ed.). St. Louis, Mo.: C. V. Mosby, 1974, pp. 1,273–1,304.
19. Rowell, L. B. Human cardiovascular adjustments to exercise and thermal stress. *Physiological Reviews*, 1974, **51**:75–159.
20. Senay, Jr., L. C., and S. Fortney. Untrained females: effects of submaximal exercise and heat on body fluids. *Journal of Applied Physiology*, 1975, **39**:643–647.
21. Tcheng, T., and C. M. Tipton. Iowa Wrestling Study: anthropometric measurements and the prediction of a "minimal" body weight for high school wrestlers. *Medicine and Science in Sports*, 1973, **5**:1–10.
22. Wyndham, C. H., N. B. Strydom, A. J. S. Benade, and A. J. Van Rensburg. Limiting rates of work for acclimatization at high wet-bulb temperatures. *Journal of Applied Physiology*, 1973, **35**:454–458.

16

Kidney and gastrointestinal responses and adaptations to exercise

In previous chapters of this book, it has been emphasized that the nature of physiological responses and adaptations to exercise is dependent in large measure upon the specific character of the exercise stimulus, that is, its intensity, duration, frequency and specific muscular involvement. This fact is perhaps best illustrated by the complex nature of the changes in kidney and gastrointestinal functions during exercise. Compared to our knowledge of such systems as the cardiovascular and respiratory systems, our understanding of kidney and gastrointestinal responses and adaptations to exercise is rudimentary. Both the complex nature of the responses and a lack of research contribute to our poor understanding of the function of these systems under exercise conditions. Accordingly, our treatment of this subject will be brief and undoubtedly oversimplified.

THE KIDNEY AT REST—A BRIEF REVIEW

Within each kidney are located a million or more compact tubules (the *nephrons*), and their associated blood vessels. A diagrammatic sketch of one such nephron and its blood supply is shown in Fig. 16.1. Nephrons such as this are responsible for the functions of the kidney, that is, filtration of blood plasma, reabsorption and retention of useful materials in the filtered liquid, and excretion of a small volume of excess water, salt, and potentially harmful substances such as ammonia and hydrogen ions (acid). Blood plasma is filtered out of the capillaries (glomerulus) into Bowman's capsule,

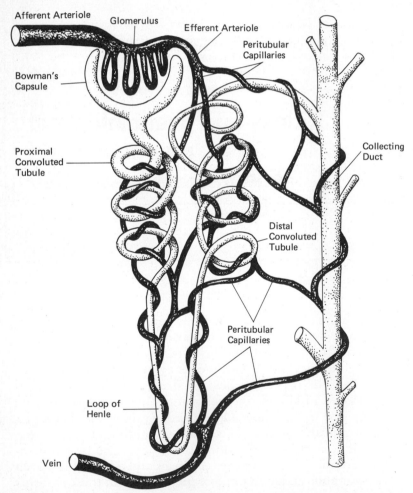

Figure 16.1. Diagrammatic sketch of a nephron and its blood supply.

the first part of the tubule (Fig. 16.1). The kidneys receive about 25 per cent of the total cardiac output at rest, that is, the renal blood flow is about 1.25 liters per minute or 1,800 liters per day. From the 1,800 liters of blood that pass into the glomerular capillaries of the kidneys each day, only about 180 liters of fluid (glomerular filtrate) are filtered into the tubules (7.5 liters per hour). This rate at which fluid is filtered out of the plasma into the nephrons is called the *glomerular filtration rate*. It is obvious that all of the 180 liters of glomerular filtrate that enter the kidney tubules are not excreted into the urine each day—only about 1–2 liters achieve this end. The remainder of the glomerular filtrate, that is, 178–179 liters, is reabsorbed from the tubules and diffuses through the interstitial fluid into the peritubular capillaries, which deliver the retained fluid back to the main circulation by way of the renal veins (Figs. 16.1, 16.2).

There are two principal mechanisms by which substances in the glomerular filtrate are reabsorbed and retained by the body—*active reabsorption* and *passive reabsorption*. Active reabsorption is a process by which the cells of the tubules move dissolved material such as sodium, potassium, glucose and amino acids out of the tubules by expending chemical energy (ATP). Passive reabsorption does not require ATP breakdown and consists of:1) simple diffusion of molecules such as urea from an area of higher concentration inside the tubules to lower concentrations in the interstitial fluid, 2) movement by the attraction of oppositely charged ions (for example, negatively charged chloride ions following positively charged sodium ions out of the tubule as the sodium ions are actively reabsorbed), and 3) osmosis of water out of the tubule because of the attraction of osmotically active substances such as sodium ions, which were previously actively reabsorbed into the interstitial fluid. Thus, passive reabsorption of water by osmosis is made possible chiefly by the active reabsorption of sodium and other osmotically active particles.

Two hormones that enhance the rate of reabsorption of materials in the glomerular filtrate are *aldosterone* and *antidiuretic hormone* (vasopressin). Aldosterone is secreted by the adrenal gland and primarily accelerates the active reabsorption of sodium; it secondarily increases the passive reabsorption of chloride, bicarbonate (HCO_3^{--}) and water. Antidiuretic hormone from the posterior pituitary gland seems to enlarge the pores of the distal convoluted tubules and collecting ducts; this allows water molecules to be passively reabsorbed by osmosis at a faster rate. In the absence of antidiuretic hormone, much more urine than normal is excreted.

Sometimes substances that may be toxic or are in excess of the body's needs accumulate in the interstitial fluid and are actively transported from the interstitial fluid through the walls of the tubules to the interior of the tubules. These potentially harmful sub-

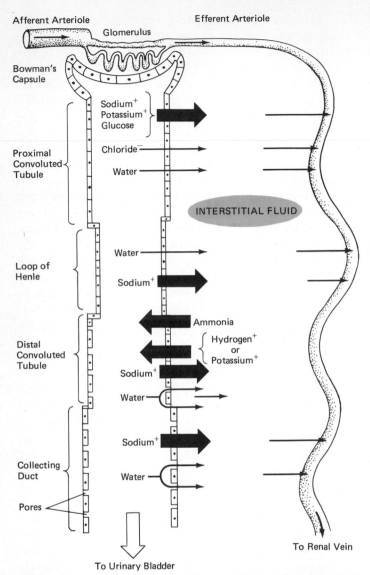

Figure 16.2. Schematic diagram illustrating transport processes in the kidney. Heavy arrows represent active reabsorption from tubule to interstitial fluid or active secretion into the tubule. Light arrows show passive reabsorption by osmosis (water), by electrical attraction (chloride) and by simple diffusion into peritubular capillary.

stances are then excreted from the body by way of the urine. The movement of materials such as ammonia, hydrogen ions and potassium from the exterior to the interior of the tubules in known as *active secretion* and is illustrated in Fig. 16.2.

KIDNEY RESPONSES TO EXERCISE

The alterations in kidney function brought on by a single exercise session are highly variable both from day to day for an individual and also between individuals. Part of this variability is a result of 1) the technical difficulties inherent in evaluating renal function and in precisely controlling fluid intake and excretion so that rest and exercise periods are strictly comparable, 2) differences in the severity and duration of the exercise, and 3) variations in temperature and physical fitness (4, 14). For example, to assure that there will be enough urine formed during a brief exercise period to make measurements of kidney function possible, it is not unusual for investigators to give subjects extra water and even tea to stimulate urine formation. But this fluid loading may create changes in kidney fuction that are not strictly related to the exercise itself. Similarly, brief, mild exercise by fit subjects in a cool environment is less apt to alter kidney function than vigorous, long duration work by unfit persons. Therefore, although it is tempting to generalize about the effects of exercise on kidney function, one should always consider the several factors described here when assessing the probable responses of the kidneys to exercise.

Renal Blood Flow

Because kidney function obviously depends upon the amount of blood delivered to the nephrons, any change in renal blood flow during exercise must have profound effects on the operation of the kidneys, for example, upon glomerular filtration rate, reabsorption and secretion, and ultimately upon urine volume. Thus, one should note that during heavy exercise, renal blood flow may be reduced by 65 per cent or more from the value found at rest (2, 4). This reduction in renal blood flow is apparently not substantial until the exercise intensity is sufficient to increase heart rate to about 135–140 beats per minute or to elevate oxygen uptake to about 50 per cent of one's maximal oxygen uptake (Fig. 16.3), (2, 4). After this threshold is reached, the reduction in blood flow to the kidneys increases in unison with further increases in workload, that is, *renal blood flow during heavy exercise is inversely related to the intensity of exercise expressed as a percentage of one's maximal oxygen uptake* (2, 4). Therefore, during a

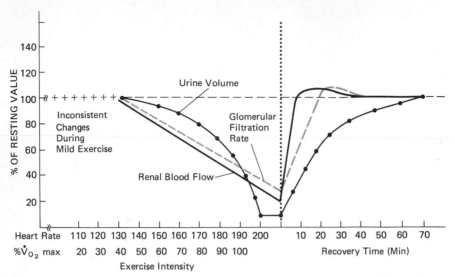

Figure 16.3. Schematic illustration of changes in renal blood flow, glomerular filtration rate and urine volume during exercise and recovery.

run or swim that requires an oxygen uptake of 3.0 liters per minute, renal blood flow might be reduced by 70 per cent in an untrained person who has a maximal oxygen uptake of 3.1 liters per minute, but by only 40 per cent in an athlete who has a maximal oxygen uptake of 5.0 liters per minute.

Even during heavy exercise rather minor decreases in renal blood flow are sometimes observed if the exercise period is of short duration, that is, 15 minutes or less (4). Accordingly, the changes in blood flow to the kidneys are related not only to the intensity of the exercise, but also to its duration, and are probably physiologically significant only in aerobic endurance exercises such as distance running or swimming. It seems that the reduction of blood flow to the kidneys serves the purposes of shifting blood to the working muscles for energy and to the skin for cooling.

Renal blood flow during severe exercise is reduced to a large extent when a subject is hypohydrated because of inadequate water intake or excessive water loss and when a subject exercises in a hot environment (4). The kidneys behave as if they knew when more water loss could be harmful to the body, but the exact mechanisms by which a hot environment and hypohydration cause reductions in renal blood flow are not clear.

Likewise, the mechanism underlying the exercise effect on renal blood flow has not been precisely determined. Blood flow to the kidneys can be diminished 1) by sympathetic nervous system activity, which constricts the afferent and/or efferent arterioles to the nephrons, 2) by greater levels of epinephrine and norepinephrine secreted by the adrenals, and 3) by local autoregulation of blood flow, whereby largely unknown chemical changes in the kidney result in arteriolar constriction. Experiments on normal, running dogs suggest that autoregulation of blood flow is more important than neural effects, but that neural stimuli are important in animals with failing hearts (7). Whether this is true for human beings remains to be demonstrated. Since dogs have a relatively greater capacity for aerobic exercise than humans, it seems likely that the results on dogs with heart failure may more accurately depict the human condition.

Glomerular Filtration Rate

As would be expected, the glomerular filtration rate during heavy exercise decreases as a function of the decreased renal blood flow, but shows highly variable changes with lighter work loads. However, the reduction in the glomerular filtration rate during severe physical activity is usually observed at slightly greater work intensities and is not as marked as the reduction in renal blood flow, that is, a greater fraction of the blood flowing into the glomerular capillaries is filtered into Bowman's capsule during severe exercise (Fig. 16.3). The explanation offered for this greater *filtration fraction* during severe exercise is that the efferent arterioles are constricted to a greater extent than the afferent arterioles; this causes a pressure rise within the glomeruli to force more fluid into Bowman's capsule (4, 14). The effects of environmental temperature, exercise duration, physical fitness, and the exerciser's hydration state on glomerular filtration rate during exercise are similar to those described for renal blood flow, and are probably direct reflections of changes in blood flow.

Urine Volume

It is not unusual for persons who have undergone prolonged heavy exercise to be unable to produce any urine whatsoever shortly after exercise (4). Part of this *anuria* is probably associated with hypohydration, but even in well-hydrated subjects, a decline in urine formation during heavy exercise is to be expected (4). This reduced urine production with severe work is mostly a function of the diminished renal blood flow, which results in decreased glomerular filtratration; that is, a reduction in glomerular filtration is usually associated with a reduction in urine volume. However, in exercisers who are also hypohydrated, it is thought that greater secretion of antidiuretic hormone increases the reabsorption of what little water is formed in the tubules (4).

Poor physical condition, hypohydration, long exercise duration and a hot environment—all enhance the *antidiuretic* effects of heavy exercise because of the role these factors play in reducing renal blood flow.

In contrast to the effects of *strenuous* exercise, mild walking has been reported to cause increased urine production (4, 5). This diuretic effect (greater urine volume) of mild exercise may be the result of a greater excretion of solutes in the urine during *mild* activity. These solutes could exert an osmotic effect to hold water in the tubules for excretion that normally would have been reabsorbed had exercise not taken place. Why the solute load is greater in urine from subjects who have exercised mildly is not known.

Excretion of Urinary Solutes

Since the volume of urine produced during heavy exercise is less than during rest or mild exercise, one might expect that the concentration of dissolved substances in this small volume of urine would be greater, so that the total amount of excreted solutes would be at least as great as the amount during rest. Although this is the usual case during hypohydration, the reverse is true during heavy exercise, that is, the concentration of urinary solutes such as sodium and chloride is *less* during heavy exercise (4). Consequently, urinary specific gravity, which reflects the concentration of dissolved substances in urine, usually *decreases* after severe exercise.

One reason why the excretion of substances such as sodium, chloride, magnesium, creatinine and urea decreases during heavy exercise is that the reduced glomerular filtration of these substances means that there are fewer ions and molecules in the tubules to be excreted (1, 3, 4). But sodium and chloride and perhaps other substances are excreted at a rate lower than would be predicted by the decreased glomerular filtration rate. Accordingly, it seems that these substances must be reabsorbed from the tubules and retained by the body at a greater rate than at rest (4). It seems likely that increased aldosterone secretion during heavy exercise serves to enhance the active reabsorption of sodium from the tubules, and that chloride ions follow the sodium out of the tubules by electrical attraction (12). The aldosterone output by the adrenal gland is apparently stimulated by the renin-angiotensin system as follows:

1) Decreased renal blood flow stimulates specialized cells of the nephrons (juxtaglomerular apparatus) to secrete an enzyme, *renin*, into the bloodstream.
2) Renin catalyzes the transormation of an inactive plasma protein, *angiotensinogen*, into *angiotensin I*.

3) Angiotensin I undergoes a further enzyme-catalyzed change into *angiotensin II*, which, in turn, stimulates the adrenal gland to release aldosterone.

Potassium excretion may be decreased, remain the same, or increase after exercise (3, 4). On the one hand, serum potassium usually rises during exercise, and one might predict that this would lead to a greater filtration and excretion of potassium in the urine. On the other hand, the rise in serum potassium might often be offset by the decreased renal blood flow observed during heavy exercise. There is at present no adequate explanation for the contradictory results achieved with similar exercise programs.

Phosphate excretion usually is diminished during exercise but rises during 30–40 minutes of recovery (14). The decrease during exercise is probably a function of the reduced glomerular filtration rate, whereas the rebound during recovery results not only from elevated glomerular filtration but also from reduced reabsorption by the kidney tubules (14).

Ammonia. Blood levels of ammonia (NH_3) increase during severe exercise in proportion to exercise intensity and remain high for about 30 minutes of recovery (8, 14). Part of this increase may be explained by a greater synthesis of ammonia from amino (NH_2) groups split from intramuscular adenosine monophosphate or amino acids in exercising muscle, and part may be explained by a reduced blood flow to the liver, where ammonia molecules are combined to form urea. Whatever the reason for elevated ammonia levels in the blood during exercise, it might be expected that this increase would lead to a greater excretion of ammonia or ammonium ions (NH_4^+) into the urine during strenuous work. Such an effect does occur and may explain the characteristic odor of postexercise urine. However, much of the increased urinary ammonia comes from the kidney tubule cells themselves. Kidney cells have a large capacity of form ammonia from amino acids. This ammonia can be actively secreted into the tubules to help carry away hydrogen ions (H^+) by forming ammonium salts such as ammonium chloride (ammonia + lactic acid + sodium chloride→ammonium chloride + sodium lactate). In this way, ammonia can help decrease the acidity of the urine by combining with the hydrogen ions of lactic acid to form ammonium ions, which, in turn, combine with negative chloride ions to form neutral salts of ammonium chloride.

In excessive amounts, ammonia in the blood can be toxic to the brain, but it has not been conclusively shown that increases in blood ammonia during exercise contribute to fatigue.

Acid Excretion. During aerobic exercise of a mild to moderate nature the excretion of acids in the urine is not consistently altered from resting conditions (4). But during anaerobic exercise, which is associated with the production of lactic acid, there is a marked increase in the excretion of acid in the urine, with a concomitant decrease in pH during exercise and for 30 minutes or longer during recovery (14). The absolute pH value of urine from exercised subjects depends upon the pre-exercise control value, but may be 1.0–1.5 units lower than at rest in previously hyperhydrated subjects (14). The excretion of more acid is obviously related to the elevated lactic acid levels in the extracellular fluids, that is, more acid is filtered out of the glomeruli into the tubules and more acid is actively secreted by the kidney cells into the tubules.

Protein Excretion and "Athletic Pseudonephritis". Nephritis is a disease of the kidney tubules characterized by a marked urinary loss of proteins, blood cells and substances from the tubular structures. Ordinarily these materials do not appear or appear only in minute amounts in the urine of normal persons at rest. During and after exercise, especially with prolonged, heavy exercise, an increase in proteins, cells and other abnormal substances can be observed in 80 per cent or more of healthy individuals (6, 9). Because these changes in excretion are similar to those seen in nephritis, but do not persist, the term "athletic pseudonephritis" has been used to describe this apparently benign effect of exercise.

The mechanism underlying "athletic pseudonephritis" has not been conclusively determined, but may include an increased permeability of the glomerular capillary membrane to large molecules resulting from hypoxia caused by reduced renal blood flow (4). Another possibility that has been considered is that higher levels of plasma proteins during exercise result in the filtration of a greater amount of proteins into the tubules; perhaps these extra proteins cannot be reabsorbed rapidly enough by the tubular cells (8). Finally, it may be that the reduced rate of renal blood flow through the glomerular capillaries during exercise simply allows large molecules more time to filter through pores in the capillary membrane; perhaps there is no actual change in the membrane structure during exercise (4).

KIDNEY FUNCTION DURING RECOVERY FROM EXERCISE

After exercise has ceased, most kidney functions return to normal resting values within an hour of recovery (14). Most of those substances which were excreted at reduced rates during exercise, as for example, sodium, chloride, magnesium and creatine, show an initial increase in excretion for 30 minutes after exercise before resting excretion rates are reestablished. This effect can be accounted for by the increased glomerular filtration of such substances following the rapid resumption of normal renal blood flow after exercise. Urine volume will also increase following the rise in the glomerular filtration rate and rehydration if the exerciser had been severely hypohydrated. Acid and ammonia excretion remain elevated after heavy exercise for 30 minutes or longer until the lactic acid levels in the body are returned to normal levels (14).

VALUE OF RENAL RESPONSES TO EXERCISE

The respones of the kidneys to heavy exercise are important because of their contributions to:1) the maintenance of adequate blood flow to the working skeletal muscles, 2) the conservation of body fluids needed for evaporative cooling, and 3) the control of pH in body fluids.

The kidneys at rest receive about 1.0–1.5 liters of cardiac output per minute, and about 65 per cent of that value or 650–975 milliliters of blood per minute can be shifted from the kidneys to the skeletal muscles during heavy exercise (4, 10). This obviously can be important to the supply of oxygen and nutrients to the muscles, and also to the maintenance of adequate blood pressure by helping to maintain venous return to the right side of the heart.

During heavy, prolonged work, particularly in a hot environment, the body can lose 1–2 liters of body water per hour by sweating. As the body becomes progressively hypohydrated under these conditions, sweat production may be retarded and evaporative cooling less effective. This diminished effectiveness of the sweating mechanism would be even more severe if the kidneys produced their normal volume of urine and contributed to greater hypohydration. Fortunately, the reduction of urine formation during heavy work tends to conserve body fluids.

Finally, although the respiratory system probably is more important quantitatively (4), the kidneys do help rid the body of excess acid and ammonia and, thus, prolong the time one can exercise without a debilitating accumulation of acid.

RENAL ADAPTATIONS TO TRAINING

Little is known about the effects of habitual exercise on kidney function, and even less is understood about the mechanisms responsible for training effects. It does appear, however, that trained persons exhibit fewer and less marked renal responses to a standard exercise bout than do untrained persons. For example, lesser reductions in renal blood flow, glomerular filtration rate and urine formation are observed in well-conditioned subjects (4). These adaptations are probably the result of a less marked vasoconstriction of afferent and efferent arterioles in the trained persons so that renal blood flow is reduced to a lesser degree. Because of these adatations in renal blood flow, it would also be expected that trained subjects would have less marked changes in excretion rates of solutes that are primarily affected by alterations in renal blood flow and glomerular filtration rate. Thus, trained subjects excrete less ammonia and protein during severe exercise than do untrained subjects (8). Also, at moderately heavy work loads trained individuals produce a greater percentage of their energy aerobically and, therefore, rely less on anaerobic glycolysis. Accordingly, less lactic acid will be excreted in the urine of the trained subjects if the exercise has become more aerobic in nature as a result of training.

GASTROINTESTINAL RESPONSES AND ADAPTATIONS TO EXERCISE

Investigations of the effects of exercise on gastrointestinal function are technically even more difficult than studies of kidney function. Consequently, it is not surprising that our knowledge of such effects is meager. Reports of gastrointestinal responses to exercise in human beings and laboratory animals can be summarized with the following conclusions: 1) *mild* exertion either slightly enhances or has no effect on gastric (stomach) emptying and acid secretion, 2) increasing rates of *heavy* work cause progressively decreasing rates of both gastric emptying and acid secretion, 3) recovery of normal gastric function after severe exercise occurs within about 1–2 hours, and 4) there is inadequate evidence that exercise has any meaningful effects on the small or large intestines (9, 11).

The fact that there is a progressive decrease in gastric movements and secretion with increasing intensities of exercise is reminiscent of the relationship between kidney function and exercise rate; this suggests that changes in the sympathetic and parasympathetic nervous system may be important mediators of the effects of exercise on the stomach. Since splanchnic blood flow, which includes gastrointestinal blood flow, is progressively diminished with increasing work loads (10), it seems probable that increased sympathetic activity and decreased parasympathetic activity are responsible for much of the reduced motility and secretion of the stomach during heavy exercise. (In the gastrointestinal tract, parasympathetic (vagus) activity stimulates and sympathetic activity depresses function.) However, because blood transfusions from exercised to rested dogs cause depression of stomach secretion in the rested dogs, it appears that some circulating factor may also play a role in the responses of the stomach to exercise (11).

Training probably reduces the depression of gastric function with any standard work task because the task after training requires a smaller percentage of the exerciser's maximal oxygen uptake. Accordingly, a smaller increase in sympathetic activity and a smaller decrease in parasympathetic activity would be expected. Thus, trained persons have a greater splanchnic blood flow during a standard exercise test than do untrained subjects (10).

Whether physical training has a protective effect on the appearance of stomach ulcers after different types of stress remains controversial (13). Studies of this question have been conducted with rats, but results have been contradictory.

Review Questions

1. Describe the effects of light and severe exercise on renal blood flow, glomerular filtration rate, and urine volume.
2. Discuss the apparent involvement of renal blood flow changes in the mechanisms of other kidney responses to exercise.
3. What role does aldosterone seem to play in mediating the effect of severe exercise on renal excretion of sodium and chloride?
4. What effect does exercise have on protein excretion in the urine? Explain a likely mechanism underlying this effect.
5. Does the effect of exercise on excretion of proteins, red blood cells, and so on, have pathological overtones? What is meant by "athletic pseudonephritis"?
6. List some of the potential benefits of the exercise response in the kidneys.
7. Describe the probable adaptations in kidney function that follow exercise training.
8. Describe and explain the effects of exercise on gastrointestinal function.

References

1. Cerny, F. Protein metabolism during two hour ergometer exercise. In H. Howald and J. R. Poortmans (Eds.), *Metabolic Adaptation to Prolonged Physical Exercise*. Basel: Birkhauser Verlag, 1975, pp. 232–237.

2. Grimby, G. Renal clearances during prolonged supine exercise at different loads. *Journal of Applied Physiology*, 1965, **20:**1294–1298.

3. Haralambi, G. Changes in electrolytes and trace elements during long-lasting exercise. In H. Howald and J. R. Poortmans (Eds.), *Metabolic Adaptation to Prolonged Physical Exercise.* Basel: Birkhauser Verlag, 1975, pp. 340–351.

4. Kachadorian, W. A. The effects of activity on renal function. In J. F. Alexander (Ed.), *Physiology of Fitness and Exercise.* Chicago: Athletic Institute, 1972, pp. 97–116.

5. Kachadorian, W. A., and R. E. Johnson. Renal responses to various rates of exercise. *Journal of Applied Physiology*, 1970, **28:**748–752.

6. Kachadorian, W. A., R. E. Johnson, R. E. Buffington, L. Lawler, J. J. Serbin, and T. Woodall. The regularity of "Athletic Pseudonephritis" after heavy exercise. *Medicine and Science in Sports*, 1970, **2:**142–145.

7. Millard, R. W., C. B. Higgins, D. Franklin, and S. F. Vatner. Regulation of the renal circulation during severe exercise in normal dogs and dogs with experimental heart failure. *Circulation Research*, 1972, **31:**881–888.

8. Poortmans, J. R. Effects of exercise and training on protein metabolism. In H. Howald and J. R. Poortmans (Eds.), *Metabolic Adaptation to Prolonged Physical Exercise.* Basel: Birkhauser Verlag, 1975, pp. 212–228.

9. Rasch, P. J., and I. D. Wilson. Other body systems and exercise. In H. B. Falls (Ed.), *Exercise Physiology.* New York: Academic Press, 1968, pp. 129–151.

10. Rowell, L. B. Human cardiovascular adjustments to exercise and thermal stress. *Physiological Reviews*, 1974, **51:**75–159.

11. Stickney, J. C., and E. J. Van Liere. The effects of exercise upon the function of the gastrointestinal tract. In W. R. Johnson (Ed.), *Science and Medicine of Exercise and Sports.* New York: Harper & Row, 1960, pp. 236–250.

12. Sundsfjord, J. A., S. B. Stromme, and A. Aakvaag. Plasma aldosterone (PA), plasma renin activity (PRA) and cortisol (PF) during exercise. In H. Howald and J. R. Poortmans (Eds.), *Metabolic Adaptation to Prolonged Physical Exercise.* Basel: Birkhauser Verlag, 1975, pp. 308–314.

13. Tharp, G. D., and J. L. Jackson. The effect of exercise training on restraint ulcers in rats. *European Journal of Applied Physiology*, 1974, **33:**285–292.

14. Wesson, L. G., Jr. Kidney function in exercise. In W. R. Johnson (Ed.), *Science and Medicine of Exercise and Sports.* New York: Harper & Row, 1960, pp. 270–284.

17

Endocrine responses and adaptations to exercise

Two organ systems, the nervous system and the endocrine system, are primarily involved in regulating the rates at which the cells of various tissues carry on their chemical activities. The nervous system is characterized by a rapid response to disturbances in cellular homeostasis, to changes in the external environment and to changing emotional circumstances. The endocrine system, on the other hand, although usually responding more slowly, often has a more profound and prolonged effect on cellular activities. Because of the widespread effects of endocrine regulation on cellular function, it is probable that changes in endocrine function are responsible for many of the physiological responses and adaptations to exercise. However, our knowledge of endocrine changes with exercise is so limited that there is little consensus concerning exactly how the endocrine system is involved in these responses and adaptations. In this chapter, therefore, we will describe what is known about the endocrine responses and adaptations to exercise and speculate on how these endocrine changes might play a role in the overall bodily reactions brought on by single or repeated bouts of exercise.

REVIEW OF ENDOCRINE SECRETIONS

An endocrine organ is imprecisely defined as a gland that secretes, directly into the bloodstream, small amounts of a substance which has specific effects on tissues somewhat distant from the endocrine gland. By this definition, a substance such as carbon dioxide is not considered an endocrine (hormone) because it is secreted in large amounts from muscles and other tissues. However, the releasing factors of the hypothalamus are generally classified as hormones, even though these substances have their effects on the pituitary gland at a distance of only a few millimeters from the hypothalamus. Table 17.1 lists the hormones deemed likely to be involved, at least indirectly, in one or more of the functional changes resulting from exercise.

MECHANISMS OF ENDOCRINE ACTION

Endocrines do not bring about *new* cellular activities but, rather, act to change the rates of specific activities already present in the cells. Endocrines are usually presumed to act in one or more of the following three ways: 1) by altering the rate of synthesis of enzyme proteins, 2) by altering the rate of synthesis of molecules such as cyclic AMP (a special type of adenosine monophosphate) or prostaglandins, which, in turn, bring about changes in enzyme activity or permeability of cell membranes to important substances, and 3) by directly altering the permeability of cell membranes. Endocrinologists are making progress in gradually specifying which types of action are most important for a given hormone, but conclusive evidence demonstrating the primary effect of most hormones is still lacking.

METHODS OF RESEARCH IN ENDOCRINOLOGY

To determine whether a given hormonal substance is involved in the responses or adaptations to exercise, physiologists use several procedures. One approach is to surgically remove the endocrine gland which is the source of the hormone and to compare the responses of such operated animals with those of unoperated control animals. A second approach is to compare the responses not only of

Table 17.1. Some Endocrines Possibly Involved in Responses and Adaptations to Exercise.

Endocrine Organ	Hormone Produced	Some Functions
Hypothalamus	Somatoliberin	Stimulates release of somatotropin from anterior pituitary
	Somatostatin	Inhibits release of somatotropin from anterior pituitary
	Thyroliberin	Stimulates release of thyrotropin from anterior pituitary
	Corticoliberin	Stimulates release of corticotropin from anterior pituitary
	Luliberin	Stimulates release of lutropin from anterior pituitary
	Prolactoliberin	Stimulates release of prolactin from anterior pituitary
	Prolactostatin	Inhibits release of prolactin from anterior pituitary
	Antidiuretic Hormone	Released from posterior pituitary, increases water retention by kidneys
Anterior Pituitary	Somatotropin	Stimulates bone growth; mobilizes fat for energy
	Thyrotropin	Stimulates production and release of thyroxine by thyroid gland
	Corticotropin	Stimulates production and release of cortisol, aldosterone, and other hormones by adrenal cortex
	Lutropin	Stimulates testes to produce testosterone; promotes development of corpus luteum in females
	Prolactin	Promotes water retention by kidneys and mobilizes fat for energy in both sexes; promotes lactation in females.
Thyroid Gland	Thyroxine	Stimulates mitochondrial function; promotes cell growth
	Calcitonin	Reduces blood calcium, phosphate levels
Adrenal Cortex	Cortisol and Others	Promotes fat utilization; conserves blood glucose; reduces inflammation
	Aldosterone and Others	Promotes sodium and water retention by kidneys
Adrenal Medulla	Adrenaline, Noradrenaline	Enhances cardiac output, vasoconstriction, glycogen breakdown, fat mobilization

(Continued)

Table 17.1.   (Continued)

Endocrine Organ	Hormone Produced	Some Functions
Pancreas	Insulin	Promotes uptake of blood glucose by cells; increases glycogen storage
	Glucagon	Promotes release of glucose from liver stores to blood; enhances cardiac output; mobilizes fat for energy
Parathyroid Glands	Parathyroid Hormone	Increases blood calcium; decreases blood phosphate levels
Testes	Testosterone	Increases muscle mass; decreases fat content of body; increases muscle glycogen and red blood cell production; responsible for male secondary sex characteristics
Liver	Somatomedin	Stimulates cartilage and bone growth upon activation by somatotropin
Many Tissues	Prostaglandins	Many activities depending upon chemistry of specific prostaglandin, e.g., increased cardiac output, vasodilatation

control animals and operated animals, but also the responses of operated animals that receive hormone injections to replace the hormone lost by the removal of the endocrine gland. A third method often used to study the importance of endocrines in exercise is to measure the levels of those hormones in urine, blood, muscle and other tissues. If the concentrations of hormones change in response to exercise, it is often assumed that the hormones must be involved in helping the body respond or adapt to the exercise. This is not necessarily so, as the discussion in the next paragraph explains.

Studies of changes in hormone levels in urine, blood and tissue in response to exercise may produce some misleading results. This is so because the concentration of a hormone at any moment in time is affected by several variables. For example, the concentration of hormone is obviously dependent upon *the rate at which the endocrine gland is producing the hormone*, but the hormone concentration is also dependent upon *the rate of hormone destruction* by enzymes in the liver, kidney, and other tissues. In addition, the concentration of hormone in blood and urine is also dependent upon *the rate at which the hormone is taken up into the tissues* in which the hormone has its effect and upon *the extent to which any changes in blood volume occur*.

Finally, it is important to know how long any change in hormone level after exercise persists; some hormones are broken down in as little as a few seconds after they are produced and have only brief effects, whereas others last for several hours and may produce effects lasting several days.

Accordingly, a rise in hormone concentration in the blood during exercise could be interpreted as an increased output of the hormone by its endocrine gland source, a decreased destruction of the hormone (perhaps because of reduced blood flow to the liver or kidneys), or a decreased uptake of the hormone by its target tissues. Even if it was proved that the rise in hormone concentration was because of increased production, the total adaptive effect of this increased hormone production may be insignificant if the production rate does not remain elevated long enough to allow the greater hormone levels to have any substantial effects on the target tissues. Thus, one must use great caution in the interpretation of changes in blood or urine levels of hormones with exercise. Such changes may indeed reflect some important alteration in endocrine function, or they may only reflect changes in blood flow either to target organs or to sites of hormone degradation. Unfortunately, most of the available data on endocrine changes with exercise consists only of reports of changes in blood or urine levels of the hormones in question. Until more complete information on other aspects of the metabolism of such hormones is available, one is probably wise not to place too much importance on observed changes in hormone concentrations in blood or urine.

HYPOTHALAMIC AND PITUITARY HORMONES AND EXERCISE

There is no direct evidence that exercise causes a change in the rates of secretion of any of the liberins (releasing hormones) or statins (release-inhibiting hormones) from the hypothalamus (Table 17.1). Logically, though, it seems that some of these hormones ought to be secreted in greater quantities to account for apparent changes in the rates of hormone secretion by the anterior pituitary and by glands such as the thyroid and adrenals. For example, exercise is generally accepted to be a stimulator of somatotropin (growth hormone) release from the anterior pituitary. If the widely held theory that somatotropin release is stimulated by hypothalamic somatoliberin is correct, then it follows that a rise in somatotropin is preceded by a rise in somatoliberin, and followed by a later rise in somatostatin, which would prevent too great a rise in somatotropin. Likewise, although there is no conclusive evidence that the secretions of thyrotropin (thyroid-stimulating hormone) or corticotropin (adrenocorticotropic

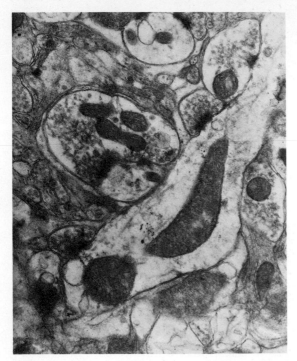

Figure 17.1. Electron micrograph of hypo-thalamus (magnification ×5,300). Large, irregu-lar shaped central structure is a nerve axon, and smaller, globular shaped structures in contact with the axon are nerve endings containing dark mitochondria and many small vesicles of acetyl-choline. (Courtesy of G. Colin Budd, Physiology Department, Medical College of Ohio, Toledo, Ohio.)

hormone) are elevated by exercise, the fact that blood levels of thy-roxine and cortisol rise with exercise suggests that the thyroid and adrenals are stimulated by thyrotropin and corticotropin, respec-tively, and that the anterior pituitary is stimulated to release these two pituitary hormones by the enhanced secretion of thyroliberin and corticoliberin from the hypothalamus.

Two explanations may account for the apparent discrepancy between the presumed need for greater secretion rates of hypothala-mic liberins and the lack of evidence that enhanced secretion does occur. First, it should be pointed out that until recently no simple reliable methods for quantifying the secretion rates of the liberins or statins existed. Accordingly, physiologists have been unable to measure any changes in liberin or statin secretion rates that might occur during exercise. Second, although higher blood levels of somatotropin, cortisol, thyroxine, and other hormones *seem* to implicate the hypothalamic hormones, it must be remembered that these higher blood levels may be accounted for by lesser rates of destruction rather than by greater rates of secretion. Thus, it may be that there is no real need for greater secretion of liberins and statins from the hypothalamus because there is no genuine increase in the rates of secretion of somatotropin, cortisol, and other hormones.

Antidiuretic Hormone

A greater secretion of antidiuretic hormone from the hypothalamus and a greater release of this hormone from the posterior pituitary may explain some of the increased retention of water by the kidneys during severe exercise, especially when the exerciser is dehydrated. (See Chapter 16). Such an increased secretion of antidiuretic hormone would be a useful response to help conserve body water during exercise, and there is evidence that such an enhanced secretion of this hormone actually takes place during heavy exercise (15).

Somatotropin (Growth Hormone)

Somatotropin elevations with exercise would seem to be useful because of the beneficial effect of somatotropin on connective tissue and muscular growth; this effect could partly account for the greater strength of tendons, ligaments and muscles, and for the greater bone thickness observed in those who are physically trained. Also, somatotropin helps to mobilize fatty acids from adipose tissue stores and to increase the fatty acid levels in the blood. This could be a useful response during exercise to help provide fuel for working muscles. Half of any newly secreted somatotropin is degraded by the liver in about 17–45 minutes, so a substantial portion of the hormone persists in the blood long enough to have significant effects on tissue growth and fatty acid mobilization. Since there is a lag period of about one hour before any effect of growth hormone on fat mobilization is observed (26), such an effect would seem important only in prolonged exercise.

Response to Exercise. Most investigations of the effects of a single bout of exercise on somatotropin levels in human blood have revealed a substantial rise that often is not seen for the first 15–20 minutes of the exercise. (See Fig. 17.2 and Refs. 11, 12, 17, 22, 25, 27). Incidentally, this response also occurs in pigs and monkeys, but not

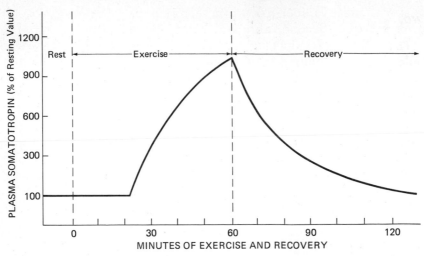

Figure 17.2. Diagram of somatotropin concentration in blood plasma during exercise and recovery.

in rats (8). Usually the increase in somatotropin is greater if the exercise is of longer duration and of greater intensity for the exerciser (22, 27), but even short-term, submaximal work can result in somatotropin increases in the blood (25).

The increase in somatotropin concentration in plasma as a response to exercise is so great that it is not likely to be totally a function of decreased hormone degradation or hormone uptake into tissues, and more probably results from an increased rate of secretion of somatotropin from the anterior pituitary (27). Although there is an association between body temperature and plasma somatotropin levels (4), there does not seem to be a strong cause-and-effect relationship between these two variables (27). It is widely recognized that somatotropin levels in blood increase in response to psychological stress, but exercise raises somatotropin concentrations even when precautions are taken to minimize psychological effects (11, 12). There have been other factors proposed as possible stimulants for somatotropin release during exercise, but the mechanism underlying this hormonal response is still unknown (22, 27).

Adaptation to Training.   There is no reproducible effect of physical training on somatotropin levels in the blood under resting conditions, but there are several reports that those who are trained tend to have less dramatic rises in blood somatotropin during exercise (12, 23, 27). Such an adaptation is perhaps in part a result of the reduced psychological stress of exercise in trained persons.

Thyrotropin (Thyroid-Stimulating Hormone)

There is reason to believe that the rate of thyrotropin secretion should be elevated during exercise because there seems to be an increased secretion of thyroxine with exercise, and secretion of thyroxine by the thyroid gland is stimulated by thyrotropin released from the pituitary. Thyrotropin secretion is increased during anticipation of exercise (21), but additional increases in thyrotropin levels in the blood because of actual physical activity have not been detected (31). Since one-half of the anticipatory rise in thyrotropin would still be present in the blood up to an hour after exercise begins, the anticipatory secretion of hormone could have an effect on thyroid function during the exercise period.

Corticotropin (Adrenocorticotropic Hormone)

The blood level of cortisol, which is secreted by the adrenal cortex, usually is increased by exhaustive exercise, and it is generally assumed that this response is triggered by a greater secretion of corticotropin from the pituitary. This assumption is based on the fact that corticotropin is a potent stimulator of adrenal hormone secretion. Corticotropin also directly enhances fat mobilization from fat stores, and this could be deemed a useful response in long duration exercise. However, perhaps because corticotropin is rapidly destroyed (half-life = 4–18 minutes) and difficult to measure, there is apparently no conclusive evidence of increased corticotropin secretion during exercise. (The half-life of a hormone is the time elapsed before one-half of a given amount of hormone is destroyed by the body.)

Corticotropin secretion does rise with emotional stress. If one can assume that anticipation of exhaustive exercise is enough of a stress to elicit an increased secretion of corticotropin, this anticipatory effect should promote cortisol secretion during exercise; corticotropin stimulates adrenal secretion within 1–2 minutes, and the cortisol is only slowly degraded (half-life = 4 hours) (27).

Lutropin (Luteinizing Hormone, Interstitial Cell-Stimulating Hormone)

Lutropin is responsible for stimulating the testes to produce testosterone. Since a rise in testosterone secretion could promote muscle hypertrophy and increased strength, an increased secretion of lutropin could be deemed a useful exercise response or adaptation. However, levels of plasma lutropin are not affected by a single bout of swimming or rowing (30), and neither lutropin nor follitropin (follicle stimulating hormone) concentrations in the blood seem to change when measured at rest after a long-term weight-training program (28).

Proclactin

Prolactin secretion during exercise could be useful both in conserving water through its antidiuretic effect on the kidneys and in mobilizing fat for energy. Some studies have shown increased prolactin levels in blood following exercise (20). Half of any newly secreted prolactin is destroyed in 15–30 minutes. This half-life should allow time for a significant effect of any increased secretion of prolactin during exercise.

THYROXINE

Thyroxine can mobilize fatty acids from adipose tissue stores and can promote cardiac hypertrophy. Both of these actions might help the body become better able to withstand the rigors of prolonged exercise, and it is, therefore, not surprising that several studies of thyroid responses to exercise have been undertaken. Thyroxine is especially interesting as a possible agent for adapting to exercise stress because it has a half-life of 6–7 days and produces effects that may be noticeable for 2 weeks or longer. Accordingly, a very small change in thyroxine availability as a result of exercise could have profound and long-lasting effects, especially on tissue growth.

Response to Exercise

The concentration of *free* thyroxine in blood is increased by about 35 per cent during a period of exercise (31). Most of the thyroxine in the blood is not "free," but is bound to circulating plasma proteins. The *total* (bound + free) thyroxine concentration in blood may actually *decrease* during exercise, because thyroxine is taken up by tissues or degraded faster than it is secreted; that is, rates of both secretion and degradation are enhanced by exercise (31, 32). However, it is the free thyroxine that is metabolically active and available for use in the tissues. But it should be pointed out that there is no apparent increase in the uptake of free thyroxine by skeletal muscles during exercise, whereas there is a greater uptake of the free hormone by the liver, the major site of breakdown of thyroxine (32). Thus, there is no clear-cut evidence that the extra free thyroxine observed in the blood of exercisers is of any particular value.

The increase in free thyroxine in the blood during exercise seems to be the result of a decreased binding of the hormone by the plasma proteins; that is, there is no change in the level of binding proteins, but only a decrease in their tendencies to bind thyroxine (32). The mechanisms underlying this decreased binding and the increased rates of secretion and degradation are unproved, but it seems likely that the greater rate of thyroxine secretion during exercise results from enhanced thyrotropin secretion, perhaps in anticipation of exercise (21). Also, the increased rate of degradation may be caused by the greater susceptibility of the larger concentrations of free thyroxine to degradation by the liver (32). (Binding to plasma proteins tends to protect thyroxine from rapid destruction, so greater amounts of free thyroxine could lead to faster destruction by the liver.)

Adaptation to Training

At rest, trained persons have reduced concentrations of *total* thyroxine and increased concentrations of *free* thyroxine. They also are characterized by higher rates of both secretion and degradation, with degradation rates being enhanced more than secretion rates. Thus, the half-lives of thyroxine for untrained and trained men are about 7 and 4 days, respectively (32). This means that half of all newly secreted thyroxine will be broken down in 7 days for untrained persons and in 4 days for trained persons. The mechanisms underlying these adaptations are probably the same as those for the acute responses.

There is no conclusive evidence that elevated concentrations of free thyroxine in the blood of trained animals have any beneficial effects. For example, most studies show no effect of physical training on basal metabolic rate, the rate at which a resting organism consumes oxygen (32). Since thyroxine is the most potent stimulus to basal metabolism, one might expect that trained animals would have greater metabolic rates, but this is not the case.

CALCITONIN AND PARATHYROID HORMONE

Calcitonin (thyrocalcitonin) from the thyroid gland and parathyroid hormone are potent regulators of calcium and phosphate levels in the blood. Since both of these minerals play important roles in muscle contraction and perhaps fatigue, it might seem reasonable to expect some changes in their hormonal regulation during exercise. Apparently no investigations of such potential changes have appeared in the literature.

HORMONES OF THE ADRENAL CORTEX

The adrenal cortex is stimulated by corticotropin from the pituitary to produce and secrete three general classes of hormones: glucocorticoids, mineralocorticoids, and sex hormones. The sex hormones are of minor significance in persons with normal testicular or ovarian functions, but the glucocorticoids and mineralocorticoids are necessary for survival in a normal stressful environment. Each of these two classes of hormones contains some 20 individual hormones, but only one in each class is of major physiological significance; cortisol represents about 95 per cent of all glucocorticoid activity, and aldosterone about 95 per cent of all mineralocorticoid activity. The half-lives of cortisol and aldosterone are about 240 and 30 minutes, respectively, so any increase of blood concentrations during exercise could have a prolonged effect.

Cortisol and the other glucocorticoids promote fat utilization in tissues by mobilizing fats and proteins and conserving carbohydrates. Under the influence of cortisol, blood glucose tends to be elevated. This conservation of blood glucose could conceivably be of some importance to help provide the brain with adequate nutrients during prolonged exercise, since nerve tissue depends heavily on glucose for energy. The mobilization of fatty acids for energy could also be useful in long duration work.

The glucocorticoids are also essential for organisms to resist stressful situations, including the stress of severe exercise training. Adrenalectomized animals are much less able to endure exercise than are normal animals (33).

The mineralocorticoids, of which aldosterone is the major representative, are involved primarily in the regulation of water, sodium, and potassium retention by the kidney. The maintenance of appropriate levels of sodium and potassium in the body fluids is vital to nerve and muscle functions because of the involvement of sodium and potassium in maintaining membrane potentials—without them nerves could not conduct impulses, and muscles could not contract. Also, aldosterone works in the kidney in cooperation with antidiuretic hormone to conserve body water, an especially important function during prolonged exercise in the heat.

Cortisol Response to Exercise

There is substantial controversy in the research literature about the effect of a single exposure to exercise on cortisol levels in the blood (26, 32). Thus, at light and moderate levels of exercise, there have been reports of increases, decreases, and no change in blood cortisol concentration. However, there is agreement that plasma cortisol concentrations and urinary excretion rates of free cortisol are enhanced by heavy, prolonged exercise (12, 22, 24, 27, 29, 33). Accordingly, it appears that the exercise must be relatively intense for a given person, and must be of long duration in order to achieve reliable increases in plasma cortisol levels and excretion rates (2, 27). Increases in plasma cortisol caused by exercise may persist for as long as 2 hours after exercise (9).

The mechanism underlying elevations in plasma cortisol probably involves increased secretion under the influence of corticotropin and is not thought to result from decreased rates of degradation or decreased uptake by tissues (27). No conclusive evidence has been presented that the output of corticotropin from the pituitary is increased during exercise.

Cortisol Adaptations to Training

In rats, whose major glucocorticoid is corticosterone rather than cortisol, the concentration of corticosterone in plasma is enhanced both at rest and after exercise in animals trained for 3–4 weeks, but these levels are returned to normal after 6 weeks of training (34). Also, the adrenals of trained rats release progressively less corticosterone upon stimulation by a standard amount of corticotropin as training progresses from 6 weeks onward. This decreased release of corticosterone has been shown to be caused by a decreased sensitivity of the adrenals to corticotropin (34).

In man, there does not seem to be any reliable effect of training on cortisol values in plasma, either at rest or after exercise (12, 27). Whether more discrete changes in adrenal glucocorticoid physiology follow physical training remains to be elucidated.

Aldosterone Response to Exercise

Plasma aldosterone concentrations rise progressively during exercise of increasing intensity with peak aldosterone levels of up to 6 times the resting value having been reported (5, 13, 19, 24, 29). This rise in aldosterone concentration may persist for 6–12 hours after completion of the exercise (5).

The mechanism underlying the aldosterone response to exercise apparently involves the renin-angiotensin system (Chapter 16) since the concentrations of both renin and angiotensin II also show substantial rises in plasma with exercise (19, 29). Thus, sympathetic nervous system activity during exercise reduces renal blood flow which, in turn, stimulates the kidney to release renin into the blood. The elevated renin activity increases the production of angiotensin which then stimulates the adrenal cortex to release aldosterone. With prolonged exercise resulting in dehydration, the initial sympathetic stimulus to the kidney may be a reduced venous pressure in the heart that is sensed by atrial volume receptors. The atrial receptors then may trigger a nerve reflex that constricts the renal arterioles (13).

Aldosterone Adaptation to Exercise

Apparently no training studies on aldosterone physiology have been conducted on human beings, but trained rats show no change in the exercise-associated rise in plasma renin activity (18).

SYMPATHOADRENAL HORMONES

All sympathetic nerve endings, including those to the adrenal glands, secrete both adrenaline (epinephrine) and noradrenaline (norepinephrine). Therefore, it is usually difficult to separate the effects of adrenal output from that of the secretion of sympathetic nerves in general when a change in plasma adrenaline or noradrenaline is observed. That is why in this discussion reference will be made to the sympathoadrenal system rather than to the adrenal glands only.

Sympathetic stimulation of blood vessels and of cardiac output is obviously important for exercise. The effect of adrenaline on increasing circulating fatty acids by activating an enzyme which degrades stored triglycerides, and on raising blood glucose by activating an enzyme which breaks down glycogen in the liver, could likewise be useful during prolonged exercise. Adrenaline and noradrenaline are quickly destroyed after their release and would not be expected to have any prolonged effects on the organism. Plasma adrenaline and noradrenaline return to resting values within 6 minutes after the end of exercise (1). About 75 per cent of the secretion of the adrenal medulla is adrenaline, whereas the sympathetic nerve endings secrete mostly noradrenaline.

Responses to Exercise

Ordinarily, one does not observe a rise in either adrenaline or noradrenaline in the blood with *mild* exercise unless that exercise is accompanied by unusual psychological stress. But as soon as the exercise intensity is great enough to elicit an oxygen uptake of more than about 60 per cent of one's maximal rate of consuming oxygen, a rise in plasma levels of both adrenaline and noradrenaline occurs (1, 6, 10, 11, 12). As exercise intensity progressively increases, so do the concentrations of these two hormones in the blood (Fig. 17.3). In-

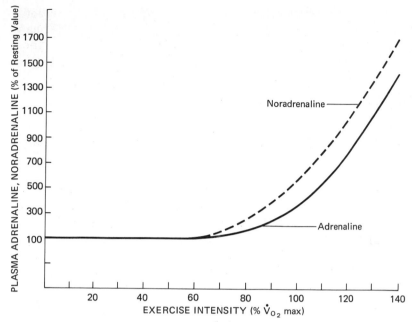

Figure 17.3. Diagram depicting rise in plasma adrenaline and noradrenaline with various intensities of exercise.

creased secretions of both sympathetic nerve endings in general, especially from nerves supplying blood vessels, and from sympathetic nerves supplying secretions of the adrenal glands are assumed to contribute to the increased blood levels of adrenaline and noradrenaline during exercise. However, the fact that more noradrenaline is released during exercise than adrenaline has led some to conclude that the sympathetic nerves are more important sources of these hormones than are the adrenal glands (12).

The mechanisms triggering the greater secretion of adrenaline and noradrenaline during exercise are not clear, but they probably include nerve reflexes originating in the cardiovascular system plus psychological effects.

Adaptations to Training

Most workers have found that with the same submaximal workload there is a somewhat lesser elevation of sympathoadrenal hormones in the blood after training (12). However, postexercise hormone excretion in the urine of trained persons is not necessarily different from that found before training (3). Any reduction in hormone elevations with submaximal exercise after training might be ac-

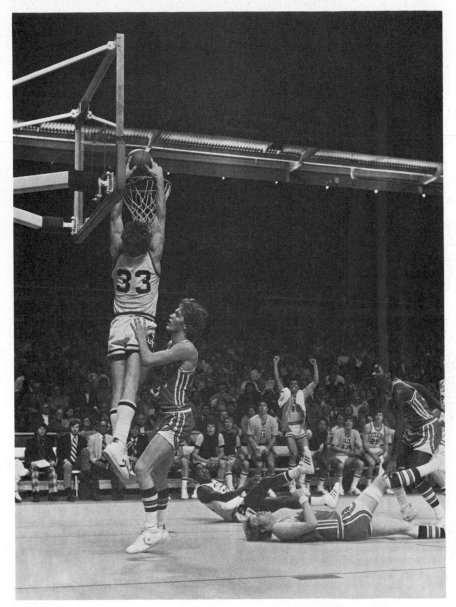

Figure 17.4. Adrenaline flows in both participants and spectators. (Courtesy of Office of Public Information, University of Toledo, Toledo, Ohio.)

counted for by the diminished psychological and physiological stresses associated with a standard exercise load after training.

HORMONES OF THE PANCREAS

Insulin and glucagon are both involved in the regulation of blood glucose levels. On the one hand, insulin tends to lower blood glucose by causing more glucose to be taken up out of the blood and across cell membranes into tissues such as skeletal muscle. On the other hand, glucagon tends to raise blood glucose by activating an enzyme that breaks down liver glycogen into glucose, which is then released into the blood. Glucagon also stimulates the heart to beat more forcefully and activates an enzyme that releases fatty acids into the blood from fat stores throughout the body. All of these hormonal actions could be important during prolonged exercise. In addition, insulin has a powerful effect on increasing glycogen stores in skeletal muscle and could conceivably be involved in the supercompensation of muscle glycogen that follows severe exercise (Chapter 4). The half-lives of glucagon and insulin are 5–10 minutes and 40 minutes, respectively.

Insulin Response to Exercise

Plasma insulin concentrations after exercise may decline to less than 50 per cent of levels observed in resting subjects (10, 12, 22, 26, 35). As with other hormonal changes during exercise, responses are apt to be greater with exercise regimens of greater intensity and greater duration (10, 12). Accordingly, one might not expect a significant fall in insulin after 5 minutes of jogging, but would be very likely to find a large decrease in plasma insulin after an exhaustive run of 2 or 3 hours. The plasma insulin concentration may not return to pre-exercise values for an hour or more after exercise (12).

It appears that the reduction in insulin found in the blood during exercise results both from a decreased secretion of insulin by the pancreas and from an increased uptake of insulin by working skeletal muscles (35).

The working muscles can get along nicely with a reduced concentration of insulin in the blood because more blood is circulating through those muscles during exercise. At the same time, blood flow to the liver is reduced so that there is less insulin circulating through the liver where insulin tends to block glucose delivery from the liver to the blood (35). Thus, the liver is free to supply additional glucose to the blood as the muscles use up glucose during exercise. It has been suggested that the decreased secretion of insulin by the pancreas during exercise is caused by elevated levels of plasma adrenaline and noradrenaline (12, 22, 26), but the fact that insulin in the plasma remains depressed for a much longer time after exercise than do adrenaline and noradrenaline speaks against this hypothesis. Since there is no reliable fall in blood glucose with most types of exercise, the decline in insulin is not caused by changes in blood glucose concentration.

Insulin Adaptation to Training

There does not seem to be a major effect of physical training on insulin in the blood of persons at rest. Trained persons do seem to have less of a reduction in insulin during work, perhaps because of a reduction in plasma adrenaline and noradrenaline during work after training (12).

Glucagon Response to Exercise

Exercise up to about 40 minutes in duration is associated with either no change or a slight increase in plasma glucagon concentrations (10, 25), but 85 minutes of exercise to exhaustion results in approximately a 3-fold increase in plasma glucagon (25). Therefore, it seems that in humans, a long duration of exercise is needed before a marked increase in plasma glucagon can be expected. This increase persists for longer than 30 minutes after exercise (25).

In dogs the increase in plasma glucagon with exercise results from greater rates of secretion of glucagon from the pancreas, but the increased glucagon is of questionable value, since a dog that has had its pancreas removed can increase the production of glucose by its liver during exercise almost as much as a normal dog (35). Because glucagon is a potent activator of glucose release from the liver, it thus seems, at least in dogs, of only minor importance during exercise.

The effect of training on glucagon secretion is unknown.

TESTOSTERONE

Prior to the age of puberty there is little difference in muscular strength between males and females. But as males begin to develop into sexual adulthood, they rapidly become stronger than females. This increased strength gives the male an advantage in many athletic events, so one might ask whether the greater strength results from the principal male sex hormone, testosterone, and whether stronger, more athletically successful males have more circulating testosterone than their weaker counterparts. A corollary question has been whether synthetic testosterone-like compounds can be administered to athletes to cause significant gains in muscular mass and strength.

Besides its relationship to muscular strength, testosterone has been implicated in the enhancement of aggressive behavior, red blood cell production, bone thickness, muscle glycogen storage, and muscle protein synthesis—all of which could theoretically be beneficial to athletic performance of various types (16). The half-life of testosterone is up to 3.4 hours, so any changes in plasma testosterone during exercise could exert effects over a considerable time.

Testosterone Response to Exercise

Testosterone levels in plasma have been reported to rise by 14–73 per cent in highly trained Olympic caliber male and female athletes and in male college-age weight lifters during strenuous work (7, 30) or to be unchanged in untrained adult males, high school-age males, and college-age females after exercise (7, 16). It is unclear to what extent any increase in plasma testosterone after exercise is the result of increased secretion of testosterone by the testes and/or adrenals or of decreased degradation of circulating testosterone as a result of diminished blood flow to the liver during heavy exercise. There is evidence that any rise in testosterone may persist for 30 minutes after exercise (30).

If testosterone were secreted at faster rates during exercise, it might be expected that levels of lutropin (interstitial cell-stimulating hormone) should also rise during exercise since lutropin stimulates the hormone-secreting cells of the testes. No such rise in lutropin has been detected (30), and this finding suggests that a rise in testosterone in plasma during exercise may be chiefly the result of a decreased rate of breakdown of testosterone in the liver.

Testosterone Adaptation to Training

There are conflicting statements in the research literature regarding whether or not regular physical training causes a change in the levels of testosterone in persons at rest (16, 28). There is at present no confirmation that training is associated with an increased level of testosterone in the blood. These is evidence that lutropin concentration in blood is not altered by 8 weeks of weight training (28).

SOMATOMEDIN

Somatomedin (sulfation factor) is produced by the liver in response to somatotropin secretion and is responsible for the effects of somatotropin on stimulating cartilage and bone growth. Since somatotropin in blood increases with exercise, it may be expected that somatomedin might also be increased with exercise. No investigations of this possibility have been conducted.

PROSTAGLANDINS

Prostaglandins are biologically active substances that are produced from polyunsaturated fatty acids. The name "prostaglandin" refers to the fact that these compounds were first found in extracts of prostate glands, but research has since shown that prostaglandins are produced in many tissues throughout the body. There are many different types of prostaglandins, each producing somewhat different actions from the others. Some are vasodilators, some, vasoconstrictors; some raise blood pressure, others lower it; some increase cardiac contractility, and some decrease fat breakdown. Thus, changes in the levels of prostaglandins or their breakdown products (thromboxanes and endoperoxides) could be involved in some of the physiological responses and adaptations to exercise.

Response to Exercise

A progressive cycling task to exhaustion, using both arms and legs, causes a modest rise in the plasma concentrations of certain types of prostaglandins (14). There have been no studies of the effects of training on prostaglandins.

SUMMARY

The study of endocrine responses and adaptations to exercise is in its infancy, but it is rapidly expanding. There are many reports describing changes in concentrations of hormones in blood during exercise, but very few comprehensive analyses of secretion rates, degradation rates and rates of uptake. Therefore, it is unclear to what extent exercise-associated increases in somatotropin, prolactin, cortisol, aldosterone, glucagon, testosterone and prostaglandins are caused by decreased rates of uptake or degradation.

It seems apparent that thyroxine secretion rates increase less than degradation rates during exercise, with the result that total plasma thyroxine levels are diminished with both exercise and training. Free thyroxine levels increase with exercise, but the physiological value of this increase is unknown. Insulin falls in the blood during exercise, whereas adrenaline and noradrenaline rise. Reliable changes in endocrine levels are most likely to be observed if the exercise is relatively intense for the exerciser and of long duration. Consequently, endocrine responses to exercise are probably of importance only during severe, prolonged exercise. Whether or not small changes in endocrines are important for long-term adaptations is unknown.

Review Questions

1. Explain the dependence of anterior pituitary hormones upon the liberins and statins of the hypothalamus.
2. Speculate on the possible value of exercise-associated increases in plasma levels of antidiuretic hormone, somatotropin, prolactin, thyroxine, cortisol, aldosterone, adrenaline and noradrenaline, glucagon, and testosterone.
3. Explain why changes in plasma concentrations of hormones do not necessarily reflect changes in hormone secretion rates.

References

1. Banister, E. W., and J. Griffiths. Blood levels of adrenergic amines during exercise. *Journal of Applied Physiology*, 1972, **33:**674–676.
2. Bonen, A. Effects of exercise on excretion rates of urinary free cortisol. *Journal of Applied Physiology*, 1976, **40:**115–158.
3. Brundin, T., and C. Cernigliaro. The effect of physical training on the sympathoadrenal response to exercise. *Scandinavian Journal of Clinical and Laboratory Investigation*, 1975, **35:**525–530.
4. Buckler, J. M. H. The relationship between changes in plasma growth hormone levels and body temperature occurring with exercise in man. *Biomedicine*, 1973, **19:**193–197.
5. Costill, D. L., R. Cote, E. Miller, T. Miller, and S. Wynder. Water and electrolyte replacement during repeated days of work in the heat. *Aviation, Space, and Environmental Medicine*, 1975, **46:**795–800.
6. Euler, U. S. von. Sympatho-adrenal activity in physical exercise. *Medicine and Science in Sports*, 1973, **6:**165–173.
7. Fahey, T. D., R. Rolph, P. Moungmee, J. Nagel, and S. Mortara. Serum testosterone, body composition, and strength of young adults. *Medicine and Science in Sports*, 1976, **8:**31–34.
8. Federspil, G., G. Udeschini, C. De Palo, and N. Sicolo. Role of

growth hormone in lipid mobilization stimulated by prolonged muscular exercise in the rat. *Hormone and Metabolic Research*, 1975, **7**:484–488.

9. Follenius, M., and G. Brandenberger. Effect of muscular exercise on daytime variations of plasma cortisol and glucose. In H. Howald and J. R. Poortmans (Eds.), *Metabolic Adaptation to Prolonged Physical Exercise*. Basel: Birkhauser Verlag, 1975, 322–325.

10. Galbo, H., J. J. Holst, and N. J. Christensen. Glucagon and plasma catecholamine responses to graded and prolonged exercise in man. *Journal of Applied Physiology*, 1975, **38**:70–76.

11. Hartley, L. H. Growth hormone and catecholamine response to exercise in relation to physical training. *Medicine and Science in Sports*, 1975, **7**:34–36.

12. Hartley, L. H., J. W. Mason, R. P. Hogan, L. G. Jones, T. A. Kotchen, E. H. Mougey, F. E. Wherry, L. L. Pennington, and P. T. Ricketts. Multiple hormonal responses to graded exercise in relation to physical training. *Journal of Applied Physiology*, 1972, **33**:602–606.

13. Kirsch, K., W. D. Risch, U. Mund, L. Rocker, and H. Stoboy. Low pressure system and blood volume regulating hormones after prolonged exercise. In H. Howald and J. R. Poortmans (Eds.), *Metabolic Adaptation to Prolonged Physical Exercise*. Basel: Birkhauser Verlag, 1975, pp. 315–321.

14. Kochan, R. G., and D. R. Lamb. Prostaglandin B equivalents in plasma of exercised men. In B. Samuelsson and R. Paoletti (Eds.), *Advances in Prostaglandin and Thromboxane Research*. New York: Raven Press, 1976, pp. 878–879.

15. Kozlowski, S., E. Szczepanska, and A. Zielinski. The hypothalamo-hypophyseal antidiuretic system in physical exercises. *Archives Internationales de Physiologie et de Biochimie*, 1967, **75**:218–228.

16. Lamb, D. R. Androgens and exercise. *Medicine and Science in Sports*, 1975, **7**:1–5.

17. Lassarre, C., F. Girard, J. Durand, and J. Raynaud. Kinetics of human growth hormone during submaximal exercise. *Journal of Applied Physiology*, 1974, **37**:826–830.

18. Leon, A. S., W. A. Pettinger, and M. A. Saviano. Enhancement of serum renin activity by exercise in the rat. *Medicine and Science in Sports*, 1973, **5**:40–43.

19. Maher, J. T., L. G. Jones, L. H. Hartley, G. H. Williams and L. I. Rose. Aldosterone dynamics during graded exercise at sea level and high altitude. *Journal of Applied Physiology*, 1975, **39**:18–22.

20. Malarkey, W. B. Recently discovered hypothalamic-pituitary hormones. *Clinical Chemistry*, 1976, **22:**5–15.
21. Mason, J. W., L. H. Hartley, T. A. Kotchen F. E. Wherry, L. L. Pennington, and L. G. Jones. Plasma thyroid-stimulating hormone response in anticipation of muscular exercise in the human. *Journal of Clinical Endocrinology and Metabolism*, 1973, **37:**403–406.
22. Metivier, G. The effects of long-lasting physical exercise and training on hormonal regulation. In H. Howald and J. R. Poortmans (Eds.), *Metabolic Adaptation to Prolonged Physical Exercise.* Basel: Birkhauser Verlag, 1975, pp. 276–292.
23. Mikulaj, L., L. Komadel, M. Vigas, R. Kvetnansky, L. Starka, P. Vencel. Some hormonal changes after different kinds of motor stress in trained and untrained young men. In H. Howald and J. R. Poortmans (Eds.), *Metabolic Adaptation to Prolonged Physical Exercise.* Basel: Birkauser Verlag, 1975, pp. 333–338.
24. Newmark, S. R., T. Himathongkam, R. P. Martin, K. H. Cooper, and L. I. Rose. Adrenocortical response to marathon running. *Journal of Clinical Endocrinology and Metabolism*, 1976, **42:**393–394.
25. Nilsson, K. O., L. G. Heding, and B. Hokfelt. The influence of short-term submaximal work on the plasma concentrations of catecholamines, pancreatic glucagon and growth hormone in man. *Acta Endocrinologica*, 1975, **79:**286–294.
26. Pruett, E. D. R. Plasma insulin concentrations during prolonged work at near-maximal oxygen intake. *Journal of Applied Physiology*, 1970, **29:**155–158.
27. Shephard, R. J., and K. H. Sidney. Effects of physical exercise on plasma growth hormone and cortisol levels in human subjects. *Exercise and Sport Sciences Reviews*, 1975, **3:**1–30.
28. Stromme, S. B., H. D. Meen, and A. Aakvaag. Effects of an androgenic–anabolic steroid on strength development and plasma testosterone levels in normal males. *Medicine and Science in Sports*, 1974, **6:**203–208.
29. Sundsfjord, J. A., S. B. Stromme, and A. Aakvaag. Plasma aldosterone, plasma renin activity and cortisol during exercise. In H. Howald and J. R. Poortmans (Eds.), *Metabolic Adaptation to Prolonged Physical Exercise.* Basel: Birkhauser Verlag, 1975, pp. 308–314.
30. Sutton, J. R., M. J. Coleman, J. Casey, and L. Lazarus. Androgen responses during physical exercise. *British Medical Journal*, 1973, **163:**520–522.
31. Terjung, R. L., and C. M. Tipton. Plasma thyroxine and thyroid–stimulating hormone levels during submaximal ex-

ercise in humans. *American Journal of Physiology*, 1971, **220**:1840–1845.

32. Terjung, R. L., and W. W. Winder. Exercise and thyroid function. *Medicine and Science in Sports*, 1975, **7**:20–26.

33. Tharp, G. D. The role of glucocorticoids in exercise. *Medicine and Science in Sports*, 1975, **7**:6–11.

34. Tharp, G. D., and R. J. Buuck. Adrenal adaptation to chronic exercise. *Journal of Applied Physiology*, 1974, **37**:720–722.

35. Vranic, M., R. Kawamori, and G. A. Wrenshall. The role of insulin and glucagon in regulating glucose turnover in dogs during exercise. *Medicine and Science in Sports*, 1975, **7**:27–33.

Exercise and health

It is widely assumed by the general public that the person who exercises regularly is healthier and less subject to disease than one who does not. This assumption is especially dear to those who enjoy regular exercise, a group including most physical educators and coaches. *Disease* is defined as a condition of the body in which there is incorrect or abnormal function of one or more of its parts. *Health,* on the other hand, is the condition of the body characterized by vigor, vitality, and freedom from disease. Although there is much scientific evidence that can be cited to support the view that those who exercise are healthier than those who do not, it is also true that much of the evidence regarding characteristics such as life span and susceptibility to coronary heart disease is inconclusive. Most of the data show that healthful characteristics are *associated* with populations of persons who exercise regularly, but such relationships are not necessarily cause-and-effect relationships. One might suspect, for example, that persons who exercise are less likely to suffer early heart attacks, not because they exercise, but because some other factor common to exercisers (for example, low body fat and superior hereditary qualities) has a protective effect on the heart.

EXPERIMENTAL AND NONEXPERIMENTAL EVIDENCE

The scientist who wishes to determine whether or not regular exercise has a beneficial effect on health has essentially two avenues of investigation open to him—experimental and nonexperimental. In an experiment, the investigator can assign subjects at random to either an exercise or a sedentary group. If the study is well-controlled, and if the subjects who exercise regularly are healthier at the end of the study, the scientist can have a relatively high degree of confidence that the difference in health between the two groups results from the exercise and not from some other factors.

With the nonexperimental approach, the investigator typically compares the health of a population of "exercisers" to that of a population of "nonexercises." However, the investigator does not assign the subjects to the exercise and nonexercise conditions; he must take the populations as they present themselves, as for example, sedentary cashiers versus active foundry workers, mail carriers versus postal clerks, executives versus laborers. Accordingly, if the active population is healthier, the scientist cannot be certain that the difference in health status is due to exercise because he is unable to control all the other possible factors (examples include diet, heredity and emotionality) that could account for the apparently beneficial effect of exercise on health.

It is unfortunate that all problems cannot be solved by experimentation. It is foolish, for example, to design an experiment to determine whether or not regular exercise enhances life span in humans; it is not reasonable to think that infants could be randomly assigned to active or sedentary living for their entire lives. Long-term experiments on humans are notoriously difficult to complete in a satisfactory manner because of uncontrollable changes in human life styles. Therefore, nonexperimental studies are vital to give us some evidence, albeit imperfect, on important questions that cannot be answered experimentally.

Criteria for Confidence in Cause and Effect
Nature of Nonexperimental Results

It is true that the results of a single nonexperimental study showing exercise to be associated with improved health should not be interpreted as proving that exercise *caused* the improved health.

On the other hand, one can have a great deal of confidence in the cause-and-effect nature of results from nonexperimental studies if the following criteria are satisfied:

1. *The association between exercise and health must be reliable.* This means that all or nearly all studies of the same association between exercise and health must show similar results. As more studies show the same association between exercise and certain health characteristics, our confidence in the cause-and-effect nature of the association increases.
2. *The association between exercise and health must be strong.* We can place much more confidence in the cause-and-effect nature of an association, for example, if it shows that 90 per cent of the exercisers are healthier than if only 51 per cent of the exercisers are healthier than the nonexercisers.
3. *The association between exercise and health must be logical.* It would be difficult to believe that regular exercise causes a reduction in the size of warts, no matter how many studies showed a strong association of this nature. There is no logical reason to think that exercise should decrease the growth of warts.
4. *The association between exercise and health must follow an appropriate chronological sequence.* For example, before one can be certain that regular aerobic endurance exercise causes a low resting heart rate, it must be shown that the low resting heart rate does not precede the exercise training. Whenever two factors A and B are related causally, it is not only possible that A causes B but also that B could conceivably cause A.
5. *The effect on health must be shown not to be caused by some obvious factor other than exercise.* One must seek out and find wanting alternative causes for the association between exercise and health. Is it exercise *per se* that causes active populations to have less body fat, or is the reduced fat simply the result of the fact that people who exercise also happen to eat less than sedentary populations? Could the same reduction in fat be caused by dietary restriction?

   Of course, it is impossible to test *all* alternative causes that might explain an association between exercise and health; many of the alternative causes are unknown. But until the obvious alternatives have been tested, one can have only limited confidence in the cause-and-effect nature of an association between exercise and health.

If the previous criteria are satisfied, one can have just as much confidence in the cause-and-effect nature of nonexperimentally discovered associations between exercise and health as one has in experimentally derived evidence. Keep these criteria in mind as you weigh the evidence presented in this chapter. Also, remember that a failure to prove absolutely that exercise has a positive effect on some health characteristics does not mean that one should abandon all physical activity performed for health purposes. There is no evidence that a properly designed exercise program is harmful to health, and there is much evidence that it may be beneficial. Thus, there is a much greater risk to health from inactivity than from appropriate regular exercise.

The remainder of this chapter is devoted to a presentation of the evidence 1) that regular exercise may influence the length and quality of human life; 2) that exercise may be useful in the prevention of disease; 3) that exercise can be useful in the treatment of disease; and 4) that improperly designed exercise programs may actually be harmful to one's health.

EXERCISE, LONGEVITY, AND QUALITY OF LIFE

As mentioned earlier, in a practical sense there can be no adequately designed experiments to test the hypothesis that regular exercise throughout life can increase longevity. Therefore, one can only compare the life spans of groups of presumably active persons with those of similar groups of presumably inactive persons. One can imagine many factors that influence life span that could easily mask any beneficial effect of lifetime exercise. Automobile accidents, wars, and infectious disease epidemics can kill many people at an early age who might otherwise have lived long, healthy lives. Accordingly, one should not expect to see a tremendous difference in the average life span of those from "active" and "sedentary" populations.

Many of the studies of exercise and longevity have included comparisons of the life spans of college athletes with those of their nonathletic classmates or of the population in general (26, 37). Those studies in which the general population was used as a control group all showed that former college athletes lived about two years longer than the general population (37). Unfortunately, the life span of all university graduates (who have better nutrition, better medical care and better jobs) tends to be longer than that of the general population, so these early studies are not very useful in determining the effect of exercise on longevity.

Comparisons of the longevity of former college athletes to that of their nonathletic counterparts are more valid, but most of these studies have shown only insignificant differences between groups (31,

37). One interesting comparison of life spans of 1,655 Japanese university athletes, 3,069 Tokyo University Medical School graduates and the general Japanese population showed that 70 per cent of the athletes, 42 per cent of the general population and only 35 per cent of the medical doctors reached the age range of 68–72 years (26).

It can be contended, of course, that college athletes do not necessarily remain active after college, and that no difference should be expected between life spans of former athletes and nonathletes. A study of 396 Finnish champion skiers (not necessarily university graduates), who tend to continue skiing for many years, showed that their average life span was 2.8 years longer than the median life expectation of the general male population (31). Perhaps future investigators will be able to amass adequate data from those who jog regularly into their later years to better judge the effect of regular endurance exercise on longevity.

Experimental evidence that exercise can increase life span in rats by 27–40 per cent has been obtained (46). Such experiments can be more readily carried out with laboratory animals than men because the animals have much shorter life spans and because their diets and living habits can be rather easily controlled. Thus, there appears to be some justification for believing that exercise may play at least a small role in increasing longevity.

Quality of Life

Regular exercise undoubtedly plays a more important role in enhancing the quality of one's life than its length. Valid experiments on this point of enhanced quality of life are difficult to come by; men and women who participate in regular exercise do so voluntarily, usually because they are convinced that physical activity does improve the quality of their lives. Again, it is impossible to assign human beings to long-term exercise or nonexercise conditions. However, it is patently obvious that one who is physically able to do more things for himself with less physical and emotional strain has a better quality of life than one who is not. There are millions of persons who find it impossible to climb a flight of stairs, carry a heavy bag of groceries, shovel snow, run to catch a bus, play tennis, go swimming, or ride a bicycle without asking someone's assistance or, at a minimum, experiencing such strain that they may be risking injury to themselves. One need only ask a person who is bedridden if he would prefer to be active to know that regular, appropriate, physical activity enhances the quality of life. A more serious question, but one that is impossible to answer for everyone, is: *How much* exercise is required to achieve the *optimal* quality of life?

REGULAR EXERCISE AND THE PREVENTION OF DISEASE

If disease is defined as the incorrect or abnormal function of a parts(s) of the body, it can be vigorously asserted that regular physical activity can prevent disease. Evidence in support of this assertion has been accumulating for more than a century. For an extensive review of the literature of the late 1800's and early 1900's the reader should consult the classic work by the late Arthur Steinhaus on the effects of chronic exercise (54).

Hypokinetic Degeneration

Hypokinesis is a relative lack of movement. An extreme case of hypokinesis would be that present in a patient placed in a total body cast for recovery from multiple bone fractures. Less extreme hypokinesis is present in office workers who sit at their desks eight hours a day and then drive to their homes where they watch 5 or 6 hours of television before retiring. Hypokinetic degeneration is a disease characterized by decreased functional capacity of many organs and systems. In those who rest in bed for several weeks or months, some or all of the following may occur (4):

1. *Osteoporosis (bone atrophy)*—Loss of bone minerals and protein makes the bones of the bed-ridden extremely susceptible to fractures.
2. *Muscle atrophy*—Gradual wasting away of skeletal muscle tissue causes progressively increasing muscular weakness. Muscle fibers assume more of the characteristics of fast-twitch fibers (14); mitochondria from atrophied muscles have a reduced capacity for aerobic metabolism (46).
3. *Loss of flexibility*—If joints are kept in improper positions for even a few days, connective tissue in tendons, ligaments, muscles and joint capsules becomes dense and shortened; eventually this connective tissue strongly resists any attempt at stretching to regain the lost range of motion of the joint. It is this connective tissue, especially that in the fascial sheaths of the muscles, that accounts for much of the limitation in range of motion of most joints in the body (11, 23).
4. *Cardiovascular degeneration*—Resting heart rate increases and stroke volume is diminished; maximal oxygen uptake is markedly lowered; the circulatory system is unable to maintain normal blood pressure responses when the patient is tilted upright; blood clots in the veins sometimes develop and may lodge in the lungs to cause death; and blood volume decreases.
5. *Respiratory problems*—Lung congestion, bronchial obstruc-

tion, and even pneumonia are more common in bedridden patients.

6. *Bladder and bowel dysfunction*—Immobilization often decreases sensitivity of the bladder and bowel so that inadequate voiding of urine and feces is common.

7. *Bed sores*—Painful ulcerations of the skin occur in those who remain motionless in bed.

There is no question that some minimal exercise program can prevent hypokinetic degenerative disease: By definition those who are reasonably active do not contract hypokinetic degenerative disease.

In earlier chapters ample discussion was presented of the efficacy of training in causing improvements in the muscular and cardiovascular system. Let us now describe briefly some of the evidence that regular exercise positively affects the characteristics of bones, ligaments, connective tissue within muscles, and nerves.

Exercise and Bone Growth. Bone tissue is constantly undergoing a process of remodeling, with minerals being removed from some parts of bones and added to others. During physical activity, stress is placed on the bone that causes an increased deposition of calcium salts along the lines of stress and removal of minerals from minimally stressed areas. In rats regular training sessions of 5 or 6 hours of light running cause few changes in either bone length or density, but more intensive exercise for shorter durations may slightly decrease bond length and increase bond density (5, 33). Also, bones from trained animals may have greater resistance to breaking and may heal faster after fracture (5). The physiological mechanism leading to stronger bones as a result of exercise is not certain (5, 33). There is no consistent evidence that training of youngsters results in shorter or taller stature.

Exercise, Ligaments, Tendons and Intramuscular Connective Tissue. Many studies of laboratory animals show that physical training strengthens the attachments of ligaments and tendons to bones (5, 58, 61). Trained ligaments are thicker and heavier, but the increased weight of the ligaments is not reflected in greater concentrations of collagen, the principal component of connective tissue fibers (5, 58). The mechanism underlying the enhanced strength of ligaments and tendons with training is unclear.

When soleus and plantaris muscles of a rat are made to work harder by surgical removal of the synergistic gastrocnemius muscle, there occurs not only a hypertrophy of the muscle fibers, but also an increase in the collagen content of the connective tissues that surround the muscle fibers (5). Perhaps the stronger connective tissue investments of the muscle allow the muscle to contract more forcefully before tears of connective tissue and capillaries result in delayed muscle soreness. The activity of an enzyme involved in collagen synthesis is increased by physical training, and this enzyme may play a part in increasing the production of collagen fibers (5). It has been speculated that lactic acid production during exercise stimulates the enzyme activity (5).

Exercise and the Nervous System. It is difficult to study neural tissue with normal biochemical and histological techniques; there are very small amounts of nerve tissue to work with, and the tissue is very easily torn or otherwise disrupted because of its delicate structure. Accordingly, it is not surprising that we know little of the adaptability of the nervous system to regular exercise. Studies of laboratory animals suggest that 1) terminal axons to muscles may be lengthened with training, 2) the area of neuromuscular junctions on trained muscles may be increased, 3) increased activity of cholinesterase enzyme may occur at neuromuscular junctions of trained muscles, especially in fast-twitch fibers, 4) the size of the cell bodies, nuclei and nucleoli of spinal motor neurons may increase with exhaustive exercise, and 5) increased activity of several enzymes of the motor neurons is present in trained animals (7, 14). Although the changes described in neural tissue are of unknown significance from a functional standpoint, it is clear that the nervous system can adapt to chronic exercise, and it seems highly probable that many of these neural adaptations are of major importance to the organism.

Coronary Heart Disease

Each year about one of every 100 American men 40 years of age or more will develop some symptom of coronary heart disease, the obstruction of one or more of the arteries that supply oxygen to the heart muscle. In about 60 per cent of these cases the obstruction of blood flow is so great that parts of the heart muscle are unable to function, cardiac output becomes inadequate, and the victims die immediately or within a few days (12). Therefore, it is clear that any significant reduction in death rate from coronary heart disease will have to be accomplished by a greater effort to *prevent* the disease rather than by attempts to treat the disease once it has manifested itself (53). Many cardiologists are of the opinion that coronary artery disease begins to develop in children and that preventive efforts, including the establishment of regular aerobic exercise habits, should be emphasized at very early ages (3, 6, 30). The principal question to be addressed in this section is: What role does regular exercise play in the prevention of premature heart disease?

Lack of Exercise as a Risk Factor in Coronary Heart Disease. Risk factors in coronary heart disease are those characteristics of persons that are associated with a large increase in susceptibility to the onset, particularly the premature onset (before age 65), of coronary heart disease (53). There are many characteristics related to coronary heart disease, but the four major risk factors seem to be: 1) consumption of a diet high in animal fat and cholesterol, 2) high levels of cholesterol and triglyceride fat in the blood, 3) hypertension (high blood pressure) and 4) cigarette smoking (53). Lack of exercise, obesity, diabetes mellitus, "high drive" personality factors and family history of heart disease are statistically less significant risk factors than the first four previously mentioned (53).

Most, but not all, comparisons of populations of presumably active workers with populations of inactive workers show that occupational physical activity predisposes one to have a lesser incidence of symptoms and early deaths from coronary heart disease. However, the active populations sometimes are reported to have a greater incidence of chest pain (angina pectoris) (19, 20, 53). Active conductors on the double-decker busses of London tended to have less coronary heart disease than the inactive bus drivers; London and Washington, D.C., postmen had less heart disease than inactive postal clerks; active workers in Israeli kibbutzim had less heart disease than their inactive counterparts; active railroad men had less heart disease than sedentary clerks; and active utility workers tended to have less heart disease than less active workers (19, 20, 53). However, some comparisons of active and inactive populations have failed to demonstrate any protective effect of occupational physical activity (20, 53). For example, Finnish workers who had physically demanding occupations had no decreased risk of heart disease, and active Los Angeles civil servants had the same risk of coronary heart disease as their less active counterparts (20, 53).

As stated earlier in this chapter, positive results of large-scale population comparisons do not prove a cause-and-effect relationship between more physical activity and less coronary heart disease. But the fact that most of these surveys implicate exercise as an independent risk factor certainly points to a high probablity that regular exercise helps prevent the early onset of coronary heart disease. Unfortunately, we need more studies of the relationship between leisure-time exercise patterns and coronary heart disease to give us better direction for prescribing preventive exercise.

Physiological Mechanism Underlying the Probable Protective Effect of Exercise. It is reasonable to ask *how* any protective effect of regular exercise against the early onset of coronary heart disease may be brought about. Many hypotheses that some single mechanism is responsible for this protective effect have been advanced, but none as yet has been proven. Most of the proposed mechanisms involve a presumed beneficial effect of regular exercise on 1) circulation to the heart muscle, 2) competency of the contractile process of the heart, 3) blood fat levels, 4) atherosclerotic lesion development, 5) blood clotting mechanisms, 6) obesity, 7) hypertension and 8) psychological well-being. Obesity and hypertension will be considered as separate diseases in subsequent discussions in this chapter.

Regular Exercise and Coronary Circulation. Because heart attacks are associated with decreased circulation of blood through the coronary arteries, one of the most obvious hypotheses to explain the beneficial effects on the risk of heart disease is that regular exercise somehow enhances coronary circulation, perhaps by enlarging the main branches of the coronary arteries, by improving the distribution of capillaries in the heart muscle, or by increasing the ability of the heart to develop new branches of healthy arteries to take over the circulation to blood-starved areas of the heart. The latter type of circulation is known as *coronary collateral circulation.* Collateral in this sense refers to the indirect, auxillary nature of the circulation.

Coronary Tree Size. It has been repeatedly demonstrated that rats physically trained from youth by swimming or treadmill running have larger coronary arteries and a greater size of the "coronary tree" than untrained control animals (2). Typically, in these studies, the coronary arteries of the animals are injected with a liquid plastic that rapidly hardens. The tissue around the plastic mold of the arteries is then digested away with chemicals, leaving a plastic model of the coronary tree which can be weighed or measured for arterial diameters. Some of the new coronary branches developed in the trained rat may serve areas of the heart already supplied from another artery and could be classified as coronary collaterals. It should be pointed out that the size of the coronary arteries of pigs is not increased by 10 minutes of treadmill running at 16 km/hr (10 mph), 5 days per week, for 22 months (35). However, each exercise regimen was of very short duration.

Cardiac Capillarization. Similarly, it has been often shown by comparing the number of capillaries filled with injected India ink or other chemicals that trained animals have more coronary capillaries, a greater number of capillaries per heart muscle fiber, and a smaller diffusion distance (half the distance between two capillaries) for oxygen than untrained animals (2). These anatomical adaptations partly account for the greater coronary blood flow in trained animals (48, 56). It is also interesting to note that rats whose mothers exercised regularly during pregnancy have greater cardiac capillarization than animals whose mothers did not exercise (44).

Coronary Collateral Circulation. A report in 1957 suggested that trained dogs had greater coronary collateral circulation after an artificial "heart attack" than did untrained controls; however, more recent experiments have failed to confirm the earlier results (2). There are no studies of coronary collateral development in *normal* human subjects, but experiments have been performed with patients who have suffered heart attacks. In these studies, the coronary circulation is viewed under x-ray after a dense material has been infused into the arteries so that the vessels will stand out under the x-ray. This process is called coronary arteriography. Most of the experiments with cardiac patients have not been able to detect a significant difference in the development of coronary collaterals between trained and untrained patients (2, 17, 49, 53). However, the experimental method of coronary arteriography may not be sensitive enough to detect meaningful changes in collateralization (2). Accordingly, it is too early to conclude with certainty whether exercise does or does not affect the development of coronary arteries, but at this point, the bulk of the evidence is in the negative direction.

If the increases in coronary tree size and capillarization that occur as a result of training in rats also occur in man, these changes should reduce the resistance and, therefore, increase the coronary blood flow at any given arterial pressure (2). Such an increased flow does occur in hearts of trained rats (48, 56). Also, the increased capillary development should result in the delivery of blood closer to the muscle fibers, so that oxygen can more effectively diffuse to the muscle cells. At the present time, however, we have no direct evidence that such changes do occur in man. If they occur, it seems likely that these circulatory adaptations are more apt to develop if training is begun in childhood.

Regular Exercise and Competency of the Cardiac Contractile Process. The oxygen uptake required by the heart to produce a given cardiac output increases with heart rate, that is, the more often the heart must contract against arterial pressure, the more oxygen must be consumed by the cardiac muscle fibers (50). Therefore, even if regular exercise has no beneficial effect on the coronary arteries, the heart of a trained person should be able to produce a given cardiac output with somewhat less coronary blood flow than the heart of an untrained person, simply because it pumps at a lower rate with a larger stroke volume (2). This contention is supported by the fact that a high resting heart rate is one of the risk factors associated with early death from coronary heart disease (53).

Greater stroke volume has been reported in trained men both with and without evidence of accompanying cardiac hypertrophy (2). If a hypertrophied heart has a greater ventricular volume at the end of diastolic filling, it makes sense that the stroke volume of larger hearts should be increased. In trained hearts where no increase in heart volume is apparent, the increased stroke volume is most likely caused by a training-induced enhancement of cardiac contractility (strength of contraction) (2, 48). Although there is little evidence that training influences cardiac contractility in man, there are several studies of this problem in rats that have produced controversial results (2, 9, 48). A majority of the evidence favors the idea that exercise has a positive effect on cardiac contractility, but there are several contradictory reports in the literature (2, 9, 48). Any increase in contractility associated with training may be related to increases in myosin ATPase activity or to a better delivery of calcium from the sarcoplasmic reticulum to troponin during the initiation of contraction (2, 9, 48, 57). There seem to be no major training-induced changes in aerobic energy production mechanisms or mitochondrial structures in the heart (2, 48).

Regardless of the mechanism involved, it is commonly observed that trained persons have greater stroke volumes and lower heart rates at rest or during a given physical load, and this training bradycardia (lower heart rate) may play an important role in the protective value of regular exercise against early death from coronary heart disease. Training bradycardia is apparently caused by an increased activity of the vagus nerves with perhaps some decrease in sympathetic stimulation to the heart (2).

Regular Exercise and Blood Fat Levels.   A victim of coronary heart disease typically has fatty deposits in the walls of the coronary arteries. These deposits narrow the arterial opening and obstruct the flow of blood. They contain a large amount of cholesterol and also some triglycerides. High levels of these fats in the blood are associated with a greater risk of early coronary heart disease (53).

Several investigators have studied the possibility that exercise might lower blood fat levels and, thereby, reduce the availability of cholesterol and triglycerides for deposit in the walls of the arteries. Unfortunately, in many of these studies, dietary fat intake and weight loss by the subjects were not adequately assessed. Because blood fat levels are affected both by diet and by weight loss, the interpretation of results of experiments in which these factors are not controlled becomes very difficult. Another problem of interpretation arises from the wide range of exercise programs used to study the relationship between exercise and blood fat levels. It may be that only very rigorous, long-term exercise programs of an aerobic endurance nature can lower blood fats with great reproducibility. From the studies that have been reported, however, we must conclude that 1) any effect of training on blood cholesterol levels is small, 2) training usually does lower triglyceride levels in the blood, and 3) the beneficial effect of training on triglycerides probably lasts for only two or three days (19, 51). Accordingly, an exercise program designed to help lower blood fats should include an exercise frequency of at least every other day.

Regular Exercise and Development of Atherosclerosis. Heart attacks are associated with the buildup of fatty deposits in the walls of the arteries, especially the coronary arteries. Atherosclerosis is the name given to this disease whereby the openings of the arteries are narrowed by the accumulation of fat in the arterial walls. The effect of regular exercise on the development of atherosclerosis has been studied in pigeons, geese, ducks, chickens, rabbits, dogs, rats and pigs (35). With a few exceptions, exercise training in these studies resulted in a reduced incidence of fatty deposits in arterial walls.

A particularly interesting experiment was done with pigs; as subjects, pigs presumably provide a good animal model for the study of atherosclerosis in humans (35). The pigs were placed on a high-fat diet that was known to produce atherosclerotic deposits similar in appearance to those in humans. The exercising animals ran 5 days per week at 16 km/hr for 10 minutes, and the study lasted 22 months. There was no demonstrable effect of this training program on blood fat levels or coronary artery size, but the exercised pigs gained less weight and had less body fat than the controls. Only 1 of 8 exercised males, and 2 of 9 exercised females, had any fatty deposits in their left coronary arteries, whereas all 9 of the male controls and all 9 of the female controls had fatty deposits. Areas of deposits of the 3 exercised animals that exhibited fatty deposits were only about 15 per cent of the average areas of fatty deposits in the nonexercised animals.

The mechanism underlying this reduction in the development of atherosclerosis in most animal models with training is not clear, but apparently these beneficial effects can occur in the absence of any lowering of blood cholesterol and triglycerides.

Regular Exercise and Blood Clotting and Fibrinolysis. The final insult to the coronary circulation that leads to a heart attack is presumably the formation of a thrombus or clot in the coronary artery that has become narrowed and roughened by the buildup of fatty deposits in its walls. If physical training could somehow reduce the probability of a clot forming in the blood vessels, or if training could increase the rate at which small clots are broken down (fibrinolysis), this could perhaps explain the protective effect of regular exercise with respect to early death or illness from coronary heart disease. However, it appears unlikely that either of these mechanisms is of particular importance in relationship to heart disease, because a single bout of vigorous exercise is associated with a faster clotting time that seems to be offset by a faster breakdown of the fibrin threads of the clots (1).

The increased coagulability of blood after heavy exercise is probably caused by the 200 per cent increase in the antihemophilic factor (Factor VIII) observed in the plasma of exercised persons (1). This factor is one of the many necessary components of the blood clotting system. The increase in the antihemophilic factor does not occur in the absence of stimulation by adrenaline, so this increase is probably caused by the activation of the sympathetic nervous system that accompanies heavy exercise (1).

As tiny clots form on the walls of arteries and veins, the fibrin threads that make up the framework of the clot can be dissolved or lysed by an enzyme called *fibrinolysin* or *plasmin*, which is the active form of *profibrinolysin* or *plasminogen*. Five minutes of *maximal* treadmill exercise results in a seven-fold increase in fibrinolytic activity, apparently by increasing the amount of a substance that converts profibrinolysin to fibrinolysin (1). There is either no increase or only a small increase in fibrinolytic activity with *submaximal* exercise of short duration, but prolongation of the exercise for many minutes or hours causes a large rise in fibrinolytic activity. The increased fibrinolytic activity during exercise is not caused by adrenaline or by temperature elevation (1).

It is not yet possible to say with certainty whether more rapid coagulation or more rapid fibrin dissolution is physiologically more important or, indeed, if either one plays any major role in the exercising person. However, it may be significant that the increased fibrinolytic response to exercise is much more reproducible than the increased coagulability (1). The fact that the changes in blood clotting and clot dissolution with exercise are no longer apparent 30–60 minutes after exercise, that is, that there is no adaptation with regular exercise (1), speaks against any important role for these changes in the prevention of early death or illness from coronary heart disease.

Regular Exercise and Psychological Well-Being. There is some evidence, albeit controversial, that certain types of psychosocial tensions, personality patterns and life styles may be significant risk factors in coronary heart disease (53). It is difficult to gather conclusive evidence in this area, and it is premature to make any final judgment concerning the impact of physical training on the risk of coronary heart disease through exercise-induced changes in psychological well–being. It is clear, however, that many, but not all, of those who participate in regular exercise programs experience improvement in their outlook on life (19).

Hypertension

Hypertension is a chronically elevated arterial blood pressure, sometimes arbitrarily defined as any resting pressure greater than 140/90 millimeters of mercury. Hypertension is responsible for 10–15 per cent of all deaths in people over 50 years of age, and is a significant risk factor not only in coronary heart disease but also in congestive heart disease, stroke and kidney disease. Hypertension can now be effectively controlled by drug therapy, but many investigators have considered the possibility that hypertension might be prevented by regular physical exercise. Most comparisons of normal physically trained or occupationally active populations with untrained or inactive groups show no differences in resting blood pressures. Also, exercise programs in those with normal blood pressure can usually be expected to cause blood pressure reductions of only a few millimeters of mercury (19, 45, 51). Thus, there is no conclusive evidence that regular exercise can prevent hypertension.

Obesity

In most developing countries in the world, undernutrition is a serious problem that is associated with an increased death rate from many diseases, but in the developed countries of North America and Europe, many persons suffer from *overnutrition* that also leads to an increased risk of early death. When food intake is in excess of the body's needs for energy, the excess energy is deposited in the form of fat. Obesity is usually defined as "excess" body fat, but there is no general agreement about how much fat is "excess." Nearly all authorities agree that normal young adult males in developed countries are about 12 per cent fat and that normal young adult females are about 23 per cent fat by weight (43). But not everyone agrees that these values are desirable; it may be that these "normal" values for the per cent of fat are too high. Regardless of whether obesity should be explicitly defined as body fat greater than 36 per cent of body weight, as the upper 10 per cent of all values for body fat in a given population, or as some other arbitrary level of fat, it is clear that obese persons have a greater risk of suffering from coronary heart disease, hypertension, diabetes and other ailments, and that they present a greater surgical risk because of the large amounts of fat that obscure blood vessels, nerves and other organs (42).

Development of Body Fat During Growth and Aging. Fat (adipose tissue) consists of many cells filled to a greater or lesser degree with triglyceride fat. The mass of fat tissue can be enlarged by increasing cell number (hyperplasia) or by increasing the size of each cell or by both processes. Fat cell number increases in human beings until 16–18 years of age and remains constant into late adulthood: There is no way other than by surgical removal to get rid of fat cells after early adulthood (42). Further gains in body fat after cell division has stopped are due to increases in fat cell size. Changes in the per cent of body fat during growth and aging are shown in Fig. 18.1. Since the amount of lean tissue in the body usually decreases after age 30 (43), it seems logical that one should attempt to maintain a constant percentage of body fat through middle and late adulthood. Therefore, one might deem *desirable* a value of no more than 12 per cent body fat for adult males and no more than 23 per cent for adult females beyond 20 years of age.

Role of Regular Exercise in Prevention of Obesity. There is evidence that physical inactivity may be a more important cause of obesity

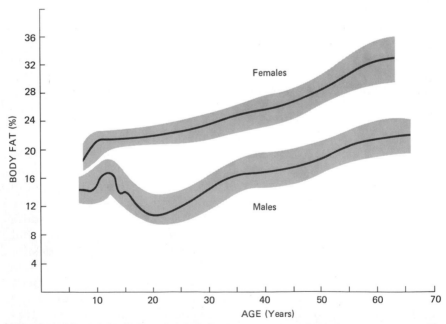

Figure 18.1 Body fat during growth and aging. Data from reference 43. Shaded areas represent one standard error above and below the means.

than excess caloric intake (35). During periods of both rest and activity obese persons tend to move less than nonobese persons and do not always eat more than those of normal weight (36). It is obvious that obesity can be prevented by exercise if food intake does not exceed the caloric expenditure during exercise plus the caloric cost of metabolism of the body in accomplishing normal daily routines. That such conditions can result from exercise is apparent when one compares the body composition of habitually active persons with that of less active individuals. Athletic populations who engage in aerobic endurance exercise, such as jogging, are characterized by lower than normal amounts of body fat, whereas weight-trained athletes may maintain a normal percentage of body fat while gaining a large amount of body weight (15). Longitudinal comparisons of trained and untrained young persons show greater lean body masses and less fat in the trained groups (43). Body weight is not substantially affected by regular exercise in growing boys and girls who do not begin training with excess body fat (38, 43). However, there is usually, but not always, less growth of fat tissue and more growth of lean muscle tissue in the trained subjects (37, 42, 43).

Exercise and Food Intake.   Since body weight does not change in growing boys and girls as a result of physical training (43), food intake must increase just enough to offset the increased caloric expenditure during exercise. However, increased appetite does not necessarily accompany increased physical activity (36). With exercise periods of about one hour, food intake sometimes does not rise and, in fact, may decrease below that of totally inactive persons (35, 42). When one regularly exercises or works vigorously for longer than one hour, food intake does increase but ordinarily only to the point where body weight is maintained (36). If one loses body weight without decreasing food intake, the weight loss must be due to the increased caloric expenditure associated with exercise and recovery from exercise, since there is no evidence that resting metabolism changes with training (42). The mechanism responsible for the increased muscle mass and decreased body fat often observed in trained individuals is not known, but it may be related to the increased concentrations of somatotropin (growth hormone) or to other endocrine changes observed as responses to exercise (42). The trained person synthesizes more protein for muscle growth and degrades fat more rapidly.

Exercise and Fat Cellularity.   Those who are extremely obese usually have a much greater number of fat cells than nonobese persons. It is conceivable that exercise early in life could reduce the number of fat cells in adulthood. Such a possibility is supported by studies on rats, which have significantly fewer fat cells at adulthood if they are physically trained at an early age than if they are sedentary throughout life (36). However, it has not yet been shown that a similar phenomenon occurs in children.

Stomach Ulcers

Many people who enjoy exercise have suggested that regular exercise provides an outlet for emotional tension and, therefore, can minimize the development of stomach ulcers. This hypothesis has received some support from the results of studies of laboratory rats. In these studies ulcers were artificially induced by restraining the animals or injecting them with ulcer-inducing drugs (29). Rats that were trained usually developed less serious ulceration of the stomach, but in one study, only treadmill running, and not swimming, was effective (29). It is thought that the protective effect, when it occurs, results from decreased acid secretion and increased mucous secretion in the stomach.

Whether the results of these studies on rats have any bearing on ulcer development in man is unknown.

Infectious Disease

Although laymen commonly assume that physically fit persons are less susceptible to viral and bacterial disease, there is neither any logic nor evidence that such is the case (28). The body's mechanisms for producing specific antibodies against disease agents is essentially unaffected by physical training.

THERAPEUTIC BENEFITS OF REGULAR EXERCISE

The advent of exercise programs for the rehabilitation of patients who have had heart attacks demonstrates a wide recognition that exercise therapy can play an important role in medical care. However, there are several types of disease in addition to heart disease for which exercise can be a useful tool to the clinician.

Exercise Therapy for Hypokinetic Degeneration

Essentially all of the adverse symptoms associated with prolonged bed rest or other inactivity can be reversed with a well-designed exercise program. Normal cardiovascular function can be regained with suitable aerobic endurance exercise (45). Flexibility can be increased with little danger of injury by a gradual program of slow, static stretching rather than ballistic, jerky movements (11, 23).

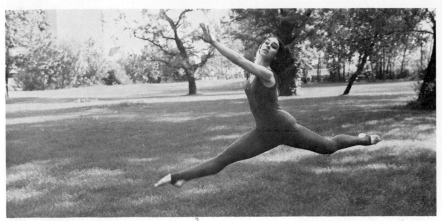

Figure 18.2. Flexibility coupled with explosive strength. (Courtesy of Office of Public Information, University of Toledo, Toledo, Ohio.)

The loss of bone minerals through osteoporosis can be reduced, if not stopped, by very moderate walking programs (52). Muscle atrophy can be reversed, bed sores eliminated, bladder and bowel dysfunction minimized, and pulmonary function improved with minimal exercise programs (4). Physical activity can also speed recovery from surgery of torn ligaments and muscles and from repair of fractured bones (5, 8, 58, 59).

Exercise Programs in Cardiac Rehabilitation

For many years patients who had suffered heart attacks were subjected to nearly total bed rest. As a result, many of the complications of prolonged bed rest (hypokinetic degeneration) occurred in these patients; their capacity to perform work was diminished; and many were unable to return to their former jobs. More and more cardiologists are now advising minimal bed rest for patients who have suffered heart attacks and are prescribing progressive exercise programs to help their patients return to normal life (21). Some rehabilitated cardiac patients have even been able to complete a marathon (32).

Although good experimental evidence that exercised cardiac patients suffer fewer repeat heart attacks and die less frequently from heart attacks is lacking, clinical comparisons of patients on exercise programs with those who do not exercise suggest that rates of reinfarction and mortality are indeed lower in exercised patients (21).

In addition to the likelihood that exercise programs may reduce the incidence of repeat heart attacks, benefits of the exercise training include the following: 1) increased physical working capacity, 2) decreased myocardial oxygen demand at rest and during submaximal exercise with a resultant decreased anginal (chest) pain, 3) decreased heart rate at rest and during submaximal work, 4) decreased symptoms of hypokinetic degeneration, 5) decreased systolic blood pressure at rest and during submaximal work, 6) decreased noradrenaline in the blood during exercise and decreased adrenaline at rest, 7) greater rate of return to gainful employment, and 8) improved psychological outlook with increased self-confidence and reduced depression (2, 21, 22, 40, 49).

It should be pointed out that patients with severe damage to the left ventricle may show little or no physiologic improvement with exercise (2). Cardiac output sometimes increases, decreases, or remains the same during submaximal work after training (2). The bulk of the evidence available suggests that physical training does not reproducibly increase the coronary collateral circulation to the hearts of cardiac patients (2, 17, 21). A decreased cardiac oxygen uptake at rest and during exercise may be the most important physiological benefit of exercise therapy in cardiac rehabilitation (2, 21, 49).

Exercise Therapy for Hypertension

Exercise is sometimes helpful in slightly reducing arterial blood pressure at rest and during submaximal exercise (22, 40, 45, 51), especially in hypertensive patients, but drug therapy is much more effective for this purpose.

Exercise Therapy for Vasoregulatory Asthenia

Vasoregulatory asthenia is a circulatory disease characterized by greater than normal sympathetic stimulation of the heart and blood vessels. Physical training has been reported to increase working capacity and markedly reduce the circulatory symptoms of vasoregulatory asthenia (24).

Regular Exercise and Occlusive Arterial Disease

Arteries of the legs that are occluded by atherosclerosis often cause severe leg pain when the affected patient walks any distance. Some studies have shown that progressive walking exercises can dramatically increase the time a patient can walk before he must stop because of severe pain (10, 51). It seems likely that this improvement is caused by enhanced blood flow in the diseased legs, but an increased tolerance to the pain should not be discounted.

Exercise Therapy for Pulmonary Disease

Patients with chronic obstructive lung disease are naturally reluctant to exercise because the increased breathing demands of exercise cause severe shortness of breath; the patient feels as though he is suffocating. This sensation results from the fact that many of the small airways in the lungs are blocked, making it extremely difficult to move an adequate volume of air through the remaining open channels. Unfortunately, physical inactivity often increases the development of airway obstruction. Therefore, patients with lung disease are usually advised to keep as active as possible to avoid hypokinetic degeneration, loss of working capacity, and loss of confidence. Exercise therapy can increase exercise tolerance and working capacity and, thereby, increase confidence and decrease the risk of hypokinetic degeneration (27, 51).

Exercise Treatment of Obesity

If obese persons can be motivated to exercise regularly, they will almost invariably lose body weight, decrease body fat, and increase lean body mass (36, 38, 42, 43, 60). Exercise has some important advantages over dietary restriction as a means of treating obesity. First, weight loss by dietary restriction results in a substantial loss of body protein, whereas weight lost by exercise consists almost entirely of fat (42). Second, as one exercises he improves the functional capacity of his cardiovascular and muscular systems and avoids the symptoms of hypokinetic degeneration. Third, exercise programs can be enjoyable recreational pursuits, whereas nobody enjoys dieting.

The preferred form of exercise in obesity therapy is that in which the trainee supports his body weight while walking, jogging, or participating in active sports. Although the caloric cost of running a given distance is about 85 per cent greater than walking (25), many obese persons are unable to run, and the longer exercise duration attained at slower speeds usually results in greater total energy expenditure. Of course, it is important to remember that weight loss by exercise is a gradual process and that the exercise program must be adhered to with regularity if one expects positive results. Also, a combination of dietary restriction and exercise usually produces the greatest weight loss.

To determine how much exercise one should perform to bring about a given weight loss, the following information must be available:

1. the subject's body weight,
2. the subject's average daily caloric intake that results in min-

imal weight fluctuation (estimated with the aid of a table of caloric values of foods such as that in Appendix A),

3. the approximate caloric cost of the exercise to be undertaken (estimated with the aid of a table such as Table 18.1), and

4. the desired weight reduction per week. Usually this should be about one pound of fat tissue or 3,500 kilocalories. More severe regimens are difficult to maintain. (Because of variable amounts of water retention during the first weeks of dieting, weight loss may not be apparent for several weeks (28).

Assume that J. Farthington Thnickersley weighed 240 pounds (109 kilograms) and wished to lose one pound per week by a combination of dietary restriction and walking at about 2.3 miles per hour. He kept track of his caloric intake for two weeks, during which time he neither gained nor lost weight. He found with the aid of a chart of caloric values of foods that he consumed an average of 3,000 kilocalories of food per day. With the aid of Table 18.1, J. Farthington determined that for each hour of walking at 2.3 mph, he would expend $240 \times 1.40 = 336$ kilocalories. Thus, if he were to walk for one hour every day, he would expend $7 \times 336 = 2,352$ kilocalories per week

Table 18.1. Approximate Energy Cost of Various Activities. Modified from Reference 28.

Activity	kcal/hr/kg body weight	kcal/hr/lb body weight
Lying in bed	1.03	0.47
Sitting, reading	1.06	0.48
Standing	1.23	0.56
Walk on level, 2.3 mph (1 mile: 26 min)	3.08	1.40
Volleyball, beginning	3.08	1.40
House painting	3.08	1.40
Table tennis	3.43	1.56
Swim back stroke, 25 yd/min	3.43	1.56
Hoeing, raking	4.09	1.86
Swim breast stroke, 20 yd/min	4.22	1.92
Slow bicycling, level roads	4.36	1.98
Gold (carry own bag)	4.75	2.16
Walk on level, 4.5 mph (1 mile: 13½ min)	5.81	2.64
Tennis	6.07	2.76
Basketball	6.20	2.82
Chopping wood	6.60	3.00
Swim crawl stroke, 45 yd/min	7.66	3.48
Swim breast stroke, 40 yd/min	8.44	3.84
Racquetball, handball, squash	9.11	4.14
Running long distance	13.20	6.00

that he would not ordinarily expend. Accordingly, to lose one pound per week by establishing a caloric deficit of 3,5000 kilocalories per week, J. F. T. must reduce his caloric intake by $3,500 - 2,352 = 1,148$ kilocalories per week or $1,148/7 = 164$ kilocalories per day. His daily caloric intake must then be reduced from 3,000 to 2,836 kilocalories. If J. Farthington decides that he cannot survive on 2,836 kilocalories, he must increase his physical activity by walking farther or faster, or by performing more vigorous types of exercise.

Other Diseases

Exercise is sometimes used as an adjunct to insulin therapy in the treatment of diabetes mellitus. It has long been recognized by physicians that diabetic patients could reduce their insulin dosage when they were physically active (16, 51). The reason for this phenomenon seems to be that the working skeletal muscles take up more glucose during exercise independently of any insulin effect (16, 51). There is no evidence that exercise affects the disease process itself; it only ameliorates the symptoms of the disease.

Chronic low back pain afflicts 70–80 per cent of the world's population at one time or another, usually between the ages of 20 and 55 (39). The cause of this aggravating pain is usually unknown, but exercise therapy is sometimes useful in relieving it. Studies of the stresses placed on the lower back with various types of exercise suggest that isometric contraction of the abdominal muscles is the preferred exercise (39). Strong abdominal muscles can counteract loads on the spine by increasing pressure in the abdominal cavity, but typical sit–ups with knees either bent or extended cause greater intradiscal pressures in the spinal column than do isometric contractions of the abdominal muscles (39).

Prolonged bed rest was often prescribed for arthritic patients as recently as 1954, but modern therapy includes mild exercise routines and passive movement of the affected joints to keep them from becoming ankylosed (frozen) (4). Inactivity makes the joints stiffer and decreases mobility in most arthritics.

POTENTIALLY HARMFUL EFFECTS OF EXERCISE

As described throughout this chapter there are many potential health benefits from regular exercise, both from a preventive and from a therapeutic standpoint. But the chapter would be incomplete without some mention of the potentially harmful effects of *poorly designed* exercise programs or the potential for injury in even well-designed programs.

Injuries to Bone, Cartilage, Ligaments, Tendons and Muscles

The best of exercise programs can occasionally result in broken bones, torn cartilages and ligaments, and ruptured tendons and muscles, to say nothing of superficial cuts, abrasions and bruises. Certain contact sports such as football and ice hockey are associated with a much greater incidence of severe injury than are other activities. Most football players who are active in the sport throughout junior and senior high school and college suffer a concussion, torn cartilage, pulled muscle, broken tooth, or fractured bone sometime in their careers. Most of these injuries do not cause any lasting harm, but there are thousands of former football players who now curse the sport they once loved, because it has left them with immobile knee joints resulting from torn cartilages or ligaments, and because these injuries have prevented them from enjoying sports such as tennis and racquetball later in life.

It has often been stated that active sports cause too much stress on bones of growing youngsters and that this stress can result in later bone deformities and osteoarthritis. Comparisons of femoral head tilt, a criterion of degenerative hip disease, between competitive male adolescent sportsmen and less active army recruits did not support this contention (41). It is true, however, that one out of ten bone fractures at the epiphyseal plate, the zone of growth in young bones, does result in some bone deformity because of the crushing of imma-

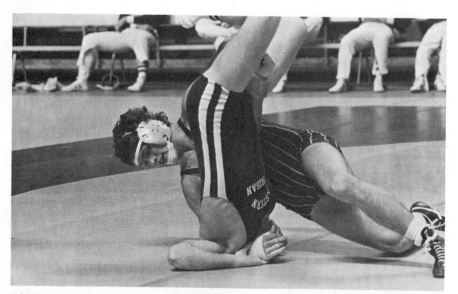

Figure 18.3.   Participation in athletics can lead to injury. (Courtesy of Office of Public Information, University of Toledo, Toledo, Ohio.)

ture bone cells and their blood supply (34). Although relatively few children suffer such deformities, this risk should be made clear to parents of children who participate in competitive sports, and especially to parents of those who play tackle football at early ages.

Minimizing Injuries in Contact Sports. There are four important principles that a coach or physical educator should stress if he wishes to minimize injuries in contact sports. First, participation should not be allowed if the appropriate protective equipment is not worn. Second, competition should be based on body weight classifications, so that small children compete against other small children. Third, safety rules should be rigidly enforced to rule out unnecessary roughness. Fourth, training should be progressive so that weak muscles and ligaments have a chance to become stronger before being subjected to severe strain. These principles are important not only to avoid injury to young bodies but also to minimize the risk of legal action being taken against the sports supervisor for failure to meet his safety responsibilities in the event of a severe injury.

Heart Attack During Exercise

Heart attack episodes during exercise stress-testing of normal subjects and cardiac patients are extremely rare (22). However, it is widely recognized by those who conduct such tests that persons who have recent or increasing chest pain, congestive heart failure, uncontrolled disturbances in heart rhythm or undue fatigue should not be subjected to strenuous exercise and that those who are tested should be carefully supervised to detect signs of impending heart problems (22). Thus, it is obvious that vigorous exercise does present some risk of heart attacks, especially for those with coronary heart disease and for those who undertake activity that is too severe for their present physical condition. The fact that some cardiac patients can eventually build up their capacities for exercise to the point where they can complete a marathon race suggests that appropriately prescribed training programs are not associated with any excessive risk of exercise-induced heart attacks. The danger arises when inappropriate exercise is undertaken by those who are not suitably prepared for the activity. For normal persons who begin a progressive exercise program, there should be little concern about suffering a heart attack during exertion; the majority of all heart attacks occur during sleep or rest (22).

Heat Illness During Exercise

As described in the chapter on temperature regulation, strenuous exercise during conditions of high environmental temperature and humidity can result in failure of the body's temperature regulating mechanisms, collapse, and even death. This risk can be minimized by consuming cool water at regular intervals during prolonged exercise or by restricting the duration of exercise under adverse environmental conditions.

Exercise-Induced Asthma

Some sensitive persons suffer attacks of asthma during vigorous exercise. Drugs can be used to minimize the severity of the attacks (18).

Review Questions

1. List the criteria that should be satisfied before one should conclude with a high level of confidence that Factor A caused Factor B in a nonexperimental research study.
2. Summarize the evidence bearing on the question of the influence of exercise on life span and the quality of life.
3. Describe the degenerative effects of prolonged physical inactivity and the evidence that regular exercise can both prevent and reverse these effects.
4. Defend the position that exercise is useful in preventing and treating coronary heart disease. Include in your discussion a description of the possible mechanisms underlying the beneficial effects of exercise.
5. Defend the position that exercise is of no significant value in preventing or treating coronary heart disease.
6. Describe the effects of vigorous exercise on body composition.
7. List some of the health hazards of regular physical activity.

References

1. Astrup, T. The effects of physical activity on blood coagulation and fibrinolysis. In J. Naughton and H. K. Hellerstein (Eds.), *Exercise Testing and Exercise Training in Coronary Heart Disease.* New York: Academic Press, 1973, pp. 169–192.
2. Barnard, R. J. Long-term effects of exercise on cardiac function. *Exercise and Sport Sciences Reviews,* 1975, **3:**113–133.
3. Blumenthal, S. Prevention of atherosclerosis. *American Journal of Cardiology,* 1973, **31:**591–594.

4. Bonner, C. D. Rehabilitation instead of bed rest? *Geriatrics*, 1969, **24**:109–118.

5. Booth, F. W., and E. W. Gould. Effects of training and disuse on connective tissue. *Exercise and Sport Sciences Reviews*, 1975, **3**:84–112.

6. Boyer, J. L. Coronary heart disease as a pediatric problem. *American Journal of Cardiology*, 1974, **33**:784–786.

7. Burke, R. E., and V. R. Edgerton. Motor unit properties and selective involvement in movement. *Exercise and Sport Sciences Reviews*, 1975, **3**:31–81.

8. Burry, H. C. Soft tissue injury in sport. *Exercise and Sport Sciences Reviews*, 1975, **3**:275–301.

9. Carey, R. A., C. M. Tipton, and D. R. Lund. Influence of training on myocardial responses of rats subjected to conditions of ischemia and hypoxia. *Cardiovascular Research*, 1976, **10**:359–367.

10. Clarke, H. H. Diet and exercise relation to peripheral vascular disease. *Physical Fitness Research Digest*, Series 6, No. 2. Washington, D.C.: President's Council on Physical Fitness and Sports, 1976.

11. deVries, H. A. *Physiology of Exercise for Physical Education and Athletics*, 2nd edition, Dubuque, Iowa: W. C. Brown Co., 1974.

12. Doyle, J. T. Can coronary heart disease be prevented? *American Journal of the Medical Sciences*, 1969, **258**:67–69.

13. Edgerton, V. R. Exercise and the growth and development of muscle tissue. In G. L. Rarick (Ed.), *Physical Activity: Human Growth and Development*. New York: Academic Press, 1973, pp. 1–31.

14. Edgerton, V. R. Neuromuscular adaptation to power and endurance work. *Canadian Journal of Applied Sport Sciences*, 1976, **1**:49–58.

15. Fahey, T. D., L. Akka, and R. Rolph. Body composition and V_{O_2} max of exceptional weight-trained athletes. *Journal of Applied Physiology*, 1975, **39**:559–561.

16. Felig, P., and J. Wahren. Fuel homeostasis in exercise. *New England Journal of Medicine*, 1975, **293**:1,078–1,084.

17. Ferguson, R. J., G. Choquette, L. Chaniotis, R. Petitclerc, R. Huot, P. Gauthier, and L. Campeau. Coronary arteriography and treadmill exercise capacity before and after 13 months physical training. *Medicine and Science in Sports*, 1973, **5**:67–68.

18. Fitch, K. D., and A. R. Morton. Cromolyn sodium in the prevention of exercise-induced asthma. *Medicine and Science in Sports*, 1973, **5**:66.

19. Fox, S. M. Relationship of activity habits to coronary heart disease. In J. Naughton and H. K. Hellerstein (Eds.), *Exercise Testing and Exercise Training in Coronary Heart Disease.* New York: Academic Press, 1973, pp. 3–21.

20. Fox, S. M., and W. L. Haskell. Population studies. *Canadian Medical Association Journal,* 1967, **96:**806–811.

21. Haskell, W. L. Physical activity after myocardial infarction. *American Journal of Cardiology,* 1974, **33:**776–783.

22. Hellerstein, H. K. Relation of exercise to acute myocardial infarction. *Circulation,* 1969, **39–40 (Supplement 4):**124–129.

23. Holland, G. The physiology of flexibility: a review of the literature. *Kinesiology Review,* 1968, **1:**49–62.

24. Holmgren, A. Vasoregulatory asthenia. *Canadian Medical Association Journal,* 1967, **96:**904–905.

25. Howley, E. T., and M. E. Glover. The caloric costs of running and walking one mile for men and women. *Medicine and Science in Sports,* 1974, **6:**235–237.

26. Ishiko, T. Commentary. *Canadian Medical Association Journal,* 1967, **96:**821.

27. Jankowski, L. W., L. Roy, R. Soucy, and J. Vallee. Aquatic exercise therapy for rehabilitation of chronic obstructive pulmonary disease. *Medicine and Science in Sports,* 1974, **6:**82.

28. Johnson, P. B., W. F. Updyke, M. Schaefer, and D. C. Stolberg. *Sport, Exercise, and You.* New York: Holt, Rinehart and Winston, 1975.

29. Johnson, T. H., and G. D. Tharp. The effect of chronic exercise on reserpine-induced gastric ulceration in rats. *Medicine and Science in Sports,* 1974, **6:**188–190.

30. Kannel, W. B., and T. R. Dawber. Atherosclerosis as a pediatric problem. *Journal of Pediatrics,* 1972, **80:**544–554.

31. Karvonen, M. J., H. Klemola, J. Virkajarvi, and A. Kekkonen. Longevity of endurance skiers. *Medicine and Science in Sports,* 1974, **6:**49–51.

32. Kavanagh, T., R. H. Shephard, and V. Pandit. Marathon running after myocardial infarction. *Journal of the American Medical Association,* 1974, **229:**1,602–1,605.

33. Lamb, D. R. Influence of exercise on bone growth and metabolism. *Kinesiology Review,* 1968, **1:**43–48.

34. Larson, R. L. Physical activity and the growth and development of bone and joint structures. In G. L. Rarick (Ed.), *Physical Activity: Human Growth and Development.* New York: Academic Press, 1973, pp. 32–59.

35. Link, R. P., W. M. Pedersoli, and A. H. Safanie. Effect of exercise on development of atherosclerosis in swine. *Atherosclerosis,* 1972, **15:**107–122.

36. Mayer, J. Exercise and weight control. In *Exercise and Fitness*, Chicago: Athletic Institute, 1960, pp. 110–122.
37. Montoye, H. J. Participation in athletics. *Canadian Medical Association Journal*, 1967, **96:**813–820.
38. Moody, D. I., J. H. Wilmore, R. N. Girandola, and J. P. Royce. The effects of a jogging program on the body composition of normal and obese high school girls. *Medicine and Science in Sports*, 1972, **4:**210–213.
39. Nachemson, A. L. Low back pain—its etiology and treatment. *Clinical Medicine*, 1971, **78:**18–24.
40. Naughton, J. The effects of acute and chronic exercise on cardiac patients. In J. Naughton and H. K. Hellerstein (Eds.), *Exercise Testing and Exercise Training in Coronary Heart Disease*. New York: Academic Press, 1973, pp. 337–346.
41. Oka, M., and S. Hatanpaa. Degenerative hip disease in adolescent athletes. *Medicine and Science in Sports*, 1976, **8:**77–80.
42. Oscai, L. B. The role of exercise in weight control. *Exercise and Sport Sciences Reviews*, 1973, **1:**103–123.
43. Parizkova, J. Body composition and exercise during growth and development. In G. L. Rarick (Ed.), *Physical Activity: Human Growth and Development*. New York: Academic Press, 1973, pp. 98–124.
44. Parizkova, J. Impact of daily work-load during pregnancy on the microstructure of the rat heart in male offspring. *European Journal of Applied Physiology*, 1975, **34:**323–326.
45. Pollock, M. L. The quantification of endurance training programs. *Exercise and Sport Sciences Reviews*, 1973, **1:**155–188.
46. Retzlaff, E. J., J. Fontaine, and W. Furuta. Effect of daily exercise on life span of albino rats. *Geriatrics*, 1966, **21:**171.
47. Rifenberick, D. H., and S. R. Max. Substrate utilization by disused rat skeletal muscles. *American Journal of Physiology*, 1974, **226:**295–297.
48. Scheuer, J. Physical training and intrinsic cardiac adaptations. *Circulation*, 1973, **47:**677–680.
49. Sim, D. N., and W. A. Neill. Investigation of the physiological basis for increased exercise threshold for angina pectoris after physical conditioning. *Journal of Clinical Investigation*, 1974, **54:**763–770.
50. Simonson, E. Evaluation of cardiac performance in exercise. *American Journal of Cardiology*, 1972, **30:**722–726.
51. Skinner, J. S. Longevity, general health, and exercise. In H. B. Falls (Ed.), *Exercise Physiology*. New York: Academic Press, 1968, pp. 219–238.
52. Smith, E. L., and S. W. Babcock. Effects of physical activity

on bone loss in the aged. *Medicine and Science in Sports,* 1973, **5:**68.

53. Stamler, J. Epidemiology of coronary heart disease. *Medical Clinics of North America,* 1973, **57:**5–46.

54. Steinhaus, A. H. Chronic effects of exercise. *Physiological Reviews,* 1933, **13:**103–147.

55. Stevenson, J. A. F. Exercise, food intake and health in experimental animals. *Canadian Medical Association Journal,* 1967, **96:**862–866.

56. Terjung, R. L., and K. Spear. Effects of exercise training on coronary blood flow of rats. *The Physiologist,* 1975, **18:**419.

57. Tibbits, G., R. J. Barnard, and N. K. Roberts. Alterations in cardiac E–C coupling induced by chronic exercise. *Medicine and Science in Sports,* 1976, **8:**55.

58. Tipton, C. M., R. D. Matthes, J. A. Maynard, and R. A. Carey. The influence of physical activity on ligaments and tendons. *Medicine and Science in Sports,* 1975, **7:**165–175.

59. Tipton, C. M., R. D. Matthes, A. C. Vailas, and P. M. Gross. Effect of immobilization, surgical repair and training on the strength of isolated knee ligaments of rats. *Medicine and Science in Sports,* 1976, **8:**61.

60. Wilmore, J. H., J. Royce, R. N. Girandola, F. I. Katch, and V. L. Katch. Body composition changes with a 10-week program of jogging. *Medicine and Science in Sports,* 1970, **2:**113–117.

61. Zuckerman, J., and G. A. Stull. Ligamentous separation force in rats as influenced by training, detraining, and cage restriction. *Medicine and Science in Sports,* 1973, **5:**44–49.

19

Aids and impediments to physical performance: fact and fiction

For hundreds and probably thousands of years athletes have ingested, injected, inhaled or applied to the skin substances that were thought to have a beneficial effect on physical performance. In earlier times it was taught that blood sucking by leeches and water deprivation would improve performance; now, some would promote the injection of blood into the veins of endurance athletes, and it is widely recognized that water supplementation rather than deprivation should be encouraged. Thus, the use of various presumed performance aids tends to wax and wane with the positive and negative testimonials of currently successful and popular athletes and coaches. If an Olympic champion in the marathon promoted a prerace potion of bat blood and buffalo saliva, one could safely predict that bats and buffaloes would soon become endangered species as thousands of distance runners attempted to get an edge on their opponents. The truth of the matter is that nothing is absolutely certain to aid athletic performance in every person; very few things are beneficial to many;

most have no effect on anyone; and some things are harmful and potentially deadly to all. It is the purpose of this chapter to describe the reasons why some substances or regimens have been presumed to be beneficial to performance and to summarize the evidence that supports or discounts such claims.

DIET

In an earlier chapter on performance and diet, it was emphasized that the important fuels for muscular exercise are carbohydrates and fats. Protein contributes insignificantly to the exercise effort from an energy standpoint. Accordingly, any promotion of protein supplementation must stand on the merit of the possible effect of extra protein on increasing the muscle mass of the athlete. This effect is unlikely unless the athlete has been deprived of adequate protein intake in his normal diet, but such deprivation could occur in athletes living in underdeveloped countries or in poverty areas of developed nations. In a normal, well-fed person, however, dietary protein supplements are not ordinarily effective in promoting extra muscular development (6).

High-Carbohydrate Diet

There does seem to be a beneficial effect of a high-carbohydrate diet on performance time in endurance events lasting longer than 30–40 minutes. With vigorous, long-duration activity, there is a severe depletion of glycogen in the working muscles that seems to limit performance. With a high-carbohydrate diet, the muscle glycogen stores can be filled to capacity so that exercise can be prolonged for as long as possible. The suggested regimen for application of the high–carbohydrate diet in a training program is described in an earlier chapter.

There is no positive effect of eating sugar several minutes or hours before athletic competition. As outlined in an earlier chapter on diet and performance, blood sugar levels are normal in all but the last minutes of the most prolonged exhaustive forms of exercise. Therefore, any beneficial effect of sugar is apt to be shown only if the sugar is eaten 30 minutes or more after the start of exercise lasting three hours or longer.

Vitamins and Minerals

There is no proven value of vitamin or mineral supplementation in the diet of persons for the purpose of enhancing athletic performance. Those persons living in poverty or consuming fad diets could possibly benefit from vitamin and mineral supplementation, but this does not seem likely for those on normal diets in well-developed countries. A more detailed discussion of performance related to vitamins and minerals is presented in an earlier chapter.

Gelatin (Glycine)

Gelatin contains high concentrations of the amino acid, glycine, which is structurally related to creatine. Believing that feeding gelatin supplements would increase the body's stores of creatine phosphate, an important energy source for intense exercise, some have recommended gelatin as an aid to athletic performance. However, well-designed studies have disclosed no beneficial effect of gelatin or glycine supplementation on performance (6, 12).

Aspartic Acid

Aspartic acid is an amino acid that is thought to be useful in reducing ammonia levels in the body. Since high levels of ammonia have been implicated in fatigue (14), it is not surprising that there have been several investigations of the influence of potassium or magnesium salts of aspartic acid on physical performance. The results of such studies on both men and laboratory animals have been contradictory (2, 6, 14). If aspartic acid is beneficial, it apparently does not work at the level of the exercising muscles, since it has been shown that levels of muscle ammonia are not reduced by the administration of aspartic acid (14). In one study the aspartic acid seemed to lower blood ammonia by increasing the liver production of urea from circulating ammonia (14). Overall, however, we must reserve judgment on whether or not aspartic acid salts can improve performance.

Dehydration

Whenever athletes are classified by weight for competition, as in such sports as wrestling, boxing and junior football, there will always be those who will attempt to gain the advantages of maturity, leverage, strength, and reach by rapidly reducing their normal body weights before weighing in so they might qualify for lower-weight classes. Much of this weight reduction is brought about by a few days of water deprivation and by water loss through sweating during exercise and exposure to heat in steam rooms, saunas, and so on. Thus, dehydration is indirectly viewed as a means by which athletic performance can be improved.

If less than about 5 per cent of the body weight is rapidly lost prior to athletic performance of short duration, it is unlikely that much of an effect on performance will be observed (2). For example, if Cedric Slumpsnuffer, whose normal weight is 140 pounds, loses 5 per cent (7 pounds) of his body weight just prior to his wrestling match with Phelonius Assult, he will not be faced with a reduction in strength or anaerobic muscular endurance, and probably will experience only a small drop in aerobic endurance. Greater percentages of weight loss through dehydration, however, are associated with performance decrements, especially in aerobic endurance (2). With prolonged work in the heat, severe dehydration can lead to marked impairment in performance and to a failure of normal temperature regulation mechanisms. As described in Chapter 15 on temperature regulation during exercise, the temperature rise in the body during prolonged heavy exercise in the heat requires that some of the blood normally distributed to working muscles must be diverted to the skin for cooling purposes. This, along with poor psychological tolerance to heat, probably accounts for the decline in performance. The precise mechanism for this increased body temperature during dehydration is unknown (2).

Because dehydration never improves and may actually diminish physical performance or even cause illness or death in certain cases, it is incorrect to consider dehydration an aid to performance. If dehydration allows an athlete to compete in a lower weight class, inappropriate to his body build, it is true that the athlete may win more contests. But this effect of dehydration should be looked upon as taking advantage of a smaller opponent, not as a means of improving athletic performance.

Water Intake Before and During Exercise

In short-term exercise during which the body is able to maintain its temperature within acceptable limits quite easily, it makes little sense to fill up with water prior to or during exercise. But with prolonged exercise of 30 minutes or more, especially in a hot environment, it has been quite conclusively shown that water intake prior to exercise allows the participant to exercise more comfortably for longer durations with lower heart rates and body temperatures (2). There is no evidence that drinking a quart or more of water a few minutes prior to athletic performance has any deleterious effect because of a full feeling in the stomach (2). Accordingly, water intake prior to prolonged exercise in the heat can often facilitate performance. It requires about 24–36 hours to voluntarily rehydrate oneself following dehydration of 4.0–7.5 per cent of body weight (2).

In a similar fashion, replenishment of body water by drinking water at intervals during prolonged exercise also has been shown to be of value for improving performance (2, 3). This beneficial effect on endurance time seems to be mostly the result of maintaining the body temperature at a lower level than is possible in a dehydrated condition. Because voluntary thirst does not drive one to refill his water stores during prolonged exercise in the heat, it may be necessary for coaches to insist that athletes drink about 200 milliliters of cool liquid approximately every 15 minutes to insure peak performance and, more importantly, to minimize the risk of heat illness.

Supplementary Salt Intake

While it is true that salt (sodium chloride) is lost in the sweat during exercise, relatively small amounts are lost compared to the loss of water. Consequently, the body fluids during prolonged exercise usually have greater than normal *concentrations* of salt. Thus, salt supplementation without adequate water supplementation can actually be harmful to salt and fluid balance. Except under the most severe, prolonged types of work in the heat, such as occurs in foundries and in hot, humid mines, it is doubtful that any extra salt is required during the work itself. Extra salt sprinkled on table food seems to be just as effective as salt supplementation in maintaining body fluid salt levels with repeated days of work in the heat (3). The effect of supplementary salt intake on most types of athletic performance is negligible and is probably more apt to be harmful than beneficial.

Commercial salt solutions containing minerals and glucose are unlikely to be detrimental to performance when taken in moderation, but athletes should not expect greater benefits from such solutions than from ordinary drinking water (2, 3). Solutions which have too much sugar and/or minerals per volume of water are only slowly emptied from the stomach during exercise, so if glucose or salts are dissolved in water to be drunk during exercise, they should be used sparingly (2).

OXYGEN

Because it has long been known that oxygen deprivation quickly brings exercise to a halt, it is not surprising that many studies have been undertaken to discover whether or not the inhalation of greater than normal concentrations of oxygen might enhance athletic performance. Such studies have investigated the breathing of oxygen-enriched gas mixtures before, during and after exercise.

Oxygen Inhalation Before Exercise

There is evidence that breathing extra oxygen just before exercise in which the breath is held allows one to perform more exercise before he must take a breath (22). Since the normal stores of oxygen in the blood and body fluids, the oxygen bound to myoglobin, and the muscle stores of creatine phosphate and glycogen should be adequate to supply energy for these short periods (usually less than a minute), it seems likely that this beneficial effect of oxygen inhalation prior to brief exercise is the result of a decreased desire to breathe. There would be a decreased stimulation to the respiratory control centers of the brain if oxygen levels in the extracellular fluids were raised and carbon dioxide levels were lowered during the period of oxygen inhalation. It is also likely to have a strong positive psychological effect on performance when exercisers know they have inhaled oxygen (22). There is little practical value in this effect to oxygen inhalation prior to performance because the oxygen breathing must take place within about one minute of the start of exercise, and in nearly all athletic competitions that much time and more is taken up by preliminary starting instructions. After a few breaths during competition, any effect of the oxygen inhalation is quickly lost.

Oxygen Inhalation During Exercise

With exercise periods shorter than 2 minutes there is no beneficial effect of breathing high concentrations of oxygen during the work (22). This is so, presumably, because anaerobic fuel reserves adequately meet the energy needs of brief exercise, because blood flow to the working muscles is not maximal until after a short period of exercise, and because it takes some time for adequate concentrations of ADP to build up in the mitochondria to spark oxygen consumption. During longer periods of exercise, oxygen inhalation usually is accompanied by better endurance, subjective feelings that the work is easier, reduced blood lactic acid levels, lower ventilation rates and lower exercise heart rates for submaximal work (16, 22). During maximal work, maximal oxygen uptake is usually increased by about 10 per cent when one breathes higher concentrations of oxygen (16). The explanation for these effects is that when one breathes high concentrations of oxygen, slightly more oxygen than normal can be bound to hemoglobin, and more oxygen can be dissolved in the plasma water so that the blood will have a higher oxygen pressure to drive oxygen into the muscle fibers. As this extra oxygen reaches the mitochondria, more ATP can be replenished aerobically so that less lactic acid need be produced from anaerobic carbohydrate metabolism. The decreased heart rates and ventilation rates can be explained by the depressing effect of high oxygen levels on the arterial chemoreceptors and on the respiratory centers of the brain (22).

In normal athletic competition the positive effect of oxygen inhalation during exercise has no use because it is impractical to wear an oxygen supply unit during competition. In noncompetitive situations, however, oxygen breathing during physical activity has great value. This is especially true for fire fighters and for those with lung disease who would remain bedridden if it were not for their portable oxygen canisters, which make possible the simple tasks of daily living that normal persons take for granted.

Oxygen Inhalation During Recovery

Oxygen inhalation during recovery would be of benefit to a performer only if he were a participant in a subsequent competition that demanded quick recovery from the previous activity. Although it is commonly asserted that oxygen breathing hastens recovery from exercise, the conclusions from the scientific literature are contradictory (22). It seems likely that any positive effects of oxygen inhalation on recovery stem from psychological, rather than physiological, factors.

HIGH-ALTITUDE TRAINING

It is known that persons who live at high altitudes generally have increased concentrations of circulating red blood cells and that such persons have much better exercise endurance at high altitudes than those who live at sea level. Some people also suspect that tissue hypoxia is an important stimulus to the adaptations in aerobic metabolism that occur after aerobic endurance training. Accordingly, it is not surprising that many have investigated the possibility that endurance athletes might have better endurance performances at sea level if they first train at high altitudes to increase the presumed hypoxia in their tissues and to bring about an increased production of red blood cells that might enhance oxygen delivery to their muscles during exercise.

Although a few early studies indicated that endurance performance at sea level was somewhat enhanced by altitude training, more recent work points out that an exercise-training effect independent of any altitude effect might have been responsible for the early results (1). Experiments in which the exercise training effect was well controlled found no beneficial effect of altitude training at 2,300 meters for 3 weeks over a similar period of training at sea level (1). It appears that any effect of high altitude training that may exist is quite small; is difficult to reproduce; and is more likely to occur at altitudes greater than 2,300 meters.

BLOOD DOPING

Some endurance athletes have attempted to increase the oxygen transport capacity of their blood by completing the following regimen. First, a pint or more of blood is withdrawn from the veins, and the red blood cells are stored. Second, the athlete resumes training, during which time the body replenishes the blood volume, including the red blood cells. Third, a short time prior to competition the stored red blood cells are injected back into the circulation to increase the number of circulating red cells. It is assumed that the increased amount of red blood cells will transfer more oxygen from the blood to the working muscles so that more ATP can be produced aerobically to give the athlete improved endurance performance.

There have been only a few scientific studies of the possibility that this "blood doping" is an effective aid to endurance performance. One of these studies showed a small improvement in maximal oxygen uptake and work time to exhaustion (4), whereas two other experiments found no such improvements (18, 21). Because the bulk of the available evidence speaks against a beneficial effect of blood doping; because there is a risk of infection, blood poisoning and intravascular blood clotting if this is attempted by medically untrained persons; and because blood letting and reinfusion go beyond the generally accepted "sportsmanlike" manipulations of normal bodily functions, such practices should be neither encouraged nor allowed.

HEAT AND COLD APPLICATIONS

The idea that applications of heat or cold to the skin might have some positive effect on muscular performance is usually based on the belief that 1) heat will increase enzyme activities in the working muscles so that ATP can be more rapidly replenished and muscle contraction can occur more quickly, 2) heat will increase blood flow to the working muscles to enhance aerobic ATP replenishment, 3) heat will decrease the viscosity or resistance of the muscles to changes in length so that less energy will have to be spent to overcome this factor, or 4) cold will decrease blood flow to the skin so that more blood can be diverted to the working muscles. At normal physiological temperatures, it seems that the latter factor is much more important than the former ones, especially with prolonged work. Over the years researchers have experimented with hot and cold baths and showers, cold sprays and cold packs on the abdominal area, cold towels over the head, and water- or air-cooled suits as possible aids to work and athletic performance.

In general, preexercise heat application that is sufficient to warm the muscles seems to have a slight (1–2 per cent) beneficial effect on the performance of athletic events such as short sprints, which have a significant anaerobic component. On the other hand, longer, aerobic events are often benefitted by the application of cold (5). However, there are contradictory reports in the literature that show no demonstrated improvement in performance with heat or cold applications, so one should expect to see many individual differences in response to these maneuvers. It is true that in certain industrial situations (work in foundries, for example) it is possible for a worker to be clothed in a water- or air-cooled suit or to have cold air directed to his head, but in ordinary athletic competitions these procedures are impractical. One exception is the use of cold towels and water sprays to cool competitors in distance events in running, cycling and rowing. Even though it may be difficult to demonstrate a significant effect of such coolants on performance time, the brief psychological lift they provide to most distance athletes makes their use commendable.

Although there are not many practical ways to apply cold during athletic competition, it is very feasible to do so in recovery periods between exercise bouts. Abdominal cold packs, cold sprays, cold towels, and even cold showers and baths can hasten recovery time and make subsequent work periods easier (5). Consequently, some of these techniques could be used in football, basketball, soccer, track, boxing, tennis, and in any other athletic event characterized by rest periods and/or substitution practices. The optimal temperature for cold water baths is 18–24°C (5). Cooling the skin to temperatures above or below this range is not likely to be effective.

ACTIVE WARM-UP

A common behavior observed in students and athletes prior to physical education classes, athletic practices and sports competitions is the participants actively "warming-up" by stretching, performing calisthenics, jogging and/or practicing the skills in which they are about to participate. The traditional reasons given for this "warm-up" include the factors related to heat application described in the previous section, plus a desire to "loosen up" the muscles, tendons and ligaments so that there will be less chance of injury to these tissues. Another reason more recently added to this list is that without warm-up, there is a greater possibility that blood flow to the heart muscle might be inadequate during the first seconds of all-out physical activity (Chapter 12).

It is unlikely that warm-up activities that increase body temperature substantially are beneficial to performance in events lasting more than a few minutes because the increased body temperature causes a shift of blood flow away from working muscles to the skin. There are, however, some reports of a beneficial effect of warm-up on sprint events, which can be performed with little blood flow to the working muscles because of the emphasis on anaerobic ATP production for such activities (7). Such a positive effect of warm-up on athletic performance is quite difficult to demonstrate; about 50 per cent of the available studies have reported that warm-up was either ineffective or, in a few cases, was actually harmful to performance (7). Any beneficial effect of warm-up is small and can be easily obscured by differences in motivation, pain tolerance, techniques of performance and strategy.

The facts that 1) there is no overwhelming evidence that warm-up is advantageous to athletic performance, and 2) there is no scientific evidence that athletes are less apt to suffer injury after warm-up do not mean that warm-up practices should be discouraged. There is minimal evidence that warm-up is harmful to performance, and the personal empirical experience of thousands of athletes and coaches suggests that warm-up does help prevent injuries. Accordingly, warm-up practices should be promoted with greatest use being made of practice of the actual physical activity in which the exerciser is about to participate. Supposedly, these preliminary trials will help to establish the appropriate neural patterns for the final performance of the activity. Warm-up is particularly to be encouraged in those who are about to participate in very heavy exercise that places sudden demands on the heart and circulation. The warm-up should minimize the risk of inadequate coronary blood flow during the first few seconds of heavy exercise.

MUSIC

Music is often part of the scene at athletic competitions. Whether the pounding bass drum or the blaring trumpets have any stimulating effect on athletic performance, or whether music arouses only the spectators, may never be proven. In any attempt to study the effects of music, one should minimize the possibility that the subjects realize that the addition or deletion of music from the performance setting is being evaluated; subjects may unconsciously respond positively to music because they assume they should. It is very difficult to accomplish this degree of experimental control when music is the variable of interest. Therefore, when a study without such control shows a beneficial effect of music on performance, the results are open to question.

Intuitively, it seems likely that rousing musical selections might be helpful to many athletes during the first minute or so of a contest

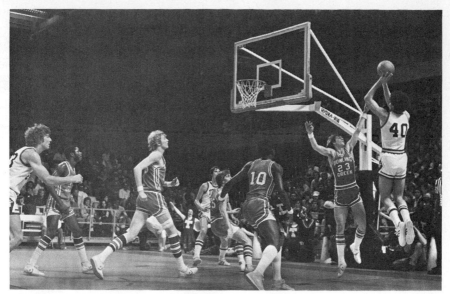

Figure 19.1. It is doubtful that these athletes would be conscious of any background music. (Courtesy of Office of Public Information, University of Toledo, Toledo, Ohio.)

because such music is associated with heightened emotions. But most athletes express the belief that once a contest is underway, they are generally oblivious to background music. This belief seems to be supported by the meager experimental evidence available: neither athletic performance nor industrial production seems to benefit from background music (15). Nevertheless, most factory workers and athletes prefer the presence of music to its absence, and performance is rarely adversely affected by music.

HYPNOSIS AND SUGGESTION

Stories of fantastic achievements in muscular performance under conditions of emotional stress, and countless examples of suddenly superior athletic performances by previously "run-of-the-mill" competitors, have led to many investigations of the role of hypnosis and suggestion on physical performance. As with most of the literature on other so-called aids to performance, the evidence regarding any beneficial effect of hypnosis and suggestion is contradictory, and much of the research suffers from inadequate controls.

The vast majority of studies dealing with the possibility that performance can be improved by suggesting to the performer that he has a great capacity, or by having the performer exercise while in a hypnotic state, have tested strength or short-duration anaerobic endurance of a few muscle groups. No strong conclusions can be stated about the effectiveness of hypnosis or suggestion on performance in tests of grip strength, dynamic elbow-flexion endurance and isometric endurance because the evidence is about equally divided between positive and negative results (16). It seems that only certain types of persons are responsive to either waking or hypnotic suggestion; the effects of such procedures are very unpredictable.

There is clinical evidence that some athletes can be helped by hypnosis if their performances are adversely affected by chronic pain or various psychological problems (17). Hypnotherapy is not always effective, however.

DRUGS

The use of most drugs as aids to performance is forbidden by athletic regulary agencies; the drugs can sometimes become physiologically and/or psychologically addictive; and they may lead to severe injury, disease or even death. Therefore, no athlete should consider the use of any agent described in this section as a potential aid to performance. The purpose of the following discussion is to provide some insight into why these drugs are ineffective or potentially harmful.

Stimulants to the Nervous System

Amphetamines. Activation of the sympathetic nervous system causes increased cardiac output, vasoconstriction of blood vessels, a rise in blood pressure, and stimulation of the psychological arousal mechanisms in the brain stem. Each of these actions should be a useful response during many types of exercise and athletic competition. Therefore, it is not surprising that drugs which mimic the effects of sympathetic stimulation are often used by athletes who wish to improve their performances. The most popular of these drugs are amphetamines, methamphetamines, and hydroxyamphetamines (trade names include: Benzedrine, Dexedrine and Isophan). It is widely recognized that the amphetamines can help one stay awake by delaying the sense of fatigue and can help persons concentrate on accomplishing long, tedious tasks. However, it is also known that these drugs are commonly abused and that this abuse often leads to psychological dependence on the drugs. In addition, excessive doses of the drug can lead to circulatory collapse and death.

Although there are many exceptions, the majority of studies

testing the effect of amphetamines on work performances such as prolonged marching, hiking, and cycling show that the drug allows the exerciser to work longer with less sense of fatigue (8). It should be pointed out, however, that there is no evidence that the work can be performed faster than in the nondrugged condition (9). As far as athletic performance is concerned, the consensus of opinion seems to be that the athlete is more emotionally aroused under the influence of the drug, but that any demonstrable effect on athletic performance is small and difficult to reproduce (6, 8, 9). The most likely types of events to be positively influenced by amphetamines are long-distance cycling and running. But it is in precisely these events that amphetamines are most dangerous. The drug can mask the sensation of oncoming circulatory collapse resulting from heat stress so that severe heat illness and even death may ensue (9).

In summary, amphetamines cause emotional arousal in many persons, but this arousal and other physiological effects are not enough to result in reproducible benefits to most types of athletic performance. When weighed against the possibility of 1) developing psychological dependence on the drug, 2) masking symptoms of potentially lethal circulatory collapse, and 3) being discovered by sports governing bodies, it seems foolish to even consider the use of amphetamines as a potential aid to athletic performance.

Cocaine. Cocaine is a highly addictive drug that acts on the brain to markedly inhibit the sensation of fatigue during prolonged work, thereby allowing substantially greater quantities of work to be performed (12). Any use of this drug is illegal and highly dangerous.

Caffeine. Coffee, tea, and cola drinks contain caffeine, with a cup of coffee containing about 150 milligrams, a cup of tea about 120 milligrams, and a glass of cola about 50 milligrams. Caffeine is noted especially for its stimulation of the brain so that the sense of fatigue is diminished, but in large doses it can also increase cardiac output and stimulate the metabolism of skeletal muscles. About 500 milligrams of caffeine seems to increase endurance to prolonged exercise (8, 12), but the drug has no effect on more anaerobic types of activities such as sprints (12).

Adrenaline

Injections of adrenaline increase heart rate, cardiac output, and blood pressure and may raise the level of blood glucose by increasing the breakdown of glycogen to glucose in the liver. There is little evidence that adrenaline injections are beneficial to endurance performance in humans (12).

Anabolic Steroids

In young boys and girls there is little difference in muscle mass and strength. But at puberty, in concert with a marked acceleration in the secretion of testosterone, males rapidly outdistance most females in muscle growth and in strength. This association between male sex hormone and strength has led to the belief that supplemental administration of drugs that have the muscle-building characteristics of testosterone might lead to improved athletic performance, especially in those events where strength and body mass are of great importance. Testosterone, besides promoting muscular development, also enhances the male secondary sex characteristics; this latter property is called the *androgenic* effect of a drug, whereas the growth promoting property is called the *anabolic* effect. Since testosterone has a structure typical of the group of chemicals called steroids, it is thus referred to as an *androgenic-anabolic steroid*. Drug manufacturers have synthesized steroid-like drugs that have strong anabolic properties, but weak androgenic properties. These synthetic drugs, the anabolic steroids, include those with the following trade names: Dianabol, Androyd, Nilevor, Maxibolen, and Winstrol. Some of these drugs have greater androgenic effects than others.

Testimonial evidence by athletes indicates that anabolic steroids are very widely used, especially by shot putters, discus throwers, hammer throwers, weight lifters, and others who must rely heavily on strength for success (9). Most of these athletes are convinced that the drug has a beneficial effect on their athletic performances. It appears that many users of anabolic steroids take the drug at several times the recommended therapeutic dose (9).

The scientific evidence regarding the effectiveness of anabolic steroids in stimulating weight gain and strength improvements is contradictory (6, 9, 11, 14, 20). Apparently well-designed studies have shown both a lack of effect and a positive effect of anabolic steroid treatment. It seems probable that one reason for the discrepancy between the negative results of many research studies and the testimonial evidence that anabolic steroids improve performance may be the differences in dosages used to obtain the two types of evidence. Because of the possibility of harmful side effects, most researchers are reluctant to use dosages as high as many athletes use routinely. On the other hand, if the presumed beneficial effect of anabolic steroid use were as substantial as many athletes believe, there should be more consistently positive results reported in the scientific literature, even with lesser doses. Because of individual differences in sensitivity and responsiveness, extreme variability in drug effects occurs. Increasing clinical evidence that long-term use of anabolic steroids may lead to leukemia and serious liver disorders, including cancer (10), shows that these drugs should be avoided.

Alcohol

Alcohol is the most widely abused drug in modern societies. Alcohol is sometimes thought to be a nervous system stimulant because it tends to remove social inhibitions by depressing the brain centers responsible for those inhibitions. In actuality, of course, alcohol is a central nervous system depressant and in large doses can produce total stupor. In small doses there is no consistent effect of alcohol on work performance, but in larger doses, such as six ounces of whiskey, athletic performance is impaired (8, 12).

Tobacco

Most people believe that tobacco smoking has a detrimental effect on athletic performance. The facts that the carbon monoxide in tobacco smoke can displace oxygen from the red blood cells and that smoking is associated with airway constriction in the small bronchioles lend some support to this possible adverse effect of smoking on athletic performance. However, there seem to be no consistent effects, positive or negative, of smoking on athletic performance (12). The common experience of young students returning to athletic training after a relatively sedentary summer is that ". . . the summer's smoking definitely cuts the wind." This experience is mostly caused by the absence of regular physical training and not by the practice of smoking.

Smoking should be actively discouraged because of its terrible long-range effects on increasing the risk of contracting lung cancer and heart disease, not because it will cause a dramatic decrement in athletic performance.

Marijuana

Marijuana smoking tends to increase heart rate and cause a feeling of relaxation and/or exhilaration. When smoked just before exercise, marijuana seems to have no effect on grip strength or on lung function, but it does require the heart to beat faster at a given submaximal workload, so that working capacity at a standard heart rate is reduced (19). Marijuana smoking does not improve athletic performance.

Review Questions

1. Explain why the following items have been thought to be potential aids to athletic performance, describe any possible harmful effects associated with their use, and state your views concerning their use in athletics: high-protein diets, high-carbohydrate diets, vitamin and mineral supplementation, gelatin, aspartic acid, dehydration, water, salt, oxygen, high-altitude training, blood doping, heat and cold applications, active warm-up, music, hypnosis and suggestion, amphetamines, cocaine, caffeine, adrenaline, alcohol, tobacco, marijuana, anabolic steroids.

2. Discuss the difference between testimonial evidence and scientific evidence pertaining to presumed aids to muscular performance. Ask your instructor or someone familiar with research design and statistics why it is so difficult to "prove" that some so-called "ergogenic aid" does not improve athletic performance. Would you always prefer scientific evidence when it conflicts with testimonial evidence? What if you are the one giving testimony?

References

1. Adams, W. C., E. M. Bernauer, D. B. Dill, and J. B. Bomar, Jr. Effects of equivalent sea-level and altitude training on V_{O_2} max and running performance. *Journal of Applied Physiology,* 1975, **39**:262–266.

2. Costill, D. L. Water and electrolytes. In W. P. Morgan (Ed.), *Ergogenic Aids and Muscular Performance.* New York: Academic Press, 1972, pp. 293–320.

3. Costill, D. L., R. Cote, E. Miller, T. Miller, and S. Wynder. Water and electrolyte replacement during repeated days of work in the heat. *Aviation, Space, and Environmental Medicine,* 1975, **46**:795–800.

4. Ekblom, B., A. N. Goldbarg, and B. Gullbring. Response to exercise after blood loss and reinfusion. *Journal of Applied Physiology,* 1972, **33**:175–180.

5. Falls, H. B. Heat and Cold Applications. In W. P. Morgan (Ed.), *Ergogenic Aids and Muscular Performance.* New York: Academic Press, 1972, pp. 119–158.

6. Fowler, W. M., Jr. The facts about ergogenic aids and sports performance. *Journal of Health, Physical Education and Recreation,* 1969, **40**:37–42.

7. Franks, B. D. Physical Warm-up. In W. P. Morgan (Ed.), *Ergogenic Aids and Muscular Performance.* New York: Academic Press, 1972, pp. 160–191.

8. Ganslen, R. V. Doping and Athletic Performance. In H. B. Falls (Ed.), *Exercise Physiology*. New York: Academic Press, 1968, pp. 198–218.

9. Golding, L. A. Drugs and Hormones. In W. P. Morgan (Ed.), *Ergogenic Aids and Muscular Performance*. New York: Academic Press, 1972, pp. 367–397.

10. Johnson, F. L. The association of oral androgenic-anabolic steroids and life-threatening disease. *Medicine and Science in Sports*, 1975, **7:**284–286.

11. Johnson, L.C., E.S. Roundy, P.E.Allsen, A.G.Fisher, and L. J. Silvester. Effect of anabolic steroid treatment on endurance. *Medicine and Science in Sports*, 1975, **7:**287–289.

12. Karpovich, P. V., and W. E. Sinning. *Physiology of Muscular Activity*. Philadelphia:W. B. Saunders, 1971, pp. 321–338.

13. Kendrick, Z. V., S. Tangsakul, A. Goldfarb, and P. A. Mole. Potassium aspartate treatment: effects on blood ammonia, urea, and exercise to exhaustion. *Medicine and Science in Sports*, 1976, **8:**70.

14. Lamb, D. R. Androgens and exercise. *Medicine and Science in Sports*, 1975, **7:**1–5.

15. Lucaccini, L. F., and L. H. Kreit. Music. In W. P. Morgan (Ed.), *Ergogenic Aids and Muscular Performance*. New York: Academic Press, 1972, pp. 235–262.

16. Margaria, R., E. Camporesi, P. Aghemo, and G. Sassi. The effect of O_2 breathing on maximal aerobic power. *Pflugers Archives*, 1972, **336:**225–235.

17. Morgan, W. P. Hypnosis and Muscular Performance. In W. P. Morgan (Ed.), *Ergogenic Aids and Muscular Performance*. New York: Academic Press, 1972, pp. 193–233.

18. Robinson, B., et al. Circulatory effects of acute expansion of blood volume. *Circulation Research*, 1966, **19:**26–32.

19. Steadward, R. D., and M. Singh. The effects of smoking marihuana on physical performance. *Medicine and Science in Sports*, 1975, **7:**309–311.

20. Stromme, S. B., H. D. Meen, and A. Aakvaag. Effects of an androgenic-anabolic steroid on strength development and plasma testosterone levels in normal males. *Medicine and Science in Sports*, 1974, **6:**203–208.

21. Williams, M. H., A. R. Goodwin, R. Perkins, and J. Bocrie. Effect of blood reinjection upon endurance capacity and heart rate. *Medicine and Science in Sports*, 1973, **5:**181–186.

22. Wilmore, J. H. Oxygen. In W. P. Morgan (Ed.), *Ergogenic Aids and Muscular Performance*. New York: Academic Press, 1972, pp. 321–342.

Appendix A

Nutritive values of the edible part of foods*

* From "Nutritive Value of Foods." U.S. Department of Agriculture, Home and Garden Bulletin No. 72, 1964.

Food, approximate measure, and weight (in grams)	Water	Food energy	Protein	Fat	Fatty acids Saturated (total)	Fatty acids Unsaturated Oleic	Fatty acids Unsaturated Linoleic	Carbohydrate	Calcium	Iron	Vitamin A value	Thiamin	Riboflavin	Niacin	Ascorbic acid
	Grams	Per cent	Calories	Grams	Grams	Grams	Grams	Grams	Grams	Milligrams	Milligrams	International units	Milligrams	Milligrams	Milligrams	Milligrams

MILK, CHEESE, CREAM, IMITATION CREAM; RELATED PRODUCTS

Milk:
Fluid:

Food	Grams	Per cent	Calories	Protein Grams	Fat Grams	Sat. Grams	Oleic Grams	Linoleic Grams	Carb. Grams	Calcium Milligrams	Iron Milligrams	Vit A Int. units	Thiamin Milligrams	Riboflavin Milligrams	Niacin Milligrams	Ascorbic Milligrams
Whole, 3.5% fat ----- 1 cup -----	244	87	160	9	9	5	3	Trace	12	288	0.1	350	0.07	0.41	0.2	2
Nonfat (skim) ----- 1 cup -----	245	90	90	9	Trace				12	296	.1	10	.09	.44	.2	2
Partly skimmed, 2% 1 cup -----	246	87	145	10	5	3	2	Trace	15	352	.1	200	.10	.52	.2	2
Cheese: Natural: Blue or Roquefort type: Ounce------ 1 oz------	28	40	105	6	9	5	3	Trace	1	89	.1	350	.01	.17	.3	0

[1] Value applies to unfortified product; value for fortified low-density product would be 1500 I.U., and the fortified high-density product would be 2290 I.U.

[Dashes in the columns for nutrients show that no suitable value could be found although there is reason to believe that a measurable amount of the nutrient may be present]

Food, approximate measure, and weight (in grams)	Water	Food energy	Protein	Fat	Fatty acids			Carbohydrate	Calcium	Iron	Vitamin A value	Thiamin	Riboflavin	Niacin	Ascorbic acid
					Saturated (total)	Unsaturated									
						Oleic	Linoleic								
	Per cent	Calories	Grams	Grams	Grams	Grams	Grams	Grams	Milligrams	Milligrams	International units	Milligrams	Milligrams	Milligrams	Milligrams
MILK, CHEESE, CREAM, IMITATION CREAM; RELATED PRODUCTS—Con.															
Cheese—Continued															
Natural—Continued	Grams														
Cheddar:															
Ounce-------- 1 oz-------- 28	37	115	7	9	5	3	Trace	1	213	.3	370	.01	.13	Trace	0
Cottage, large or small curd:															
Creamed:															
Package of 12-oz., net wt. 1 pkg-------- 340	78	360	46	14	8	5	Trace	10	320	1.0	580	.10	.85	.3	0
Cream:															
Package of 8-oz., net wt. 1 pkg-------- 227	51	850	18	86	48	28	3	5	141	.5	3,500	.05	.54	.2	0
Parmesan, grated:															
Tablespoon------ 1 tbsp------ 5	17	25	2	2	1	Trace	Trace	Trace	68	Trace	60	Trace	.04	Trace	0
Swiss:															
Ounce-------- 1 oz-------- 28	39	105	8	8	4	3	Trace	1	262	.3	320	Trace	.11	Trace	0

Food, approximate measure, and weight		Grams	Water (pct)	Food energy (cal.)	Protein (g)	Fat (g)	Saturated (total) (g)	Unsaturated — Oleic (g)	Unsaturated — Linoleic (g)	Carbohydrate (g)	Calcium (mg)	Iron (mg)	Vitamin A (I.U.)	Thiamin (mg)	Riboflavin (mg)	Niacin (mg)	Ascorbic acid (mg)
Pasteurized processed cheese:																	
American: Ounce	1 oz.	28	40	105	7	9	5	3	Trace	1	198	.3	350	.01	.12	Trace	0
Cubic inch	1 cu. in.	18	40	65	4	5	3	2	Trace	Trace	122	.2	210	Trace	.07	Trace	0
Swiss: Ounce	1 oz.	28	40	100	8	8	4	3	Trace	1	251	.3	310	Trace	.11	Trace	0
Cream:																	
Half-and-half (cream and milk)	1 cup	242	80	325	8	28	15	9	1	11	261	.1	1,160	.07	.39	.1	2
	1 tbsp.	15	80	20	1	2	1	1	Trace	1	16	Trace	70	Trace	.02	Trace	Trace
Light, coffee or table	1 cup	240	72	505	7	49	27	16	1	10	245	.1	2,020	.07	.36	.1	2
	1 tbsp.	15	72	30	1	3	2	1	Trace	1	15	Trace	130	Trace	.02	Trace	Trace
Sour	1 cup	230	72	485	7	47	26	16	1	10	235	.1	1,930	.07	.35	.1	2
	1 tbsp.	12	72	25	Trace	2	1	1	Trace	1	12	Trace	100	Trace	.02	Trace	Trace
Whipped topping (pressurized)	1 cup	60	62	155	2	14	8	5	Trace	6	67	—	570	—	.04	—	1
	1 tbsp.	3	62	10	Trace	1	Trace	Trace	—	Trace	3	—	30	—	Trace	—	—
Whipping, unwhipped (volume about double when whipped):																	
Light	1 cup	239	62	715	6	75	41	25	2	9	203	.1	3,060	.05	.29	.1	2
	1 tbsp.	15	62	45	Trace	5	3	2	Trace	1	13	Trace	190	Trace	.02	Trace	Trace
Heavy	1 cup	238	57	840	5	90	50	30	3	7	179	.1	3,670	.05	.26	.1	2
	1 tbsp.	15	57	55	Trace	6	3	2	Trace	1	11	Trace	230	Trace	.02	Trace	Trace
Imitation cream products (made with vegetable fat):																	
Creamers: Powdered	1 cup	94	2	505	4	33	31	1	0	52	21	.6	²200	Trace	Trace	Trace	0
	1 tsp.	2	2	10	Trace	1	1	Trace	0	1	1	Trace	²Trace	0	0	—	0
Liquid (frozen)	1 cup	245	77	345	3	27	25	1	Trace	25	29	—	²100	0	0	—	0
	1 tbsp.	15	77	20	Trace	2	1	Trace	0	2	2	—	10	0	0	—	0
Sour dressing (imitation sour cream) made with nonfat dry milk.	1 cup	235	72	440	9	38	35	1	Trace	17	277	.1	—	.07	.38	.2	1
	1 tbsp.	12	72	20	Trace	2	2	Trace	Trace	1	14	Trace	Trace	Trace	.02	Trace	Trace
Whipped topping: Pressurized	1 cup	70	61	190	1	17	15	1	0	9	5	—	²340	0	0	—	0
	1 tbsp.	4	61	10	Trace	1	1	Trace	0	Trace	Trace	—	²20	0	0	—	0

² Contributed largely from beta-carotene used for coloring.

MILK, CHEESE, CREAM, IMITATION CREAM; RELATED PRODUCTS—Con.

Food, approximate measure, and weight (in grams)	Water	Food energy	Protein	Fat	Fatty acids			Carbo-hydrate	Cal-cium	Iron	Vita-min A value	Thia-min	Ribo-flavin	Niacin	Ascor-bic acid
					Satu-rated (total)	Unsaturated									
						Oleic	Lin-oleic								
	Per-cent	*Calo-ries*	*Grams*	*Grams*	*Grams*	*Grams*	*Grams*	*Grams*	*Milli-grams*	*Milli-grams*	*Inter-national units*	*Milli-grams*	*Milli-grams*	*Milli-grams*	*Milli-grams*
Whipped topping—Continued															
Frozen———— 1 cup———— 75	52	230	1	20	18	Trace	0	15	5		²560		0		
1 tbsp———— 4	52	10	Trace	1	1	Trace	0	1	Trace		²30		0		
Powdered, made with 1 cup———— 75 whole milk.	58	175	3	12	10	1	Trace	15	62	Trace	²330	.02	.08	.1	Trace
1 tbsp———— 4	58	10	Trace	1	1	Trace	Trace	1	3	Trace	²20	Trace	Trace	Trace	Trace
Milk beverages:															
Cocoa, homemade———— 1 cup———— 250	79	245	10	12	7	4	Trace	27	295	1.0	400	.10	.45	.5	3
Chocolate-flavored drink made with skim milk and 2% added butterfat. 1 cup———— 250	83	190	8	6	3	2	Trace	27	270	.5	210	.10	.40	.3	3
Malted milk:															
Dry powder, approx. 1 oz.———— 28 3 heaping tea-spoons per ounce.	3	115	4	2				20	82	.6	290	.09	.15	.1	0
Beverage———— 1 cup———— 235	78	245	11	10	7	5	1	28	317	.7	590	.14	.49	.2	2
Milk desserts:															
Custard, baked———— 1 cup———— 265	77	305	14	15	7	5	1	29	297	1.1	930	.11	.50	.3	1
Ice cream:															
Regular (approx. 10% fat). ½ gal.———— 1,064	63	2,055	48	113	62	37	3	221	1,553	.5	4,680	.43	2.23	1.1	11
1 cup———— 133	63	255	6	14	8	5	Trace	28	194	.1	590	.05	.28	.1	1
3 fl. oz. cup——— 50	63	95	2	5	3	2	Trace	10	73	Trace	220	.02	.11	.1	1
Rich (approx. 16% fat). ½ gal.———— 1,188	63	2,635	31	191	105	63	6	214	927	.2	7,840	.24	1.31	1.2	12
1 cup———— 148	63	330	4	24	13	8	1	27	115	Trace	980	.03	.16	.1	1
Ice milk:															
Hardened———— ½ gal.———— 1,048	67	1,595	50	53	29	17	2	235	1,635	1.0	2,200	.52	2.31	1.0	10
1 cup———— 131	67	200	6	7	4	2	Trace	29	204	.1	280	.07	.29	.2	1
Soft-serve———— 1 cup———— 175	67	265	8	9	5	3	Trace	39	273	.2	370	.09	.39	.2	2

Food	Measure	g	Water	Cal.	Prot.	Fat	Sat.	Oleic	Lino.	Carb.	Ca	Fe	Vit. A	Thia.	Ribo.	Niacin	Asc.
Yoghurt:																	
Made from partially skimmed milk.	1 cup	245	89	125	8	4	2	1	Trace	13	294	.1	170	.10	.44	.2	2
Made from whole milk.	1 cup	245	88	150	7	8	5	3	Trace	12	272	.1	340	.07	.39	.2	2
EGGS																	
Eggs, large, 24 ounces per dozen:																	
Raw or cooked in shell or with nothing added:																	
Whole, without shell.	1 egg	50	74	80	6	6	2	3	Trace	Trace	27	1.1	590	.05	.15	Trace	0
White of egg.	1 white	33	88	15	4	Trace				Trace	3	Trace	0	Trace	.09	Trace	0
Yolk of egg.	1 yolk	17	51	60	3	5	2	2	Trace	Trace	24	.9	580	.04	.07	Trace	0
Scrambled with milk and fat.	1 egg	64	72	110	7	8	3	3	Trace	1	51	1.1	690	.05	.18	Trace	0
MEAT, POULTRY, FISH, SHELLFISH; RELATED PRODUCTS																	
Bacon, (20 slices per lb. raw), broiled or fried, crisp.	2 slices	15	8	90	5	8	3	4	1	1	2	.5	0	.08	.05	.8	
Beef,[3] cooked:																	
Cuts braised, simmered, or pot-roasted:																	
Lean and fat.	3 ounces	85	53	245	23	16	8	7	Trace	0	10	2.9	30	.04	.18	3.5	
Lean only.	2.5 ounces	72	62	140	22	5	2	2	Trace	0	10	2.7	10	.04	.16	3.3	
Hamburger (ground beef), broiled:																	
Lean.	3 ounces	85	60	185	23	10	5	4	Trace	0	10	3.0	20	.08	.20	5.1	
Regular.	3 ounces	85	54	245	21	17	8	8	Trace	0	9	2.7	30	.07	.18	4.6	
Roast, oven-cooked, no liquid added:																	
Relatively fat, such as rib:																	
Lean and fat.	3 ounces	85	40	375	17	34	16	15	1	0	8	2.2	70	.05	.13	3.1	
Lean only.	1.8 ounces	51	57	125	14	7	3	3	Trace	0	6	1.8	10	.04	.11	2.6	
Relatively lean, such as heel of round:																	
Lean and fat.	3 ounces	85	62	165	25	7	3	3	Trace	0	11	3.2	10	.06	.19	4.5	
Lean only.	2.7 ounces	78	65	125	24	3	1	1	Trace	0	10	3.0	Trace	.06	.18	4.3	
Steak, broiled:																	
Relatively, fat, such as sirloin:																	
Lean and fat.	3 ounces	85	44	330	20	27	13	12	1	0	9	2.5	50	.05	.16	4.0	
Lean only.	2.0 ounces	56	59	115	18	4	2	2	Trace	0	7	2.2	10	.05	.14	3.6	
Relatively, lean, such as round:																	
Lean and fat.	3 ounces	85	55	220	24	13	6	6	Trace	0	10	3.0	20	.07	.19	4.8	
Lean only.	2.4 ounces	68	61	130	21	4	2	2	Trace	0	9	2.5	10	.06	.16	4.1	
Beef, canned:																	
Corned beef.	3 ounces	85	59	185	22	10	5	4	Trace	0	17	3.7	20	.01	.20	2.9	
Corned beef hash.	3 ounces	85	67	155	7	10	5	4	Trace	9	11	1.7		.01	.08	1.8	
Beef, dried or chipped.	2 ounces	57	48	115	19	4	2	2	Trace	0	11	2.9		.04	.18	2.2	
Beef and vegetable stew.	1 cup	235	82	210	15	15		5	Trace	15	28	2.8	2,310	.13	.17	4.4	15

[2] Contributed largely from beta-carotene used for coloring.

[3] Outer layer of fat on the cut was removed to within approximately ½-inch of the lean. Deposits of fat within the cut were not removed.

Food, approximate measure, and weight (in grams)		Water	Food energy	Protein	Fat	Fatty acids Saturated (total)	Fatty acids Unsaturated Oleic	Fatty acids Unsaturated Linoleic	Carbohydrate	Calcium	Iron	Vitamin A value	Thiamin	Riboflavin	Niacin	Ascorbic acid
	Grams	Percent	Calories	Grams	Grams	Grams	Grams	Grams	Grams	Milligrams	Milligrams	International units	Milligrams	Milligrams	Milligrams	Milligrams
MEAT, POULTRY, FISH, SHELLFISH; RELATED PRODUCTS—Continued																
Beef potpie, baked, 4¼-inch diam., weight before baking about 8 ounces. 1 pie	227	55	560	23	33	9	20	2	43	32	4.1	1,860	0.25	0.27	4.5	7
Chicken, cooked:																
Flesh only, broiled 3 ounces	85	71	115	20	3	1	1	1	0	8	1.4	80	.05	.16	7.4	---
Breast, fried, ½ breast:																
With bone 3.3 ounces	94	58	155	25	5	1	2	1	1	9	1.3	70	.04	.17	11.2	---
Flesh and skin only 2.7 ounces	76	58	155	25	5	1	2	1	1	9	1.3	70	.04	.17	11.2	---
Drumstick, fried:																
With bone 2.1 ounces	59	55	90	12	4	1	2	1	Trace	6	.9	50	.03	.15	2.7	---
Flesh and skin only 1.3 ounces	38	55	90	12	4	1	2	1	Trace	6	.9	50	.03	.15	2.7	---
Chicken, canned, boneless 3 ounces	85	65	170	18	10	3	4	2	0	18	1.3	200	.03	.11	3.7	3
Chicken potpie, baked 4¼-inch diam., weight before baking about 8 ounces. 1 pie	227	57	535	23	31	10	15	3	42	68	3.0	3,020	.25	.26	4.1	5
Chili con carne, canned:																
With beans 1 cup	250	72	335	19	15	7	7	Trace	30	80	4.2	150	.08	.18	3.2	---
Without beans 1 cup	255	67	510	26	38	18	17	1	15	97	3.6	380	.05	.31	5.6	---
Heart, beef, lean, braised 3 ounces	85	61	160	27	5	---	---	---	1	5	5.0	20	.21	1.04	6.5	1
Lamb, cooked:																
Chop, thick, with bone, 1 chop, broiled. 4.8 ounces	137	47	400	25	33	18	12	1	0	10	1.5	---	.14	.25	5.6	---
Lean and fat 4.0 ounces	112	47	400	25	33	18	12	1	0	10	1.5	---	.14	.25	5.6	---
Lean only 2.6 ounces	74	62	140	21	6	3	2	Trace	0	9	1.5	---	.11	.20	4.5	---
Leg, roasted:																
Lean and fat 3 ounces	85	54	235	22	16	9	6	Trace	0	9	1.4	---	.13	.23	4.7	---
Lean only 2.5 ounces	71	62	130	20	5	3	2	Trace	0	9	1.4	---	.12	.21	4.4	---
Shoulder, roasted:																
Lean and fat 3 ounces	85	50	285	18	23	13	8	1	0	9	1.0	---	.11	.20	4.0	---
Lean only 2.3 ounces	64	61	130	17	6	3	2	Trace	0	8	1.0	---	.10	.18	3.7	---

Food and approximate measure	Grams														
Liver, beef, fried — 2 ounces	57	130	15	6	—	—	—	3	6	5.0	30,280	.15	2.37	9.4	15
Pork, cured, cooked:															
Ham, light cure, lean and fat, roasted. — 3 ounces	85	245	18	19	7	8	2	0	8	2.2	0	.40	.16	3.1	—
Luncheon meat:															
Boiled ham, sliced — 2 ounces	57	135	11	10	4	4	1	0	6	1.6	0	.25	.09	1.5	—
Canned, spiced or unspiced. — 2 ounces	57	165	8	14	5	6	1	1	5	1.2	0	.18	.12	1.6	—
Pork, fresh,³ cooked:															
Chop, thick, with bone. 1 chop, 3.5 ounces.	98	260	16	21	8	9	2	0	8	2.2	0	.63	.18	3.8	—
Lean and fat — 2.3 ounces	66	260	16	21	8	9	2	0	8	2.2	0	.63	.18	3.8	—
Lean only — 1.7 ounces	48	130	15	7	2	3	1	0	7	1.9	0	.54	.16	3.3	—
Roast, oven-cooked, no liquid added:															
Lean and fat — 3 ounces	85	310	21	24	9	10	2	0	9	2.7	0	.78	.22	4.7	—
Lean only — 2.4 ounces	68	175	20	10	3	4	1	0	9	2.6	0	.73	.21	4.4	—
Cuts, simmered:															
Lean and fat — 3 ounces	85	320	20	26	9	11	2	0	8	2.5	0	.46	.21	4.1	—
Lean only — 2.2 ounces	63	135	18	6	2	3	1	0	8	2.3	0	.42	.19	3.7	—
Sausage:															
Bologna, slice, 3-in. diam. by ⅛ inch. — 2 slices	26	80	3	7	—	—	—	Trace	2	.5	—	.04	.06	.7	—
Braunschweiger, slice 2-in. diam. by ¼ inch. — 2 slices	20	65	3	5	—	—	—	Trace	2	1.2	1,310	.03	.29	1.6	—
Deviled ham, canned — 1 tbsp.	13	45	2	4	2	2	Trace	0	1	.3	—	.02	.01	.2	—
Frankfurter, heated (8 per lb. purchased pkg.). — 1 frank	56	170	7	15	—	—	—	1	3	.8	—	.08	.11	1.4	—
Pork links, cooked (16 links per lb. raw). — 2 links	26	125	5	11	4	5	1	Trace	2	.6	0	.21	.09	1.0	—
Salami, dry type — 1 oz.	28	130	7	11	—	—	—	Trace	4	1.0	—	.10	.07	1.5	—
Salami, cooked — 1 oz.	28	90	5	7	—	—	—	Trace	3	.7	—	.07	.07	1.2	—
Vienna, canned (7 sausages per 5-oz. can). — 1 sausage	16	40	2	3	—	—	—	Trace	1	.3	—	.01	.02	.4	—
Veal, medium fat, cooked, bone removed:															
Cutlet — 3 oz.	85	185	23	9	5	4	Trace	0	9	2.7	—	.06	.21	4.6	—
Roast — 3 oz.	85	230	23	14	7	6	Trace	0	10	2.9	—	.11	.26	6.6	—
Fish and shellfish:															
Bluefish, baked with table fat. — 3 oz.	85	135	22	4	—	—	—	0	25	.6	40	.09	.08	1.6	—
Clams:															
Raw, meat only — 3 oz.	85	65	11	1	—	—	—	2	59	5.2	90	.08	.15	1.1	—
Canned, solids and liquid. — 3 oz.	85	45	7	1	—	—	—	2	47	3.5	—	.01	.09	.9	—
Crabmeat, canned — 3 oz.	85	85	15	2	—	—	—	1	38	.7	—	.07	.07	1.6	8

³ Outer layer of fat on the cut was removed to within approximately ½-inch of the lean. Deposits of fat within the cut were not removed.

[Dashes in the columns for nutrients show that no suitable value could be found although there is reason to believe that a measurable amount of the nutrient may be present]

Food, approximate measure, and weight (in grams)	Water	Food energy	Protein	Fat	Fatty acids			Carbohydrate	Calcium	Iron	Vitamin A value	Thiamin	Riboflavin	Niacin	Ascorbic acid
					Saturated (total)	Unsaturated									
						Oleic	Linoleic								
	Grams	Percent	Calories	Grams	Grams	Grams	Grams	Grams	Grams	Milligrams	Milligrams	International units	Milligrams	Milligrams	Milligrams	Milligrams

MEAT, POULTRY, FISH, SHELLFISH; RELATED PRODUCTS—Continued

Food, approximate measure, and weight (in grams)	Grams	Percent	Calories	Protein Grams	Fat Grams	Sat. Grams	Oleic Grams	Linoleic Grams	Carbo. Grams	Calcium mg	Iron mg	Vit A IU	Thiamin mg	Riboflavin mg	Niacin mg	Ascorbic mg
Fish and shellfish—Continued																
Fish sticks, breaded, cooked, frozen; stick 3¾ by 1 by ½ inch. 10 sticks or 8 oz. pkg. — 227	66	400	38	20	5	4	10	15	25	0.9	—	0.09	0.16	3.6	—
Haddock, breaded, fried 3 oz. — 85	66	140	17	5	1	3	Trace	5	34	1.0	—	.03	.06	2.7	2
Ocean perch, breaded, fried. 3 oz. — 85	59	195	16	11	—	—	—	6	28	1.1	—	.08	.09	1.5	
Oysters, raw, meat only (13–19 med. selects). 1 cup — 240	85	160	20	4				8	226	13.2	740	.33	.43	6.0	
Salmon, pink, canned 3 oz. — 85	71	120	17	5	1	1	Trace	0	⁴167	.7	60	.03	.16	6.8	
Sardines, Atlantic, canned in oil, drained solids. 3 oz. — 85	62	175	20	9				0	372	2.5	190	.02	.17	4.6	
Shad, baked with table fat and bacon. 3 oz. — 85	64	170	20	10				0	20	.5	20	.11	.22	7.3	
Shrimp, canned, meat 3 oz. — 85	70	100	21	1				1	98	2.6	50	.01	.03	1.5	
Swordfish, broiled with butter or margarine. 3 oz. — 85	65	150	24	5				0	23	1.1	1,750	.03	.04	9.3	
Tuna, canned in oil, drained solids. 3 oz. — 85	61	170	24	7	2	1	1	0	7	1.6	70	.04	.10	10.1	
MATURE DRY BEANS AND PEAS, NUTS, PEANUTS; RELATED PRODUCTS																
Almonds, shelled, whole kernels. 1 cup — 142	5	850	26	77	6	52	15	28	332	6.7	0	.34	1.31	5.0	Trace
Beans, dry: Common varieties as Great Northern, navy, and others: Cooked, drained: Great Northern 1 cup — 180	69	210	14	1				38	90	4.9	0	.25	.13	1.3	0

Food, approximate measure		Weight (g)	Water (%)	Food energy (cal.)	Protein (g)	Fat (g)	Saturated (total) (g)	Oleic (g)	Linoleic (g)	Carbohydrate (g)	Calcium (mg)	Iron (mg)	Vitamin A (I.U.)	Thiamine (mg)	Riboflavin (mg)	Niacin (mg)	Ascorbic acid (mg)
Navy (pea)	1 cup	190	69	225	15	1				40	95	5.1	0	.27	.13	1.3	0
Canned, solids and liquid:																	
White with—																	
Frankfurters (sliced).	1 cup	255	71	365	19	18				32	94	4.8	330	.18	.15	3.3	Trace
Pork and tomato sauce.	1 cup	255	71	310	16	7	2	3	1	49	138	4.6	330	.20	.08	1.5	5
Pork and sweet sauce.	1 cup	255	66	385	16	12	4	5	1	54	161	5.9	10	.15	.10	1.3	
Red kidney.	1 cup	255	76	230	15	1				42	74	4.6		.13	.10	1.5	
Lima, cooked, drained.	1 cup	190	64	260	16	1				49	55	5.9		.25	.11	1.3	
Cashew nuts, roasted.	1 cup	140	5	785	24	64	11	45	4	41	53	5.3	140	.60	.35	2.5	
Coconut, fresh, meat only:																	
Pieces, approx. 2 by 2 by ½ inch.	1 piece	45	51	155	2	16	14	1	Trace	4	6	.8	0	.02	.01	.2	1
Shredded or grated, firmly packed.	1 cup	130	51	450	5	46	39	3	Trace	12	17	2.2	0	.07	.03	.7	4
Cowpeas or blackeye peas, dry, cooked.	1 cup	248	80	190	13	1				34	42	3.2	20	.41	.11	1.1	Trace
Peanuts, roasted, salted, halves.	1 cup	144	2	840	37	72	16	31	21	27	107	3.0		.46	.19	24.7	0
Peanut butter.	1 tbsp.	16	2	95	4	8	2	4	2	3	9	.3		.02	.02	2.4	0
Peas, split, dry, cooked.	1 cup	250	70	290	20	1				52	28	4.2	100	.37	.22	2.2	
Pecans, halves.	1 cup	108	3	740	10	77	5	48	15	16	79	2.6	140	.93	.14	1.0	2
Walnuts, black or native, chopped.	1 cup	126	3	790	26	75	4	26	36	19	Trace	7.6	380	.28	.14	.9	
VEGETABLES AND VEGETABLE PRODUCTS																	
Asparagus, green:																	
Cooked, drained:																	
Spears, ½-in. diam. at base.	4 spears	60	94	10	1	Trace				2	13	.4	540	.10	.11	.8	16
Pieces, 1½ to 2-in. lengths.	1 cup	145	94	30	3	Trace				5	30	.9	1,310	.23	.26	2.0	38
Canned, solids and liquid.	1 cup	244	94	45	5	1				7	44	4.1	1,240	.15	.22	2.0	37
Beans:																	
Lima, immature seeds, cooked, drained.	1 cup	170	71	190	13	1				34	80	4.3	480	.31	.17	2.2	29
Green:																	
Snap:																	
Cooked, drained.	1 cup	125	92	30	2	Trace				7	63	.8	680	.09	.11	.6	15
Canned, solids and liquid.	1 cup	239	94	45	2	Trace				10	81	2.9	690	.07	.10	.7	10

[4] If bones are discarded, value will be greatly reduced.

[Dashes in the columns for nutrients show that no suitable value could be found although there is reason to believe that a measurable amount of the nutrient may be present]

Food, approximate measure, and weight (in grams)	Water	Food energy	Protein	Fat	Fatty acids			Carbohydrate	Calcium	Iron	Vitamin A value	Thiamin	Riboflavin	Niacin	Ascorbic acid
					Saturated (total)	Unsaturated Oleic	Linoleic								
	Grams	Percent	Calories	Grams	Grams	Grams	Grams	Grams	Grams	Milligrams	Milligrams	International units	Milligrams	Milligrams	Milligrams	Milligrams
VEGETABLES AND VEGETABLE PRODUCTS—Continued																
Beans—Continued																
Snap—Continued																
Yellow or wax:																
Cooked, drained... 1 cup	125	93	30	2	Trace			6	63	0.8	290	0.09	0.11	0.6	16
Canned, solids and liquid. 1 cup	239	94	45	2	1			10	81	2.9	140	.07	.10	.7	12
Sprouted mung beans, cooked, drained. 1 cup	125	91	35	4	Trace			7	21	1.1	30	.11	.13	.9	8
Beets:																
Cooked, drained, peeled:																
Whole beets, 2-in. diam. 2 beets	100	91	30	1	Trace			7	14	.5	20	.03	.04	.3	6
Diced or sliced. 1 cup	170	91	55	2	Trace			12	24	.9	30	.05	.07	.5	10
Canned, solids and liquid. 1 cup	246	90	85	2	Trace			19	34	1.5	20	.02	.05	.2	7
Beet greens, leaves and stems, cooked, drained. 1 cup	145	94	25	3	Trace			5	144	2.8	7,400	.10	.22	.4	22
Blackeye peas. See Cowpeas.																
Broccoli, cooked, drained:																
Whole stalks, medium size. 1 stalk	180	91	45	6	1			8	158	1.4	4,500	.16	.36	1.4	162
Stalks cut into ½-in. pieces. 1 cup	155	91	40	5	1			7	136	1.2	3,880	.14	.31	1.2	140
Chopped, yield from 10-oz. frozen pkg. 1⅓ cups	250	92	65	7	1			12	135	1.8	6,500	.15	.30	1.3	143
Brussels sprouts, 7-8 sprouts (1¼ to 1½ in. diam.) per cup, cooked. 1 cup	155	88	55	7	1			10	50	1.7	810	.12	.22	1.2	135
Cabbage:																
Common varieties:																

Food, approximate measure, and weight (in grams)													
Raw:													
Coarsely shredded or sliced. 1 cup	70	92	15	1	Trace	4	34	.3	90	.04	.04	.2	33
Finely shredded or chopped. 1 cup	90	92	20	1	Trace	5	44	.4	120	.05	.05	.3	42
Cooked. 1 cup	145	94	30	2	Trace	6	64	.4	190	.06	.06	.4	48
Red, raw, coarsely shredded. 1 cup	70	90	20	1	Trace	5	29	.6	30	.06	.04	.3	43
Savoy, raw, coarsely shredded. 1 cup	70	92	15	2	Trace	3	47	.6	140	.04	.06	.2	39
Cabbage, celery or Chinese, raw, cut in 1-in. pieces. 1 cup	75	95	10	1	Trace	2	32	.5	110	.04	.03	.5	19
Cabbage, spoon (or pakchoy), cooked. 1 cup	170	95	25	2	Trace	4	252	1.0	5,270	.07	.14	1.2	26
Carrots:													
Raw:													
Whole, 5½ by 1 inch (25 thin strips). 1 carrot	50	88	20	1	Trace	5	18	.4	5,500	.03	.03	.3	4
Grated. 1 cup	110	88	45	1	Trace	11	41	.8	12,100	.06	.06	.7	9
Cooked, diced. 1 cup	145	91	45	1	Trace	10	48	.9	15,220	.08	.07	.7	9
Canned, strained or chopped (baby food). 1 ounce	28	92	10	Trace	Trace	2	7	.1	3,690	.01	.01	.1	1
Cauliflower, cooked, flowerbuds. 1 cup	120	93	25	3	Trace	5	25	.8	70	.11	.10	.7	66
Celery, raw:													
Stalk, large outer, 8 by about 1½ inches, at root end. 1 stalk	40	94	5	Trace	Trace	2	16	.1	100	.01	.01	.1	4
Pieces, diced. 1 cup	100	94	15	1	Trace	4	39	.3	240	.03	.03	.3	9
Collards, cooked. 1 cup	190	91	55	5	1	9	289	1.1	10,260	.27	.37	2.4	87
Corn, sweet:													
Cooked, ear 5 by 1¾ inches.[5] 1 ear	140	74	70	3	1	16	2	.5	[6]310	.09	.08	1.0	7
Canned, solids and liquid. 1 cup	256	81	170	5	2	40	10	1.0	[6]690	.07	.12	2.3	13
Cowpeas, cooked, immature seeds. 1 cup	160	72	175	13	1	29	38	3.4	560	.49	.18	2.3	28
Cucumbers, 10-ounce; 7½ by about 2 inches:													
Raw, pared. 1 cucumber	207	96	30	1	Trace	7	35	.6	Trace	.07	.09	.4	23
Raw, pared, center slice ⅛-inch thick. 6 slices	50	96	5	Trace	Trace	2	8	.2	Trace	.02	.02	.1	6
Dandelion greens, cooked. 1 cup	180	90	60	4	1	12	252	3.2	21,060	.24	.29		32

[5] Measure and weight apply to entire vegetable or fruit including parts not usually eaten.

[6] Based on yellow varieties; white varieties contain only a trace of cryptoxanthin and carotenes, the pigments in corn that have biological activity.

VEGETABLES AND VEGETABLE PRODUCTS—Continued

Food, approximate measure, and weight (in grams)		Water	Food energy	Protein	Fat	Fatty acids Saturated (total)	Fatty acids Unsaturated Oleic	Fatty acids Unsaturated Linoleic	Carbo-hydrate	Cal-cium	Iron	Vita-min A value	Thia-min	Ribo-flavin	Niacin	Ascor-bic acid
	Grams	Per-cent	Calo-ries	Grams	Grams	Grams	Grams	Grams	Grams	Milli-grams	Milli-grams	Inter-national units	Milli-grams	Milli-grams	Milli-grams	Milli-grams
Endive, curly (including escarole). 2 ounces	57	93	10	1	Trace	------	------	------	2	46	1.0	1,870	0.04	0.08	0.3	6
Kale, leaves including stems, cooked. 1 cup	110	91	30	4	1	------	------	------	4	147	1.3	8,140	------	.13	.6	68
Lettuce, raw: Butterhead, as Boston types; head, 4-inch diameter. 1 head	220	95	30	3	Trace	------	------	------	6	77	4.4	2,130	.14	.13	1.3	18
Crisphead, as Iceberg; 1 head, 4¾-inch diameter.	454	96	60	4	Trace	------	------	------	13	91	2.3	1,500	.29	.27	.2	29
Looseleaf, or bunching varieties, leaves. 2 large	50	94	10	1	Trace	------	------	------	2	34	.7	950	.03	.04	.2	9
Mushrooms, canned, solids and liquid. 1 cup	244	93	40	5	Trace	------	------	------	6	15	1.2	Trace	.04	.60	4.8	4
Mustard greens, cooked. 1 cup	140	93	35	3	1	------	------	------	6	193	2.5	8,120	.11	.19	.9	68
Okra, cooked, pod 3 by ⅝ inch. 8 pods	85	91	25	2	Trace	------	------	------	5	78	.4	420	.11	.15	.8	17
Onions: Mature: Raw, onion 2½-inch diameter. 1 onion	110	89	40	2	Trace	------	------	------	10	30	.6	40	.04	.04	.2	11
Cooked. 1 cup	210	92	60	3	Trace	------	------	------	14	50	.8	80	.06	.06	.4	14
Young green, small, without tops. 6 onions	50	88	20	1	Trace	------	------	------	5	20	.3	Trace	.02	.02	.2	12
Parsley, raw, chopped. 1 tablespoon	4	85	Trace	Trace	Trace	------	------	------	Trace	8	.2	340	Trace	.01	Trace	7
Parsnips, cooked. 1 cup	155	82	100	2	1	------	------	------	23	70	.9	50	.11	.12	.2	16
Peas, green: Cooked. 1 cup	160	82	115	9	1	------	------	------	19	37	2.9	860	.44	.17	3.7	33
Canned, solids and liquid. 1 cup	249	83	165	9	1	------	------	------	31	50	4.2	1,120	.23	.13	2.2	22

Food	Measure	Grams	Water (%)	Food energy (cal.)	Protein (g)	Fat (g)	Saturated (g)	Oleic (g)	Linoleic (g)	Carbohydrate (g)	Calcium (mg)	Iron (mg)	Vitamin A (I.U.)	Thiamine (mg)	Riboflavin (mg)	Niacin (mg)	Ascorbic acid (mg)
Canned, strained (baby food).	1 ounce	28	86	15	1	Trace				3	8	.4	140	.02	.02	.4	3
Peppers, hot, red, without seeds, dried (ground chili powder, added seasonings).	1 tablespoon	15	8	50	2	2				8	40	2.3	9,750	.03	.17	1.3	2
Peppers, sweet:																	
Raw, about 5 per pound: Green pod without stem and seeds.	1 pod	74	93	15	1	Trace				4	7	.5	310	.06	.06	.4	94
Cooked, boiled, drained	1 pod	73	95	15	1	Trace				3	7	.4	310	.05	.05	.4	70
Potatoes, medium (about 3 per pound raw):																	
Baked, peeled after baking.	1 potato	99	75	90	3	Trace				21	9	.7	Trace	.10	.04	1.7	20
Boiled:																	
Peeled after boiling	1 potato	136	80	105	3	Trace				23	10	.8	Trace	.13	.05	2.0	22
Peeled before boiling	1 potato	122	83	80	2	Trace				18	7	.6	Trace	.11	.04	1.4	20
French-fried, piece 2 by ½ by ½ inch: Cooked in deep fat	10 pieces	57	45	155	2	7	2	2	4	20	9	.7	Trace	.07	.04	1.8	12
Frozen, heated	10 pieces	57	53	125	2	5	1	1	2	19	5	1.0	Trace	.08	.01	1.5	12
Mashed: Milk added	1 cup	195	83	125	4	1				25	47	.8	50	.16	.10	2.0	19
Milk and butter added	1 cup	195	80	185	4	8	4	3	Trace	24	47	.8	330	.16	.10	1.9	18
Potato chips, medium, 2-inch diameter.	10 chips	20	2	115	1	8	2	2	4	10	8	.4	Trace	.04	.01	1.0	3
Pumpkin, canned	1 cup	228	90	75	2	1				18	57	.9	14,590	.07	.12	1.3	12
Radishes, raw, small, without tops.	4 radishes	40	94	5	Trace	Trace				1	12	.4	Trace	.01	.01	.1	10
Sauerkraut, canned, solids and liquid.	1 cup	235	93	45	2	Trace				9	85	1.2	120	.07	.09	.4	33
Spinach: Cooked	1 cup	180	92	40	5	1				6	167	4.0	14,580	.13	.25	1.0	50
Canned, drained solids	1 cup	180	91	45	5	1				6	212	4.7	14,400	.03	.21	.6	24
Squash: Cooked: Summer, diced	1 cup	210	96	30	2	Trace				7	52	.8	820	.10	.16	1.6	21
Winter, baked, mashed.	1 cup	205	81	130	4	1				32	57	1.6	8,610	.10	.27	1.4	27
Sweetpotatoes: Cooked, medium, 5 by 2 inches, weight raw about 6 ounces: Baked, peeled after baking.	1 sweetpotato	110	64	155	2	1				36	44	1.0	8,910	.10	.07	1.0	24
Boiled, peeled after boiling.	1 sweetpotato	147	71	170	2	1				39	47	1.0	11,610	.13	.09	.9	25

[Dashes in the columns for nutrients show that no suitable value could be found although there is reason to believe that a measurable amount of the nutrient may be present]

Food, approximate measure, and weight (in grams)		Water	Food energy	Protein	Fat	Fatty acids			Carbohydrate	Calcium	Iron	Vitamin A value	Thiamin	Riboflavin	Niacin	Ascorbic acid
						Saturated (total)	Unsaturated									
							Oleic	Linoleic								
		Per cent	*Calories*	*Grams*	*Grams*	*Grams*	*Grams*	*Grams*	*Grams*	*Milligrams*	*Milligrams*	*International units*	*Milligrams*	*Milligrams*	*Milligrams*	*Milligrams*
VEGETABLES AND VEGETABLE PRODUCTS—Continued																
Sweetpotatoes—Continued																
Candied, 3½ by 2¼ inches.	1 sweetpotato.	*Grams* 175	60	295	2	6	2	3	1	60	65	1.6	11,030	0.10	0.08	0.8	17
Canned, vacuum or solid pack.	1 cup	218	72	235	4	Trace				54	54	1.7	17,000	.10	.10	1.4	30
Tomatoes:																	
Raw, approx. 3-in. diam. 2⅛ in. high; wt., 7 oz.	1 tomato	200	94	40	2	Trace				9	24	.9	1,640	.11	.07	1.3	[7]42
Canned, solids and liquid.	1 cup	241	94	50	2	1				10	14	1.2	2,170	.12	.07	1.7	41
Tomato catsup:																	
Cup	1 cup	273	69	290	6	1				69	60	2.2	3,820	.25	.19	4.4	41
Tablespoon	1 tbsp.	15	69	15	Trace	Trace				4	3	.1	210	.01	.01	.2	2
Tomato juice, canned:																	
Cup	1 cup	243	94	45	2	Trace				10	17	2.2	1,940	.12	.07	1.9	39
Glass (6 fl. oz.)	1 glass	182	94	35	2	Trace				8	13	1.6	1,460	.09	.05	1.5	29
Turnips, cooked, diced	1 cup	155	94	35	1	Trace				8	54	.6	Trace	.06	.08	.5	34
Turnip greens, cooked	1 cup	145	94	30	3	Trace				5	252	1.5	8,270	.15	.33	.7	68
FRUITS AND FRUIT PRODUCTS																	
Apples, raw (about 3 per lb.)[3]	1 apple	150	85	70	Trace	Trace				18	8	.4	50	.04	.02	.1	3
Apple juice, bottled or canned.	1 cup	248	88	120	Trace	Trace				30	15	1.5	------	.02	.05	.2	2
Applesauce, canned:																	
Sweetened	1 cup	255	76	230	1	Trace				61	10	1.3	100	.05	.03	.1	[8]3
Unsweetened or artificially sweetened.	1 cup	244	88	100	1	Trace				26	10	1.2	100	.05	.02	.1	[8]2

Food	Measure	Grams	Water (%)	Food energy (cal.)	Protein (g)	Fat (g)	Saturated fatty acids (g)	Unsaturated oleic (g)	Unsaturated linoleic (g)	Carbo-hydrate (g)	Calcium (mg)	Iron (mg)	Vitamin A (I.U.)	Thiamine (mg)	Riboflavin (mg)	Niacin (mg)	Ascorbic acid (mg)
Apricots:																	
Raw (about 12 per lb.) [5]	3 apricots	114	85	55	1	Trace	-	-	-	14	18	.5	2,890	.03	.04	.7	10
Canned in heavy sirup	1 cup	259	77	220	2	Trace	-	-	-	57	28	.8	4,510	.05	.06	.9	10
Dried, uncooked (40 halves per cup).	1 cup	150	25	390	8	1	-	-	-	100	100	8.2	16,350	.02	.23	4.9	19
Cooked, unsweetened, fruit and liquid.	1 cup	285	76	240	5	1	-	-	-	62	63	5.1	8,550	.01	.13	2.8	8
Apricot nectar, canned	1 cup	251	85	140	1	Trace	-	-	-	37	23	.5	2,380	.03	.03	.5	[8]8
Avocados, whole fruit, raw: [5]																	
California (mid- and late-winter; diam. 3⅛ in.).	1 avocado	284	74	370	5	37	7	17	5	13	22	1.3	630	.24	.43	3.5	30
Florida (late summer, fall; diam. 3⅝ in.).	1 avocado	454	78	390	4	33	7	15	4	27	30	1.8	880	.33	.61	4.9	43
Bananas, raw, medium size. [5]	1 banana	175	76	100	1	Trace	-	-	-	26	10	.8	230	.06	.07	.8	12
Banana flakes	1 cup	100	3	340	4	1	-	-	-	89	32	2.8	760	.18	.24	2.8	7
Blackberries, raw	1 cup	144	84	85	2	1	-	-	-	19	46	1.3	290	.05	.06	.5	30
Blueberries, raw	1 cup	140	83	85	1	1	-	-	-	21	21	1.4	140	.04	.08	.6	20
Cantaloups, raw; medium, 5-inch diameter about 1⅔ pounds. [5]	½ melon	385	91	60	1	Trace	-	-	-	14	27	.8	[9]6,540	.08	.06	1.2	63
Cherries, canned, red, sour, pitted, water pack.	1 cup	244	88	105	2	Trace	-	-	-	26	37	.7	1,660	.07	.05	.5	12
Cranberry juice cocktail, canned.	1 cup	250	83	165	Trace	Trace	-	-	-	42	13	.8	Trace	.03	.03	.1	[10]40
Cranberry sauce, sweetened, canned, strained.	1 cup	277	62	405	Trace	1	-	-	-	104	17	.6	60	.03	.03	.1	6
Dates, pitted, cut	1 cup	178	22	490	4	1	-	-	-	130	105	5.3	90	.16	.17	3.9	0
Figs, dried, large, 2 by 1 in.	1 fig	21	23	60	1	Trace	-	-	-	15	26	.6	20	.02	.02	.1	0
Fruit cocktail, canned, in heavy sirup.	1 cup	256	80	195	1	Trace	-	-	-	50	23	1.0	360	.05	.03	1.3	5

[5] Measure and weight apply to entire vegetable or fruit including parts not usually eaten.

[7] Year-round average. Samples marketed from November through May, average 20 milligrams per 200-gram tomato; from June through October, around 52 milligrams.

[8] This is the amount from the fruit. Additional ascorbic acid may be added by the manufacturer. Refer to the label for this information.

[9] Value for varieties with orange-colored flesh; value for varieties with green flesh would be about 540 I.U.

[10] Value listed is based on products with label stating 30 milligrams per 6 fl. oz. serving.

387

[Dashes in the columns for nutrients show that no suitable value could be found although there is reason to believe that a measurable amount of the nutrient may be present]

Food, approximate measure, and weight (in grams)		Water	Food energy	Protein	Fat	Fatty acids			Carbohydrate	Calcium	Iron	Vitamin A value	Thiamin	Riboflavin	Niacin	Ascorbic acid
						Saturated (total)	Unsaturated									
							Oleic	Linoleic								
	Grams	Percent	Calories	Grams	Grams	Grams	Grams	Grams	Grams	Milligrams	Milligrams	International units	Milligrams	Milligrams	Milligrams	Milligrams
FRUITS AND FRUIT PRODUCTS—Con.																
Grapefruit:																
Raw, medium, 3¾-in. diam.[5]																
White --- ½ grapefruit.	241	89	45	1	Trace	---			12	19	0.5	10	0.05	0.02	0.2	44
Pink or red --- ½ grapefruit.	241	89	50	1	Trace	---			13	20	0.5	540	0.05	0.02	0.2	44
Canned, sirup pack --- 1 cup	254	81	180	2	Trace	---			45	33	.8	30	.08	.05	.5	76
Grapefruit juice:																
Fresh --- 1 cup	246	90	95	1	Trace	---			23	22	.5	(11)	.09	.04	.4	92
Canned, white:																
Unsweetened --- 1 cup	247	89	100	1	Trace	---			24	20	1.0	20	.07	.04	.4	84
Sweetened --- 1 cup	250	86	130	1	Trace	---			32	20	1.0	20	.07	.04	.4	78
Frozen, concentrate, unsweetened:																
Undiluted, can, 6 fluid ounces.	207	62	300	4	1	---			72	70	.8	60	.29	.12	1.4	286
Diluted with 3 parts water, by volume. --- 1 cup	247	89	100	1	Trace	---			24	25	.2	20	.10	.04	.5	96
Dehydrated crystals --- 4 oz.	113	1	410	6	1	---			102	100	1.2	80	.40	.20	2.0	396
Prepared with water --- 1 cup (1 pound yields about 1 gallon).	247	90	100	1	Trace	---			24	22	.2	20	.10	.05	.5	91
Grapes, raw:[5]																
American type (slip skin). --- 1 cup	153	82	65	1	1	---			15	15	.4	100	.05	.03	.2	3
European type (adherent skin). --- 1 cup	160	81	95	1	Trace	---			25	17	.6	140	.07	.04	.4	6
Grapejuice:																
Canned or bottled --- 1 cup	253	83	165	1	Trace	---			42	28	.8	---	.10	.05	.5	Trace
Frozen concentrate, sweetened:																
Undiluted, can, 6 fluid ounces. --- 1 can	216	53	395	1	Trace	---			100	22	.9	40	.13	.22	1.5	(13)

Food	Measure	Grams	Water (%)	Food energy (cal.)	Protein	Fat	Saturated	Unsaturated (oleic)	Unsaturated (linoleic)	Carbohydrate	Calcium	Iron	Vitamin A	Thiamine	Riboflavin	Niacin	Ascorbic acid
Diluted with 3 parts water, by volume.	1 cup	250	86	135	1	Trace				33	8	.3	10	.05	.03	.5	(¹²)
Grapejuice drink, canned.	1 cup	250	86	135	Trace	Trace				35	8	.3	--	.03	.03	.3	(¹²)
Lemons, raw, 2⅛-in. diam., size 165.⁵ Used for juice.	1 lemon	110	90	20	1	Trace				6	19	.4	10	.03	.01	.1	39
Lemon juice, raw	1 cup	244	91	60	1	Trace				20	17	.5	50	.07	.02	.2	112
Lemonade concentrate: Frozen, 6 fl. oz. per can.	1 can	219	48	430	Trace	Trace				112	9	.4	40	.04	.07	.7	66
Diluted with 4⅓ parts water, by volume.	1 cup	248	88	110	Trace	Trace				28	2	Trace	Trace	Trace	.02	.2	17
Lime juice: Fresh.	1 cup	246	90	65	1	Trace				22	22	.5	20	.05	.02	.2	79
Canned, unsweetened	1 cup	246	90	65	1	Trace				22	22	.5	20	.05	.02	.2	52
Limeade concentrate, frozen: Undiluted, can, 6 fluid ounces.	1 can	218	50	410	Trace	Trace				108	11	.2	Trace	.02	.02	.2	26
Diluted with 4⅓ parts water, by volume.	1 cup	247	90	100	Trace	Trace				27	2	Trace	Trace	Trace	Trace	Trace	5
Oranges, raw, 2⅝-in. diam., all commercial, varieties.⁵	1 orange	180	86	65	1	Trace				·16	54	.5	260	.13	.05	.5	66
Orange juice, fresh, all varieties.	1 cup	248	88	110	2	Trace				26	27	.5	500	.22	.07	1.0	124
Canned, unsweetened	1 cup	249	87	120	2	Trace				28	25	1.0	500	.17	.05	.7	100
Frozen concentrate: Undiluted, can, 6 fluid ounces.	1 can	213	55	360	5	Trace				87	75	.9	1,620	.68	.11	2.8	360
Diluted with 3 parts water, by volume.	1 cup	249	87	120	2	Trace				29	25	.2	550	.22	.02	1.0	120
Dehydrated crystals	4 oz.	113	1	430	6	2				100	95	1.9	1,900	.76	.24	3.3	408
Prepared with water (1 pound yields about 1 gallon).	1 cup	248	88	115	2	1				27	25	.5	500	.20	.07	1.0	109
Orange-apricot juice drink	1 cup	249	87	125	1	Trace				32	12	.2	1,440	.05	.02	.5	¹⁰ 40

⁵ Measure and weight apply to entire vegetable or fruit including parts not usually eaten.

¹⁰ Value listed is based on product with label stating 30 milligrams per 6 fl. oz. serving.

¹¹ For white-fleshed varieties value is about 20 I.U. per cup; for red-fleshed varieties, 1,080 I.U. per cup.

¹² Present only if added by the manufacturer. Refer to the label for this information.

[Dashes in the columns for nutrients show that no suitable value could be found although there is reason to believe that a measurable amount of the nutrient may be present]

Food, approximate measure, and weight (in grams)		Water	Food energy	Protein	Fat	Fatty acids Saturated (total)	Unsaturated Oleic	Unsaturated Linoleic	Carbohydrate	Calcium	Iron	Vitamin A value	Thiamin	Riboflavin	Niacin	Ascorbic acid
	Grams	Per cent	Calories	Grams	Grams	Grams	Grams	Grams	Grams	Milligrams	Milligrams	International units	Milligrams	Milligrams	Milligrams	Milligrams
FRUITS AND FRUIT PRODUCTS—Con.																
Orange and grapefruit juice:																
Frozen concentrate:																
Undiluted, can, 6 fluid ounces. 1 can	210	59	330	4	1	---	---	---	78	61	0.8	800	0.48	0.06	2.3	302
Diluted with 3 parts water, by volume. 1 cup	248	88	110	1	Trace	---	---	---	26	20	.2	270	.16	.02	.8	102
Papayas, raw, ½-inch cubes. 1 cup	182	89	70	1	Trace	---	---	---	18	36	.5	3,190	.07	.08	.5	102
Peaches:																
Raw:																
Whole, medium, 2-inch diameter, about 4 per pound.[5] 1 peach	114	89	35	1	Trace	---	---	---	10	9	.5	[11]1,320	.02	.05	1.0	7
Sliced. 1 cup	168	89	65	1	Trace	---	---	---	16	15	.8	[12]2,230	.03	.08	1.6	12
Canned, yellow-fleshed, solids and liquid:																
Sirup pack, heavy:																
Halves or slices. 1 cup	257	79	200	1	Trace	---	---	---	52	10	.8	1,100	.02	.06	1.4	7
Water pack. 1 cup	245	91	75	1	Trace	---	---	---	20	10	.7	1,100	.02	.06	1.4	7
Dried, uncooked. 1 cup	160	25	420	5	1	---	---	---	109	77	9.6	6,240	.02	.31	8.5	28
Cooked, unsweetened, 10–12 halves and juice. 1 cup	270	77	220	3	1	---	---	---	58	41	5.1	3,290	.01	.15	4.2	6
Frozen:																
Carton, 12 ounces, not thawed. 1 carton	340	76	300	1	Trace	---	---	---	77	14	1.7	2,210	.03	.14	2.4	[14]185
Pears:																
Raw, 3 by 2½-inch diameter.[5] 1 pear	182	83	100	1	1	---	---	---	25	13	.5	30	.04	.07	.2	7
Canned, solids and liquid:																
Sirup pack, heavy:																
Halves or slices. 1 cup	255	80	195	1	1	---	---	---	50	13	.5	Trace	.03	.05	.3	4

390

Food, approximate measure, and weight (in grams)			Water (percent)	Food energy (calories)	Protein (grams)	Fat (grams)	Carbohydrate (grams)	Calcium (mg)	Iron (mg)	Vitamin A (I.U.)	Thiamine (mg)	Riboflavin (mg)	Niacin (mg)	Ascorbic acid (mg)
Pineapple:														
Raw, diced	1 cup	140	85	75	1	Trace	19	24	.7	100	.12	.04	.3	24
Canned, heavy sirup pack, solids and liquid:														
Crushed	1 cup	260	80	195	1	Trace	50	29	.8	120	.20	.06	.5	17
Sliced, slices and juice.	2 small or 1 large.	122	80	90	Trace	Trace	24	13	.4	50	.09	.03	.2	8
Pineapple juice, canned..	1 cup	249	86	135	1	Trace	34	37	.7	120	.12	.04	.5	*22
Plums, all except prunes:														
Raw, 2-inch diameter, 1 plum about 2 ounces.⁵		60	87	25	Trace	Trace	7	7	.3	140	.02	.02	.3	3
Canned, sirup pack (Italian prunes):														
Plums (with pits) and juice.⁵	1 cup	256	77	205	1	Trace	53	22	2.2	2,970	.05	.05	.9	4
Prunes, dried, "softenized", medium:														
Uncooked.⁵	4 prunes	32	28	70	1	Trace	18	14	1.1	440	.02	.04	.4	1
Cooked, unsweetened, 17–18 prunes and ⅓ cup liquid.⁵	1 cup	270	66	295	2	1	78	60	4.5	1,860	.08	.18	1.7	2
Prune juice, canned or bottled.	1 cup	256	80	200	1	Trace	49	36	10.5		.03	.03	1.0	*5
Raisins, seedless:														
Packaged, ½ oz. or 1½ tbsp. per pkg.	1 pkg.	14	18	40	Trace	Trace	11	9	.5	Trace	.02	.01	.1	Trace
Cup, pressed down..	1 cup	165	18	480	4	Trace	128	102	5.8	30	.18	.13	.8	2
Raspberries, red:														
Raw	1 cup	123	84	70	1	1	17	27	1.1	160	.04	.11	1.1	31
Frozen, 10-ounce carton, not thawed.	1 carton.	284	74	275	2	1	70	37	1.7	200	.06	.17	1.7	59
Rhubarb, cooked, sugar added.	1 cup	272	63	385	1	Trace	98	212	1.6	220	.06	.15	.7	17
Strawberries:														
Raw, capped	1 cup	149	90	55	1	1	13	31	1.5	90	.04	.10	1.0	88
Frozen, 10-ounce carton, not thawed.	1 carton.	284	71	310	1	1	79	40	2.0	90	.06	.17	1.5	150
Tangerines, raw, medium, 2⅜-in. diam., size 176.⁵	1 tangerine.	116	87	40	1	Trace	10	34	.3	360	.05	.02	.1	27
Tangerine juice, canned, sweetened.	1 cup	249	87	125	1	1	30	45	.5	1,050	.15	.05	.2	55
Watermelon, raw, wedge, 4 by 8 inches (⅛ of 10 by 16-inch melon, about 2 pounds with rind).⁵	1 wedge	925	93	115	2	1	27	30	2.1	2,510	.13	.13	.7	30

⁵ Measure and weight apply to entire vegetable or fruit including parts not usually eaten.

⁵ This is the amount from the fruit. Additional ascorbic acid may be added by the manufacturer. Refer to the label for this information.

¹³ Based on yellow-fleshed varieties; for white-fleshed varieties value is about 50 I.U. per 114-gram peach and 80 I.U. per cup of sliced peaches.

¹⁴ This value includes ascorbic acid added by manufacturer.

[Dashes in the columns for nutrients show that no suitable value could be found although there is reason to believe that a measurable amount of the nutrient may be present]

Food, approximate measure, and weight (in grams)			Water	Food energy	Protein	Fat	Fatty acids			Carbohydrate	Calcium	Iron	Vitamin A value	Thiamin	Riboflavin	Niacin	Ascorbic acid
							Saturated (total)	Unsaturated Oleic	Linoleic								
		Grams	Percent	Calories	Grams	Grams	Grams	Grams	Grams	Grams	Milligrams	Milligrams	International units	Milligrams	Milligrams	Milligrams	Milligrams
GRAIN PRODUCTS																	
Bagel, 3-in. diam.:																	
Egg	1 bagel	55	32	165	6	2	---	---	---	28	9	1.2	30	0.14	0.10	1.2	0
Water	1 bagel	55	29	165	6	2	---	1	1	30	8	1.2	0	.15	.11	1.4	0
Barley, pearled, light, uncooked.	1 cup	200	11	700	16	2	Trace	1	1	158	32	4.0	0	.24	.10	6.2	0
Biscuits, baking powder from home recipe with enriched flour, 2-in. diam.	1 biscuit	28	27	105	2	5	1	2	1	13	34	.4	Trace	.06	.06	.1	Trace
Biscuits, baking powder from mix, 2-in. diam.	1 biscuit	28	28	90	2	3	1	1	1	15	19	.6	Trace	.08	.07	.6	Trace
Bran flakes (40% bran), added thiamin and iron.	1 cup	35	3	105	4	1				28	25	12.3	0	.14	.06	2.2	0
Bran flakes with raisins, added thiamin and iron.	1 cup	50	7	145	4	1				40	28	13.5	Trace	.16	.07	2.7	0
Breads:																	
Boston brown bread, slice 3 by ¾ in.	1 slice	48	45	100	3	1				22	43	.9	0	.05	.03	.6	0
Cracked-wheat bread:																	
Loaf, 1 lb.	1 loaf	454	35	1,190	40	10	2	5	2	236	399	5.0	Trace	.53	.41	5.9	Trace
Slice, 18 slices per loaf.	1 slice	25	35	65	2	1	---	---	---	13	22	.3	Trace	.03	.02	.3	Trace
French or vienna bread:																	
Enriched, 1 lb. loaf.	1 loaf	454	31	1,315	41	14	3	8	2	251	195	10.0	Trace	1.27	1.00	11.3	Trace
Unenriched, 1 lb. loaf.	1 loaf	454	31	1,315	41	14	3	8	2	251	195	3.2	Trace	.36	.36	3.6	Trace
Italian bread:																	
Enriched, 1 lb. loaf.	1 loaf	454	32	1,250	41	4	Trace	1	2	256	77	10.0	0	1.32	.91	11.8	0
Unenriched, 1 lb. loaf.	1 loaf	454	32	1,250	41	4	Trace	1	2	256	77	3.2	0	.41	.27	3.6	0
Raisin bread:																	
Loaf, 1 lb.	1 loaf	454	35	1,190	30	13	3	8	2	243	322	5.9	Trace	.23	.41	3.2	Trace

Slice, 18 slices per loaf.	25	35	65	2	1				13	18	.3	Trace	.01	.02	.2	Trace
Rye bread:																
American, light (⅓ rye, ⅔ wheat):																
Loaf, 1 lb.	454	36	1,100	41	5				236	340	7.3	0	.82	.32	6.4	0
Slice, 18 slices per loaf.	25	36	60	2	Trace				13	19	.4	0	.05	.02	.4	0
Pumpernickel, loaf, 1 lb.	454	34	1,115	41	5				241	381	10.9	0	1.04	.64	5.4	0
White bread, enriched: [15]																
Soft-crumb type:																
Loaf, 1 lb.	454	36	1,225	39	15	3	8	2	229	381	11.3	Trace	1.13	.95	10.9	Trace
Slice, 18 slices per loaf.	25	36	70	2	1				13	21	.6	Trace	.06	.05	.6	Trace
Slice, toasted.	22	25	70	2	1				13	21	.6	Trace	.06	.05	.6	Trace
Slice, 22 slices per loaf.	20	36	55	2	1				10	17	.5	Trace	.05	.04	.5	Trace
Slice, toasted.	17	25	55	2	1				10	17	.5	Trace	.05	.04	.5	Trace
Loaf, 1½ lbs.	680	36	1,835	59	22	5	12	3	343	571	17.0	Trace	1.70	1.43	16.3	Trace
Slice, 24 slices per loaf.	28	36	75	2	1				14	24	.7	Trace	.07	.06	.7	Trace
Slice, toasted.	24	25	75	2	1				14	24	.7	Trace	.07	.06	.7	Trace
Slice, 28 slices per loaf.	24	36	65	2	1				12	20	.6	Trace	.06	.05	.6	Trace
Slice, toasted.	21	25	65	2	1				12	20	.6	Trace	.06	.05	.6	Trace
Firm-crumb type:																
Loaf, 1 lb.	454	35	1,245	41	17	4	10	2	228	435	11.3	Trace	1.22	.91	10.9	Trace
Slice, 20 slices per loaf.	23	35	65	2	1				12	22	.6	Trace	.06	.05	.6	Trace
Slice, toasted.	20	24	65	2	1				12	22	.6	Trace	.06	.05	.6	Trace
Loaf, 2 lbs.	907	35	2,495	82	34	8	20	4	455	871	22.7	Trace	2.45	1.81	21.8	Trace
Slice, 34 slices per loaf.	27	35	75	2	1				14	26	.7	Trace	.07	.05	.6	Trace
Slice, toasted.	23	35	75	2	1				14	26	.7	Trace	.07	.05	.6	Trace
Whole-wheat bread, soft-crumb type:																
Loaf, 1 lb.	454	36	1,095	41	12	2	6	2	224	381	13.6	Trace	1.36	.45	12.7	Trace
Slice, 16 slices per loaf.	28	36	65	3	1				14	24	.8	Trace	.09	.03	.8	Trace
Slice, toasted.	24	24	65	3	1				14	24	.8	Trace	.09	.03	.8	Trace

[15] Values for iron, thiamin, riboflavin, and niacin per pound of unenriched white bread would be as follows:

	Iron Milligrams	Thiamin Milligrams	Riboflavin Milligrams	Niacin Milligrams
Soft crumb	3.2	.31	.39	5.0
Firm crumb	3.2	.32	.59	4.1

[Dashes in the columns for nutrients show that no suitable value could be found although there is reason to believe that a measurable amount of the nutrient may be present]

Food, approximate measure, and weight (in grams)	Water	Food energy	Protein	Fat	Fatty acids Saturated (total)	Fatty acids Unsaturated Oleic	Fatty acids Unsaturated Linoleic	Carbohydrate	Calcium	Iron	Vitamin A value	Thiamin	Riboflavin	Niacin	Ascorbic acid
	Grams	Per cent	Calories	Grams	Grams	Grams	Grams	Grams	Grams	Milligrams	Milligrams	International units	Milligrams	Milligrams	Milligrams	Milligrams

Note: the column units row reads: Grams (weight); Per cent (Water); Calories (Food energy); Grams (Protein, Fat, Fatty acids, Carbohydrate); Milligrams (Calcium, Iron); International units (Vitamin A value); Milligrams (Thiamin, Riboflavin, Niacin, Ascorbic acid).

GRAIN PRODUCTS—Continued

Food	Weight (g)	Water (%)	Food energy (Cal.)	Protein (g)	Fat (g)	Saturated (total) (g)	Oleic (g)	Linoleic (g)	Carbohydrate (g)	Calcium (mg)	Iron (mg)	Vitamin A value (IU)	Thiamin (mg)	Riboflavin (mg)	Niacin (mg)	Ascorbic acid (mg)
Bread—Continued																
Whole-wheat bread, firm-crumb type:																
Loaf, 1 lb____ 1 loaf____	454	36	1,100	48	14	3	6	3	216	449	13.6	Trace	1.18	0.54	12.7	Trace
Slice, 18 slices per loaf.____ 1 slice____	25	36	60	3	1	----	----	----	12	25	.8	Trace	.06	.03	.7	Trace
Slice, toasted____ 1 slice____	21	24	60	3	1	----	----	----	12	25	.8	Trace	.06	.03	.7	Trace
Breadcrumbs, dry, grated. 1 cup____	100	6	390	13	5	1	2	1	73	122	3.6	Trace	.22	.30	3.5	Trace
Buckwheat flour, light, sifted. 1 cup____	98	12	340	6	1	----	----	----	78	11	1.0	0	.08	.04	.4	0
Bulgur, canned, seasoned. 1 cup____	135	56	245	8	4				44	27	1.9	0	.08	.05	4.1	0
Cakes made from cake mixes:																
Angelfood:																
Whole cake.____ 1 cake____	635	34	1,645	36	1				377	603	1.9	0	.03	.70	.6	0
Piece, ½ of 10-in. diam. cake.____ 1 piece____	53	34	135	3	Trace				32	50	.2	0	Trace	.06	.1	0
Cupcakes, small, 2½ in. diam.:																
Without icing____ 1 cupcake__	25	26	90	1	3	1	1	1	14	40	.1	40	.01	.03	.1	Trace
With chocolate icing.__ 1 cupcake__	36	22	130	2	5	2	2	1	21	47	.3	60	.01	.04	.1	Trace
Devil's food, 2-layer, with chocolate icing:																
Whole cake.____ 1 cake____	1,107	24	3,755	49	136	54	58	16	645	653	8.9	1,660	.33	.89	3.3	1
Piece, ⅟₁₆ of 9-in. diam. cake.____ 1 piece____	69	24	235	3	9	3	4	1	40	41	.6	100	.02	.06	.2	Trace
Cupcake, small, 2½ in. diam.____ 1 cupcake__	35	24	120	2	4	1	2	Trace	20	21	.3	50	.01	.03	.1	Trace
Gingerbread:																
Whole cake.____ 1 cake____	570	37	1,575	18	39	10	19	9	291	513	9.1	Trace	.17	.51	4.6	2
Piece, ⅑ of 8-in. square cake.____ 1 piece____	63	37	175	2	4	1	2	1	32	57	1.0	Trace	.02	.06	.5	Trace
White, 2-layer, with chocolate icing:																
Whole cake.____ 1 cake____	1,140	21	4,000	45	122	45	54	17	716	1,129	5.7	680	.23	.91	2.3	2

Food	Measure																
Piece, 1/16 of 9-in. diam. cake.	1 piece	71	21	250	3	8	3	3	1	45	70	.4	40	.01	.06	.1	Trace
Cakes made from home recipes:[16]																	
Boston cream pie; piece 1/12 of 8-in. diam.	1 piece	69	35	210	4	6	2	2	1	34	46	.3	140	.02	.08	.1	Trace
Fruitcake, dark, made with enriched flour:																	
Loaf, 1-lb.	1 loaf	454	18	1,720	22	69	15	37	13	271	327	11.8	540	.59	.64	3.6	2
Slice, 1/30 of 8-in. loaf.	1 slice	15	18	55	1	2	Trace	1	Trace	9	11	.4	20	.02	.02	.1	Trace
Plain sheet cake:																	
Without icing:																	
Whole cake.	1 cake	777	25	2,830	35	108	30	52	21	434	497	3.1	1,320	.16	.70	1.6	2
Piece, 1/9 of 9-in. square cake.	1 piece	86	25	315	4	12	3	6	2	48	55	.3	150	.02	.08	.2	Trace
With boiled white icing, piece, 1/9 of 9-in. square cake.	1 piece	114	23	400	4	12	3	6	2	71	56	.3	150	.02	.08	.2	Trace
Pound:																	
Loaf, 8½ by 3½ by 3in.	1 loaf	514	17	2,430	29	152	34	68	17	242	108	4.1	1,440	.15	.46	1.0	0
Slice, ½-in. thick.	1 slice	30	17	140	2	9	2	4	1	14	6	.2	80	.01	.03	.1	0
Sponge:																	
Whole cake.	1 cake	790	32	2,345	60	45	14	20	4	427	237	9.5	3,560	.40	1.11	1.6	Trace
Piece, 1/12 of 10-in. diam. cake.	1 piece	66	32	195	5	4	1	2	Trace	36	20	.8	300	.03	.09	.1	Trace
Yellow, 2-layer, without icing:																	
Whole cake.	1 cake	870	24	3,160	39	111	31	53	22	506	618	3.5	1,310	.17	.70	1.7	2
Piece, 1/16 of 9-in. diam. cake.	1 piece	54	24	200	2	7	2	3	1	32	39	.2	80	.01	.04	.1	Trace
Yellow, 2-layer, with chocolate icing:																	
Whole cake.	1 cake	1,203	21	4,390	51	156	55	69	23	727	818	7.2	1,920	.24	.96	2.4	Trace
Piece, 1/16 of 9-in. diam. cake.	1 piece	75	21	275	3	10	3	4	1	45	51	.5	120	.02	.06	.2	Trace
Cake icings. See Sugars, Sweets.																	
Cookies:																	
Brownies with nuts:																	
Made from home recipe with enriched flour.	1 brownie	20	10	95	1	6	1	3	1	10	8	.4	40	.04	.02	.1	Trace
Made from mix.	1 brownie	20	11	85	1	4	1	2	1	13	9	.4	20	.03	.02	.1	Trace

[16] Unenriched cake flour used unless otherwise specified.

[Dashes in the columns for nutrients show that no suitable value could be found although there is reason to believe that a measurable amount of the nutrient may be present]

Food, approximate measure, and weight (in grams)		Water	Food energy	Protein	Fat	Fatty acids			Carbohydrate	Calcium	Iron	Vitamin A value	Thiamin	Riboflavin	Niacin	Ascorbic acid
						Saturated (total)	Unsaturated									
							Oleic	Linoleic								
	Grams	Percent	Calories	Grams	Grams	Grams	Grams	Grams	Grams	Milligrams	Milligrams	International units	Milligrams	Milligrams	Milligrams	Milligrams
GRAIN PRODUCTS—Continued																
Cookies—Continued																
Chocolate chip:																
Made from home recipe with enriched flour. 1 cookie	10	3	50	1	3	1	1	1	6	4	0.2	10	0.01	0.01	0.1	Trace
Commercial 1 cookie	10	3	50	1	2	1	1	Trace	7	4	.2	10	Trace	Trace	Trace	Trace
Fig bars, commercial 1 cookie	14	14	50	1	1				11	11	.2	20	Trace	.01	.1	Trace
Sandwich, chocolate or vanilla, commercial. 1 cookie	10	2	50	1	2	1	1	Trace	7	2	.1	0	Trace	Trace	.1	0
Corn flakes, added nutrients:																
Plain 1 cup	25	4	100	2	Trace				21	4	.4	0	.11	.02	.5	0
Sugar-covered 1 cup	40	2	155	2	Trace				36	5	.4	0	.16	.02	.8	0
Corn (hominy) grits, degermed, cooked:																
Enriched 1 cup	245	87	125	3	Trace				27	2	.7	[17] 150	.10	.07	1.0	0
Unenriched 1 cup	245	87	125	3	Trace				27	2	.2	[17] 150	.05	.02	.5	0
Cornmeal:																
Whole-ground, unbolted, dry. 1 cup	122	12	435	11	5	1	2	2	90	24	2.9	[17] 620	.46	.13	2.4	0
Bolted (nearly whole-grain) dry. 1 cup	122	12	440	11	4	Trace	1	2	91	21	2.2	[17] 590	.37	.10	2.3	0
Degermed, enriched:																
Dry form 1 cup	138	12	500	11	2				108	8	4.0	[17] 610	.61	.36	4.8	0
Cooked 1 cup	240	88	120	3	1				26	2	1.0	[17] 140	.14	.10	1.2	0
Degermed, unenriched:																
Dry form 1 cup	138	12	500	11	2				108	8	1.5	[17] 610	.19	.07	1.4	0
Cooked 1 cup	240	88	120	3	1				26	2	.5	[17] 140	.05	.02	.2	0
Corn muffins, made with enriched degermed cornmeal and enriched flour; muffin 2⅜-in. diam. 1 muffin	40	33	125	3	4	2	2	Trace	19	42	.7	[17] 120	.08	.09	.6	Trace

Food	Measure																
Corn muffins, made with mix, egg, and milk; muffin 2⅜-in. diam.	1 muffin	40	30	130	3	4	1	2	1	20	96	.6	[17]100	.07	.08	.6	Trace
Corn, puffed, presweetened, added nutrients	1 cup	30	2	115	1	Trace				27	3	.5	0	.13	.05	.6	0
Corn, shredded, added nutrients	1 cup	25	3	100	2	Trace				22	1	.6	0	.11	.05	.5	0
Crackers:																	
Graham, 2½-in. square	4 crackers	28	6	110	2	3				21	11	.4	0	.01	.06	.4	0
Saltines	4 crackers	11	4	50	1	1				8	2	.1	0	Trace	Trace	.1	0
Danish pastry, plain (without fruit or nuts):																	
Packaged ring, 12 ounces	1 ring	340	22	1,435	25	80	24	37	15	155	170	3.1	1,050	.24	.51	2.7	Trace
Round piece, approx. 4¼-in. diam. by 1 in.	1 pastry	65	22	275	5	15	5	7	3	30	33	.6	200	.05	.10	.5	Trace
Ounce	1 oz.	28	22	120	2	7	2	3	3	13	14	.3	90	.02	.04	.2	Trace
Doughnuts, cake type	1 doughnut	32	24	125	1	6	1	4	Trace	16	13	[18].4	30	[18].05	[18].05	[18].4	Trace
Farina, quick-cooking, enriched, cooked	1 cup	245	89	105	3	Trace				22	147	[19].7	0	[19].12	[19].07	[19]1.0	0
Macaroni, cooked:																	
Enriched:																	
Cooked, firm stage (undergoes additional cooking in a food mixture)	1 cup	130	64	190	6	1				39	14	[19]1.4	0	[19].23	[19].14	[19]1.8	0
Cooked until tender	1 cup	140	72	155	5	1				32	8	[19]1.3	0	[19].20	[19].11	[19]1.5	0
Unenriched:																	
Cooked, firm stage (undergoes additional cooking in a food mixture)	1 cup	130	64	190	6	1				39	14	.7	0	.03	.03	.5	0
Cooked until tender	1 cup	140	72	155	5	1				32	11	.6	0	.01	.01	.4	0
Macaroni (enriched) and cheese, baked	1 cup	200	58	430	17	22	10	9	2	40	362	1.8	860	.20	.40	1.8	Trace
Canned	1 cup	240	80	230	9	10	4	3	1	26	199	1.0	260	.12	.24	1.0	Trace
Muffins, with enriched white flour; muffin, 3-inch diam.	1 muffin	40	38	120	3	4	1	2	1	17	42	.6	40	.07	.09	.6	Trace
Noodles (egg noodles), cooked:																	
Enriched	1 cup	160	70	200	7	2	1	1	Trace	37	16	[19]1.4	110	[19].22	[19].13	[19]1.9	0
Unenriched	1 cup	160	70	200	7	2	1	1	Trace	37	16	1.0	110	.05	.03	.6	0

[17] This value is based on product made from yellow varieties of corn; white varieties contain only a trace.

[18] Based on product made with enriched flour. With unenriched flour, approximate values per doughnut are: Iron, 0.2 milligram; thiamin, 0.01 milligram; riboflavin, 0.03 milligram; niacin, 0.2 milligram.

[19] Iron, thiamin, riboflavin, and niacin are based on the minimum levels of enrichment specified in standards of identity promulgated under the Federal Food, Drug, and Cosmetic Act.

[Dashes in the columns for nutrients show that no suitable value could be found although there is reason to believe that a measurable amount of the nutrient may be present]

Food, approximate measure, and weight (in grams)		Water	Food energy	Protein	Fat	Fatty acids			Carbohydrate	Calcium	Iron	Vitamin A value	Thiamin	Riboflavin	Niacin	Ascorbic acid
						Saturated (total)	Unsaturated									
							Oleic	Linoleic								
	Grams	*Percent*	*Calories*	*Grams*	*Grams*	*Grams*	*Grams*	*Grams*	*Grams*	*Milligrams*	*Milligrams*	*International units*	*Milligrams*	*Milligrams*	*Milligrams*	*Milligrams*
GRAIN PRODUCTS—Continued																
Oats (with or without corn) puffed, added nutrients. 1 cup	25	3	100	3	1	--	--	--	19	44	1.2	0	0.24	0.04	0.5	0
Oatmeal or rolled oats, cooked. 1 cup	240	87	130	5	2	--	--	--	23	22	1.4	0	.19	.05	.2	0
Pancakes, 4-inch diam.:																
Wheat, enriched flour (home recipe). 1 cake	27	50	60	2	2	Trace	1	1	9	27	.4	30	.05	.06	.4	Trace
Buckwheat (made from mix with egg and milk). 1 cake	27	58	55	2	2	1	1	Trace	6	59	.4	60	.03	.04	.2	Trace
Plain or buttermilk (made from mix with egg and milk). 1 cake	27	51	60	2	2	1	1	Trace	9	58	.3	70	.04	.06	.2	Trace
Pie (piecrust made with unenriched flour):																
Sector, 4-in., 1/7 of 9-in. diam. pie:																
Apple (2-crust). 1 sector	135	48	350	3	15	4	7	3	51	11	.4	40	.03	.03	.5	1
Butterscotch (1-crust). 1 sector	130	45	350	6	14	5	6	2	50	98	1.2	340	.04	.13	.3	Trace
Cherry (2-crust). 1 sector	135	47	350	4	15	4	7	3	52	19	.4	590	.03	.03	.7	Trace
Custard (1-crust). 1 sector	130	58	285	8	14	5	6	2	30	125	.8	300	.07	.21	.4	0
Lemon meringue (1-crust). 1 sector	120	47	305	4	12	4	6	2	45	17	.6	200	.04	.10	.2	4
Mince (2-crust). 1 sector	135	43	365	3	16	4	8	3	56	38	1.4	Trace	.09	.05	.5	1
Pecan (1-crust). 1 sector	118	20	490	6	27	4	16	5	60	55	3.3	190	.19	.08	.4	Trace
Pineapple chiffon (1-crust). 1 sector	93	41	265	6	11	3	5	2	36	22	.8	320	.04	.08	.4	1
Pumpkin (1-crust). 1 sector	130	59	275	5	15	5	6	2	32	66	.7	3,210	.04	.13	.7	Trace
Piecrust, baked shell for pie made with:																
Enriched flour. 1 shell	180	15	900	11	60	16	28	12	79	25	3.1	0	.36	.25	3.2	0
Unenriched flour. 1 shell	180	15	900	11	60	16	28	12	79	25	.9	0	.05	.05	.9	0

Food, approximate measure	Measure	g	Water %	Food energy	Protein	Fat	Sat.	Oleic	Linoleic	Carbohydrate	Calcium	Iron	Vit. A	Thiamin	Riboflavin	Niacin	Ascorbic acid
Piecrust mix including stick form: Package, 10-oz., for double crust.	1 pkg.	284	9	1,480	20	93	23	46	21	141	131	1.4	0	.11	.11	2.0	0
Pizza (cheese) 5½-in. sector; ⅛ of 14-in. diam. pie.	1 sector	75	45	185	7	6	2	3	Trace	27	107	.7	290	.04	.12	.7	4
Popcorn, popped: Plain, large kernel	1 cup	6	4	25	1	Trace	—	—	—	5	1	.2	—	—	.01	.1	0
With oil and salt	1 cup	9	3	40	1	2	1	Trace	Trace	5	1	.2	—	—	.01	.2	0
Sugar coated	1 cup	35	4	135	2	1	—	—	—	30	2	.5	—	—	.02	.4	0
Pretzels: Dutch, twisted	1 pretzel	16	5	60	2	1	—	—	—	12	4	.2	0	Trace	Trace	.1	0
Thin, twisted	1 pretzel	6	5	25	1	Trace	—	—	—	5	1	.1	0	Trace	Trace	Trace	0
Stick, small, 2¼ inches	10 sticks	3	5	10	Trace	Trace	—	—	—	2	1	Trace	0	Trace	Trace	Trace	0
Stick, regular, 3⅛ inches	5 sticks	3	5	10	Trace	Trace	—	—	—	2	1	Trace	0	Trace	Trace	Trace	0
Rice, white: Enriched: Raw	1 cup	185	12	670	12	1	—	—	—	149	44	[20]5.4	0	[20].81	[20].06	[20]6.5	0
Cooked	1 cup	205	73	225	4	Trace	—	—	—	50	21	[20]1.8	0	[20].23	[20].02	[20]2.1	0
Instant, ready-to-serve	1 cup	165	73	180	4	Trace	—	—	—	40	5	[20]1.3	0	[20].21	[20]—	[20]1.7	0
Unenriched, cooked	1 cup	205	73	225	4	Trace	—	—	—	50	21	.4	0	.04	.02	.8	0
Parboiled, cooked	1 cup	175	73	185	4	Trace	—	—	—	41	33	[20]1.4	0	[20].19	[20]—	[20]2.1	0
Rice, puffed, added nutrients	1 cup	15	4	60	1	Trace	—	—	—	13	3	.3	0	.07	.01	.7	0
Rolls, enriched: Cloverleaf or pan: Home recipe	1 roll	35	26	120	3	3	1	1	1	20	16	.7	30	.09	.09	.8	Trace
Commercial	1 roll	28	31	85	2	2	Trace	1	Trace	15	21	.5	Trace	.08	.05	.6	Trace
Frankfurter or hamburger	1 roll	40	31	120	3	2	1	1	1	21	30	.8	Trace	.11	.07	.9	Trace
Hard, round or rectangular	1 roll	50	25	155	5	2	1	1	Trace	30	24	1.2	Trace	.13	.12	1.4	Trace
Rye wafers, whole-grain, 1⅞ by 3½ inches	2 wafers	13	6	45	2	Trace	—	—	—	10	7	.5	0	.04	.03	.2	0
Spaghetti, cooked, tender stage, enriched	1 cup	140	72	155	5	1	—	—	—	32	11	[19]1.3	0	[19].20	[19].11	[19]1.5	0

[19] Iron, thiamin, riboflavin, and niacin are based on the minimum levels of enrichment specified in standards of identity promulgated under the Federal Food, Drug, and Cosmetic Act.

[20] Iron, thiamin, and niacin are based on the minimum levels of enrichment specified in standards of identity promulgated under the Federal Food, Drug, and Cosmetic Act. Riboflavin is based on unenriched rice. When the minimum level of enrichment for riboflavin specified in the standards of identity becomes effective the value will be 0.12 milligram per cup of parboiled rice and of white rice.

[Dashes show that no basis could be found for imputing a value although there was some reason to believe that a measurable amount of the constituent might be present]

Food, approximate measure, and weight (in grams)	Water	Food energy	Protein	Fat	Fatty acids Saturated (total)	Fatty acids Unsaturated Oleic	Fatty acids Unsaturated Linoleic	Carbohydrate	Calcium	Iron	Vitamin A value	Thiamin	Riboflavin	Niacin	Ascorbic acid
	Grams	Percent	Calories	Grams	Grams	Grams	Grams	Grams	Grams	Milligrams	Milligrams	International units	Milligrams	Milligrams	Milligrams	Milligrams

GRAIN PRODUCTS—Continued

Food, approximate measure, and weight (in grams)	Grams	Water Percent	Food energy Calories	Protein Grams	Fat Grams	Saturated (total) Grams	Unsaturated Oleic Grams	Unsaturated Linoleic Grams	Carbohydrate Grams	Calcium Milligrams	Iron Milligrams	Vitamin A value International units	Thiamin Milligrams	Riboflavin Milligrams	Niacin Milligrams	Ascorbic acid Milligrams
Spaghetti with meat balls, and tomato sauce:																
Home recipe _____ 1 cup_____	248	70	330	19	12	4	6	1	39	124	3.7	1,590	0.25	0.30	4.0	22
Canned _____ 1 cup_____	250	78	260	12	10	2	3	4	28	53	3.3	1,000	.15	.18	2.3	5
Spaghetti in tomato sauce with cheese:																
Home recipe _____ 1 cup_____	250	77	260	9	9	2	5	1	37	80	2.3	1,080	.25	.18	2.3	13
Canned _____ 1 cup_____	250	80	190	6	2	1	1	1	38	40	2.8	930	.35	.28	4.5	10
Waffles, with enriched flour, 7-in. diam. 1 waffle.	75	41	210	7	7	2	4	1	28	85	1.3	250	.13	.19	1.0	Trace
Waffles, made from mix, enriched, egg and milk added, 7-in. diam. 1 waffle_____	75	42	205	7	8	3	3	1	27	179	1.0	170	.11	.17	.7	Trace
Wheat, puffed, added nutrients. 1 cup_____	15	3	55	2	Trace	_____	_____	_____	12	4	.6	0	.08	.03	1.2	0
Wheat, shredded, plain__ 1 biscuit__	25	7	90	2	1	_____	_____	_____	20	11	.9	0	.06	.03	1.1	0
Wheat flakes, added nutrients. 1 cup_____	30	4	105	3	Trace	_____	_____	_____	24	12	1.3	0	.19	.04	1.5	0
Wheat flours:																
Whole-wheat, from hard wheats, stirred. 1 cup_____	120	12	400	16	2	Trace	1	1	85	49	4.0	0	.66	.14	5.2	0
All-purpose or family flour, enriched:																
Sifted _____ 1 cup_____	115	12	420	12	1	_____	_____	_____	88	18	[19]3.3	0	[19].51	[19].30	[19]4.0	0
Unsifted _____ 1 cup_____	125	12	455	13	1	_____	_____	_____	95	20	[19]3.6	0	[19].55	[19].33	[19]4.4	0
Self-rising, enriched__ 1 cup_____	125	12	440	12	1	_____	_____	_____	93	331	[19]3.6	0	[19].55	[19].33	[19]4.4	0
Cake or pastry flour, sifted. 1 cup_____	96	12	350	7	1	_____	_____	_____	76	16	.5	0	.03	.03	.7	0

FATS, OILS

	Grams	Water Percent	Food energy Calories	Protein Grams	Fat Grams	Saturated (total) Grams	Unsaturated Oleic Grams	Unsaturated Linoleic Grams	Carbohydrate Grams	Calcium Milligrams	Iron Milligrams	Vitamin A value International units	Thiamin Milligrams	Riboflavin Milligrams	Niacin Milligrams	Ascorbic acid Milligrams
Butter:																
Regular, 4 sticks per pound:																
Stick _____ ½ cup_____	113	16	810	1	92	51	30	3	1	23	0	[23]3,750	_____	_____	_____	0

Food	Measure	Grams	Water (%)	Food energy (cal)	Protein (g)	Fat (g)	Saturated fatty acids (g)	Oleic (g)	Linoleic (g)	Carbo-hydrate (g)	Calcium (mg)	Iron (mg)	Vitamin A (I.U.)	Thiamin (mg)	Ribo-flavin (mg)	Niacin (mg)	Ascorbic acid (mg)
Tablespoon (approx. 1/8 stick)	1 tbsp	14	16	100	Trace	12	6	4	Trace	Trace	3	0	[21]470	—	—	—	0
Pat (1-in. sq. 1/3-in. high; 90 per lb.)	1 pat	5	16	35	Trace	4	2	1	Trace	Trace	1	0	[21]170	—	—	—	0
Whipped, 6 sticks or 2, 8-oz. containers per pound:																	
Stick	1/2 cup	76	16	540	1	61	34	20	2	Trace	15	0	[21]2,500	—	—	—	0
Tablespoon (approx. 1/8 stick)	1 tbsp	9	16	65	Trace	8	4	3	Trace	Trace	2	0	[21]310	—	—	—	0
Pat (1 1/4-in. sq. 1/3-in. high; 120 per lb.)	1 pat	4	16	25	Trace	3	2	1	Trace	Trace	1	0	[21]130	—	—	—	0
Fats, cooking:																	
Lard	1 cup	205	0	1,850	0	205	78	94	20	0	0	0	0	0	0	0	0
	1 tbsp	13	0	115	0	13	5	6	1	0	0	0	0	0	0	0	0
Vegetable fats	1 cup	200	0	1,770	0	200	50	100	44	0	0	0	—	0	0	0	0
	1 tbsp	13	0	110	0	13	3	6	3	0	0	0	—	0	0	0	0
Margarine:																	
Regular, 4 sticks per pound:																	
Stick	1/2 cup	113	16	815	1	92	17	46	25	Trace	23	0	[22]3,750	0	0	0	0
Tablespoon (approx. 1/8 stick)	1 tbsp	14	16	100	Trace	12	2	6	3	Trace	3	0	[22]470	0	0	0	0
Pat (1-in. sq. 1/3-in. high; 90 per lb.)	1 pat	5	16	35	Trace	4	1	2	1	Trace	1	0	[22]170	0	0	0	0
Whipped, 6 sticks per pound:																	
Stick	1/2 cup	76	16	545	1	61	11	31	17	Trace	15	0	[22]2,500	0	0	0	0
Soft, 2 8-oz. tubs per pound:																	
Tub	1 tub	227	16	1,635	1	184	34	68	68	Trace	45	0	[22]7,500	0	0	0	0
Tablespoon	1 tbsp	14	16	100	Trace	11	2	4	4	Trace	3	0	[22]470	0	0	0	0
Oils, salad or cooking:																	
Corn	1 cup	220	0	1,945	0	220	22	62	117	0	0	0	0	0	0	0	0
	1 tbsp	14	0	125	0	14	1	4	7	0	0	0	0	0	0	0	0
Cottonseed	1 cup	220	0	1,945	0	220	55	46	110	0	0	0	0	0	0	0	0
	1 tbsp	14	0	125	0	14	4	3	7	0	0	0	0	0	0	0	0
Olive	1 cup	220	0	1,945	0	220	24	167	15	0	0	0	0	0	0	0	0
	1 tbsp	14	0	125	0	14	2	11	1	0	0	0	0	0	0	0	0
Peanut	1 cup	220	0	1,945	0	220	40	103	64	0	0	0	0	0	0	0	0
	1 tbsp	14	0	125	0	14	3	7	4	0	0	0	0	0	0	0	0
Safflower	1 cup	220	0	1,945	0	220	18	37	165	0	0	0	0	0	0	0	0
	1 tbsp	14	0	125	0	14	1	2	10	0	0	0	0	0	0	0	0
Soybean	1 cup	220	0	1,945	0	220	33	44	114	0	0	0	0	0	0	0	0
	1 tbsp	14	0	125	0	14	2	3	7	0	0	0	0	0	0	0	0

[19] Iron, thiamin, riboflavin, and niacin are based on the minimum levels of enrichment specified in standards of identity promulgated under the Federal Food, Drug, and Cosmetic Act.

[21] Year-round average.

[22] Based on the average vitamin A content of fortified margarine. Federal specifications for fortified margarine require a minimum of 15,000 I.U. of vitamin A per pound.

Food, approximate measure, and weight (in grams)	Water	Food energy	Protein	Fat	Fatty acids			Carbohydrate	Calcium	Iron	Vitamin A value	Thiamin	Riboflavin	Niacin	Ascorbic acid
					Saturated (total)	Unsaturated									
						Oleic	Linoleic								
	Grams	Per cent	Calories	Grams	Grams	Grams	Grams	Grams	Grams	Milligrams	Milligrams	International units	Milligrams	Milligrams	Milligrams	Milligrams

FATS, OILS—Continued

Food, approximate measure, and weight (in grams)	Grams	Per cent	Calories	Grams	Grams	Grams	Grams	Grams	Grams	Milligrams	Milligrams	International units	Milligrams	Milligrams	Milligrams	Milligrams
Salad dressings:																
Blue cheese_____ 1 tbsp_____	15	32	75	1	8	2	2	4	1	12	Trace	30	Trace	0.02	Trace	Trace
Commercial, mayonnaise type:																
Regular_____ 1 tbsp_____	15	41	65	Trace	6	1	1	3	2	2	Trace	30	Trace	Trace	Trace	------
Special dietary, low-calorie. 1 tbsp_____	16	81	20	Trace	2	Trace	Trace	1	1	3	Trace	40	Trace	Trace	Trace	------
French:																
Regular_____ 1 tbsp_____	16	39	65	Trace	6	1	1	3	3	2	.1	------	------	------	------	------
Special dietary, low-fat with artificial sweeteners. 1 tbsp_____	15	95	Trace	Trace	Trace	------	------	------	Trace	2	.1	------	------	------	------	------
Home cooked, boiled_____ 1 tbsp_____	16	68	25	1	2	1	1	Trace	2	14	.1	80	.01	.03	Trace	Trace
Mayonnaise_____ 1 tbsp_____	14	15	100	Trace	11	2	2	6	Trace	3	.1	40	Trace	.01	Trace	------
Thousand island_____ 1 tbsp_____	16	32	80	Trace	8	1	2	4	3	2	.1	50	Trace	Trace	Trace	Trace
SUGARS, SWEETS																
Cake icings:																
Chocolate made with milk and table fat. 1 cup_____	275	14	1,035	9	38	21	14	1	185	165	3.3	580	.06	.28	.6	1
Coconut (with boiled icing). 1 cup_____	166	15	605	3	13	11	1	Trace	124	10	.8	0	.02	.07	.3	0
Creamy fudge from mix with water only. 1 cup_____	245	15	830	7	16	5	8	3	183	96	2.7	Trace	.05	.20	.7	Trace
White, boiled_____ 1 cup_____	94	18	300	1	0	------	------	------	76	2	Trace	0	Trace	.03	Trace	0
Candy:																
Caramels, plain or chocolate. 1 oz_____	28	8	115	1	3	2	1	Trace	22	42	.4	Trace	.01	.05	.1	Trace
Chocolate, milk, plain_ 1 oz_____	28	1	145	2	9	5	3	Trace	16	65	.3	80	.02	.10	.1	Trace
Chocolate-coated peanuts. 1 oz_____	28	1	160	5	12	3	6	2	11	33	.4	Trace	.10	.05	2.1	Trace

Fondant; mints, uncoated; candy corn.	1 oz	28	8	105	Trace	Trace	—	—	—	25	4	.3	0	Trace	Trace	Trace	0
Fudge, plain.	1 oz	28	8	115	1	4	2	1	Trace	21	22	.3	Trace	.01	.03	.1	Trace
Gum drops.	1 oz	28	12	100	Trace	Trace	—	—	—	25	2	.1	0	0	Trace	Trace	0
Hard.	1 oz	28	1	110	0	Trace	—	—	—	28	6	.5	0	0	0	0	0
Marshmallows.	1 oz	28	17	90	1	Trace	—	—	—	23	5	.5	0	0	Trace	Trace	0
Chocolate-flavored sirup or topping:																	
Thin type.	1 fl. oz	38	32	90	1	1	Trace	Trace	Trace	24	6	.6	Trace	.01	.03	.2	0
Fudge type.	1 fl. oz	38	25	125	2	5	3	2	Trace	20	48	.5	60	.02	.08	.2	Trace
Chocolate-flavored beverage powder (approx. 4 heaping teaspoons per oz.):																	
With nonfat dry milk.	1 oz	28	2	100	5	1	Trace	Trace	Trace	20	167	.5	10	.04	.21	.2	1
Without nonfat dry milk.	1 oz	28	1	100	1	1	Trace	Trace	Trace	25	9	.6	0	.01	.03	.1	0
Honey, strained or extracted.	1 tbsp.	21	17	65	Trace	0	—	—	—	17	1	.1	0	Trace	.01	.1	Trace
Jams and preserves.	1 tbsp.	20	29	56	Trace	Trace	—	—	—	14	4	.2	Trace	Trace	.01	Trace	Trace
Jellies.	1 tbsp.	18	29	50	Trace	Trace	—	—	—	13	4	.3	Trace	Trace	.01	Trace	1
Molasses, cane:																	
Light (first extraction).	1 tbsp.	20	24	50	—	—	—	—	—	13	33	.9	—	.01	.01	Trace	—
Blackstrap (third extraction).	1 tbsp.	20	24	45	—	—	—	—	—	11	137	3.2	—	.02	.04	.4	—
Sirups:																	
Sorghum.	1 tbsp.	21	23	55	—	—	—	—	—	14	35	2.6	—	.02	—	Trace	—
Table blends, chiefly corn, light and dark.	1 tbsp.	21	24	60	0	0	—	—	—	15	9	.8	0	0	0	0	0
Sugars:																	
Brown, firm packed.	1 cup	220	2	820	0	0	—	—	—	212	187	7.5	0	.02	.07	.4	0
White:																	
Granulated.	1 cup	200	Trace	770	0	0	—	—	—	199	0	.2	0	0	0	0	0
Granulated.	1 tbsp.	11	Trace	40	0	0	—	—	—	11	0	Trace	0	0	0	0	0
Powdered, stirred before measuring.	1 cup	120	Trace	460	0	0	—	—	—	119	0	.1	0	0	0	0	0

MISCELLANEOUS ITEMS

Barbecue sauce	1 cup	250	81	230	4	17	2	5	9	20	53	2.0	900	.03	.03	.8	13
Beverages, alcoholic:																	
Beer	12 fl. oz	360	92	150	1	0	—	—	—	14	18	Trace	—	.01	.11	2.2	—
Gin, rum, vodka, whiskey:																	
80-proof	1½ fl. oz. jigger.	42	67	100	—	—	—	—	—	Trace	—	—	—	—	—	—	—
86-proof	1½ fl. oz. jigger.	42	64	105	—	—	—	—	—	Trace	—	—	—	—	—	—	—
90-proof	1½ fl. oz. jigger.	42	62	110	—	—	—	—	—	Trace	—	—	—	—	—	—	—

[Dashes in the columns for nutrients show that no suitable value could be found although there is reason to believe that a measurable amount of the nutrient may be present]

Food, approximate measure, and weight (in grams)	Water	Food energy	Protein	Fat	Fatty acids Saturated (total)	Fatty acids Unsaturated Oleic	Fatty acids Unsaturated Linoleic	Carbohydrate	Calcium	Iron	Vitamin A value	Thiamin	Riboflavin	Niacin	Ascorbic acid
	Grams	Per cent	Calories	Grams	Grams	Grams	Grams	Grams	Grams	Milligrams	Milligrams	International units	Milligrams	Milligrams	Milligrams	Milligrams

(Units row — Grams, Per cent, Calories, then Grams for Protein/Fat/Fatty acids/Carbohydrate, Milligrams for Calcium/Iron, International units for Vitamin A, Milligrams for Thiamin/Riboflavin/Niacin/Ascorbic acid)

Food, approximate measure, and weight (in grams)	Grams	Per cent	Calories	Protein (Grams)	Fat (Grams)	Saturated (total) (Grams)	Unsat. Oleic (Grams)	Unsat. Linoleic (Grams)	Carbohydrate (Grams)	Calcium (mg)	Iron (mg)	Vit. A (I.U.)	Thiamin (mg)	Riboflavin (mg)	Niacin (mg)	Ascorbic acid (mg)
MISCELLANEOUS ITEMS—Continued																
Beverages, alcoholic—Continued																
Gin, rum, vodka, whiskey—Con.																
94-proof ... 1½ fl. oz. jigger	42	60	115	---					Trace							
100-proof ... 1½ fl. oz. jigger	42	58	125	---					Trace							
Wines:																
Dessert ... 3½ fl. oz. glass	103	77	140	Trace	0				8	8			.01	.02	.2	---
Table ... 3½ fl. oz. glass	102	86	85	Trace	0				4	9	.4		Trace	.01	.1	---
Beverages, carbonated, sweetened, nonalcoholic:																
Carbonated water ... 12 fl. oz.	366	92	115	0	0				29			0	0	0	0	0
Cola type ... 12 fl. oz.	369	90	145	0	0				37			0	0	0	0	0
Fruit-flavored sodas and Tom Collins mixes ... 12 fl. oz.	372	88	170	0	0				45			0	0	0	0	0
Ginger ale ... 12 fl. oz.	366	92	115	0	0				29			0	0	0	0	0
Root beer ... 12 fl. oz.	370	90	150	0	0				39			0	0	0	0	0
Bouillon cubes, approx. ½ in. ... 1 cube	4	4	5	1	Trace				Trace							
Chocolate:																
Bitter or baking ... 1 oz.	28	2	145	3	15	8	6	Trace	8	22	1.9	20	.01	.07	.4	0
Semi-sweet, small pieces ... 1 cup	170	1	860	7	61	34	22	1	97	51	4.4	30	.02	.14	.9	0
Gelatin:																
Plain, dry powder in envelope ... 1 envelope	7	13	25	6	Trace				0							
Dessert powder, 3-oz. package ... 1 pkg.	85	2	315	8	0				75							
Gelatin dessert, prepared with water ... 1 cup	240	84	140	4	0				34							

Food, approximate measure	Measure	Grams	Water (%)	Food energy (Cal.)	Protein (g)	Fat (g)	Saturated (g)	Oleic (g)	Linoleic (g)	Carbohydrate (g)	Calcium (mg)	Iron (mg)	Vitamin A (I.U.)	Thiamine (mg)	Riboflavin (mg)	Niacin (mg)	Ascorbic acid (mg)
Olives, pickled:																	
Green	4 medium or 3 extra large or 2 giant.	16	78	15	Trace	2	Trace	2	Trace	Trace	8	.2	40	—	Trace	Trace	—
Ripe: Mission	3 small or 2 large.	10	73	15	Trace	2	Trace	2	Trace	Trace	9	.1	10	Trace	Trace	Trace	—
Pickles, cucumber:																	
Dill, medium, whole, 3¾ in. long, 1¼ in. diam.	1 pickle	65	93	10	1	Trace	—	—	—	1	17	.7	70	Trace	Trace	Trace	4
Fresh, sliced, 1½ in. diam., ¼ in. thick.	2 slices	15	79	10	Trace	Trace	—	—	—	3	5	.3	20	Trace	Trace	Trace	1
Sweet, gherkin, small, whole, approx. 2½ in. long, ¾ in. diam.	1 pickle	15	61	20	Trace	Trace	—	—	—	6	2	.2	10	Trace	Trace	Trace	1
Relish, finely chopped, sweet.	1 tbsp.	15	63	20	Trace	Trace	—	—	—	5	3	.1	—	—	—	—	—
Popcorn. See Grain Products.																	
Popsicle, 3 fl. oz. size.	1 popsicle.	95	80	70	0	0	0	0	0	18	0	Trace	0	0	0	0	0
Pudding, home recipe with starch base:																	
Chocolate	1 cup	260	66	385	8	12	7	4	Trace	67	250	1.3	390	.05	.36	.3	1
Vanilla (blanc mange)	1 cup	255	76	285	9	10	5	3	Trace	41	298	Trace	410	.08	.41	.3	2
Pudding mix, dry form, 4-oz. package.	1 pkg.	113	2	410	3	2	1	1	Trace	103	23	1.8	Trace	.02	.08	.5	0
Sherbet	1 cup	193	67	260	2	2	—	—	—	59	31	Trace	120	.02	.06	Trace	4
Soups:																	
Canned, condensed, ready-to-serve:																	
Prepared with an equal volume of milk:																	
Cream of chicken	1 cup	245	85	180	7	10	3	3	3	15	172	.5	610	.05	.27	.7	2
Cream of mushroom	1 cup	245	83	215	7	14	4	5	4	16	191	.5	250	.05	.34	.7	1
Tomato	1 cup	250	84	175	7	7	3	2	1	23	168	.8	1,200	.10	.25	1.3	15
Prepared with an equal volume of water:																	
Bean with pork	1 cup	250	84	170	8	6	1	2	2	22	63	2.3	650	.13	.08	1.0	3
Beef broth, bouillon consomme.	1 cup	240	96	30	5	0	0	0	0	3	Trace	.5	Trace	Trace	.02	1.0	—
Beef noodle	1 cup	240	93	70	4	3	1	1	1	7	7	1.0	50	.05	.07	1.0	Trace
Clam chowder, Manhattan type (with tomatoes, without milk).	1 cup	245	92	80	2	3	—	—	—	12	34	1.0	880	.02	.02	1.0	—
Cream of chicken	1 cup	240	92	95	3	6	1	2	1	8	24	.5	410	.02	.05	.5	Trace
Cream of mushroom	1 cup	240	90	135	2	10	2	3	3	10	41	.5	70	.02	.12	.7	Trace
Minestrone	1 cup	245	90	105	5	3	—	—	—	14	37	1.0	2,350	.07	.05	1.0	—

[Dashes in the columns for nutrients show that no suitable value could be found although there is reason to believe that a measurable amount of the nutrient may be present]

Food, approximate measure, and weight (in grams)		Water	Food energy	Protein	Fat	Fatty acids			Carbohydrate	Calcium	Iron	Vitamin A value	Thiamin	Riboflavin	Niacin	Ascorbic acid
						Saturated (total)	Unsaturated Oleic	Unsaturated Linoleic								
	Grams	Percent	Calories	Grams	Grams	Grams	Grams	Grams	Grams	Milligrams	Milligrams	International units	Milligrams	Milligrams	Milligrams	Milligrams
MISCELLANEOUS ITEMS—Continued																
Soups—Continued																
Canned, condensed, ready-to-serve—Con.																
Prepared with an equal volume of water—Con.																
Split pea	1 cup	245	85	145	9	3	1	2	Trace	21	29	1.5	440	0.25	0.15	1.5	1
Tomato	1 cup	245	90	90	2	3	Trace	1	1	16	15	.7	1,000	.05	.05	1.2	12
Vegetable beef	1 cup	245	92	80	5	2	Trace	1	—	10	12	.7	2,700	.05	.05	1.0	—
Vegetarian	1 cup	245	92	80	2	2	—	—	—	13	20	1.0	2,940	.05	.05	1.0	—
Dehydrated, dry form:																
Chicken noodle (2-oz. package)	1 pkg	57	6	220	8	6	2	3	1	33	34	1.4	190	.30	.15	2.4	3
Onion mix (1½-oz. package)	1 pkg	43	3	150	6	5	1	2	1	23	42	.6	30	.05	.03	.3	6
Tomato vegetable with noodles (2½-oz. pkg.)	1 pkg	71	4	245	6	6	2	3	1	45	33	1.4	1,700	.21	.13	1.8	18
Frozen, condensed:																
Clam chowder, New England type (with milk, without tomatoes):																
Prepared with equal volume of milk	1 cup	245	83	210	9	12	—	—	—	16	240	1.0	250	.07	.29	.5	Trace
Prepared with equal volume of water	1 cup	240	89	130	4	8	—	—	—	11	91	1.0	50	.05	.10	.5	—
Cream of potato:																
Prepared with equal volume of milk	1 cup	245	83	185	8	10	5	3	Trace	18	208	1.0	590	.10	.27	.5	Trace
Prepared with equal volume of water	1 cup	240	90	105	3	5	3	2	Trace	12	58	1.0	410	.05	.05	.5	—

Food	Measure	Weight (g)	Water (%)	Food energy (cal.)	Protein (g)	Fat (g)	Sat. fatty acids (g)	Oleic (g)	Linoleic (g)	Carbohydrate (g)	Calcium (mg)	Iron (mg)	Vit. A (I.U.)	Thiamine (mg)	Riboflavin (mg)	Niacin (mg)	Ascorbic acid (mg)
Cream of shrimp:																	
Prepared with equal volume of milk.	1 cup	245	82	245	9	16	---	---	---	15	189	.5	290	.07	.27	.5	Trace
Prepared with equal volume of water.	1 cup	240	88	160	5	12	---	---	---	8	38	.5	120	.05	.05	.5	---
Oyster stew:																	
Prepared with equal volume of milk.	1 cup	240	83	200	10	12	---	---	---	14	305	1.4	410	.12	.41	.5	Trace
Prepared with equal volume of water.	1 cup	240	90	120	6	8	---	---	---	8	158	1.4	240	.07	.19	.5	---
Tapioca, dry, quick-cooking.	1 cup	152	13	535	1	Trace	---	---	---	131	15	.6	0	0	0	0	0
Tapioca desserts:																	
Apple.	1 cup	250	70	295	1	Trace	---	---	---	74	8	.5	30	Trace	Trace	Trace	Trace
Cream pudding.	1 cup	165	72	220	8	8	4	3	Trace	28	173	.7	480	.07	.30	.2	2
Tartar sauce.	1 tbsp.	14	34	75	Trace	8	1	3	4	1	3	.1	30	Trace	Trace	Trace	Trace
Vinegar.	1 tbsp.	15	94	Trace	Trace	0	---	---	---	1	1	.1	---	Trace	Trace	Trace	---
White sauce, medium.	1 cup	250	73	405	10	31	16	10	1	22	288	.5	1,150	.10	.43	.5	2
Yeast:																	
Baker's, dry, active.	1 pkg.	7	5	20	3	Trace	---	---	---	3	3	1.1	Trace	.16	.38	2.6	Trace
Brewer's, dry.	1 tbsp.	8	5	25	3	Trace	---	---	---	3	17	1.4	Trace	1.25	.34	3.0	Trace
Yoghurt. See Milk, Cheese, Cream, Imitation Cream.																	

Appendix B

Estimation of O₂ deficit during nonsteady-state exercise

Because oxygen deficit is the difference between the amount of energy (in units of oxygen) required to perform a given amount of work and the amount of oxygen actually consumed during the work, it is necessary to first estimate oxygen cost of the work. This can be done satisfactorily only if the subject performs mechanical work (force times distance) which can be accurately measured, for example, on a bicycle ergometer or on a treadmill set at a grade greater than horizontal. Next, one subtracts from the oxygen cost of the work the amount of oxygen actually consumed during the work as measured by the usual methods. The procedure is as follows:

A. Estimation of oxygen cost:
   1. Determine the caloric equivalent of the units of mechanical work performed. For example, 100 kgm of work equal 0.23427 kcal; 1,000 ft.-lb. of work equal 0.32389 kcal; and 1,000 joules equal 0.23889 kcal.

2. Estimate the kcal of energy actually expended to produce the mechanical work determined in the preceding paragraph by assuming the subject has a mechanical efficiency of 22 per cent and substituting in the following equation:

Energy Cost (kcal =
    100 × Work Performed (kcal)/Mechanical Efficiency (%)

3. Assume the caloric equivalent of a liter of oxygen to be 5.0 kcal and convert the energy cost from kcal to liters of oxygen by dividing by 5.0.

SUMMARY:

$$O_2 \text{ Cost (l)} = \frac{100 \times \text{Energy Cost of Work Produced (kcal)}}{\text{Mechanical Efficiency (\%)} \times 5.0}$$

B. Subtract from the oxygen cost the actual oxygen consumed during the work.

Appendix C

Conversion factors

Temperature
$$°C = (°F - 32) \times {}^5/_9$$
$$°F = ({}^9/_5°C) + 32$$
Weight
1 kilogram = 1,000 grams = 2.2046 pounds
1 pound = 454 grams
1 gram = 0.035 ounces
Length
1 meter = 100 centimeters = 1,000 millimeters = 39.37 inches = 1.09 yards
1 kilometer = 1,000 meters = 0.62137 miles
1 inch = 2.54 centimeters = 25.4 millimeters
Volume
1 liter = 1.0567 U.S. quarts
1 milliliter = 0.03381 fluid ounces

410

Velocity

1 kilometer/hour = 16.7 meters/minute = 0.62137 miles/hour

1 mile/hour = 26.8 meters/minute = 1.61 kilometers/hour

Work/Energy

1 kilocalorie = 426.85 kilogram-meters = 426.85 kilopond*-meters = 3.9680 British Thermal Units (B.T.U.) = 3087.4 foot-pounds = 4,186 joules

1 kilogram-meter = 0.0023427 kilocalories = 1 kilopond-meter = 7.2330 foot-pounds = 9.8066 joules

1 foot-pound = 0.00032389 kilocalories = 0.13825 kilogram-meters = 1.3558 joules

Power (Work/Time)

1 watt = 3.41304 British Thermal Units/hour = 6.12 kilopond-meters/minute = 0.01433 kilocalories/minute = 0.73756 foot-pounds/second = 0.001341 horsepower = 1 joule/second

1 kilocalorie/minute = 3.9685 B.T.U. = 51.457 foot-pounds/second = 426.974 kilopond-meters/minute = 0.093557 horsepower = 69.767 watts

1 horsepower = 75 kilopond-meters/minute = 745.7 watts = 550 foot-pounds/second

Pressure

1 atmosphere = 10.33 meters of water = 14.7 pounds per square inch = 760 millimeters of mercury = 29.92 inches of mercury

---

* A *kilopond* is the force acting upon a mass of one kilogram at normal acceleration of gravity. This force is slightly greater as one moves from the equator toward the poles. For practical purposes, 1 kilopond-meter = 1 kilogram-meter.

Appendix D

Standard symbols in pulmonary gas exchange

	Symbol	Definition	Example
Quantitative variables	P	Gas pressure	$P_{O_2} = 100$ mm Hg
	V	Gas volume	$V_{Tidal} = 500$ ml
	$\dot{V}$	Gas volume (flow) per unit time	$\dot{V}_{Expired} = 6$ L/min
	f	Frequency of respiration	$f = 10$ breaths/min
	F	Fractional concentration of gas in dry gas phase	F_{O_2} in air $= 0.2094$
	C	Concentration in blood or other aqueous phase	$C_{O_2 Arterial} = 0.3$ vol%
	$\dot{Q}$	Blood volume flow per unit time	$\dot{Q}_{Bronchial} = 100$ ml/min
	R	Respiratory exchange ratio (RQ)	$\dot{V}_{CO_2}/\dot{V}_{O_2} = 0.80$
	D	Diffusing capacity	$D_{LO_2} = 50$ ml O_2/min/mm Hg ΔP_{O_2}
Qualifying terms			
Gas	A	Alveolar	$P_{O_2 A} = 100$ mm Hg
	D	Dead space	$V_D = 150$ ml
	T	Tidal	$V_T = 500$ ml
	I	Inspired	$F_I O_2 = 0.2094$
	E	Expired	$F_E CO_2 = 0.045$
Blood	a	Arterial	$P_{O_2 a} = 95$
	v	Venous	$P_{O_2 v} = 40$
	c	Capillary	$P_{O_2 c} = 60$
	b	Unspecified site	

Appendix E

STPD (standard temperature, pressure, dry) correction factors

Tabled values are multiplication factors used to correct volumes of moist gas to volumes occupied by dry gas at 0°C, 760 mm Hg. Values in the left hand column are observed barometric pressures at the time of gas collection, whereas values across the top are observed temperatures of gas collected.

Observed Barometric Reading, Uncorrected for Temperature	15°	16°	17°	18°	19°	20°	21°	22°	23°	24°	25°	26°	27°	28°	29°	30°	31°	32°
700	0.855	851	847	842	838	834	829	825	821	816	812	807	802	797	793	788	783	778
702	857	853	849	845	840	836	832	827	823	818	814	809	805	800	795	790	785	780
704	860	856	852	847	843	839	834	830	825	821	816	812	807	802	797	792	787	783
706	862	858	854	850	845	841	837	832	828	823	819	814	810	804	800	795	790	785
708	865	861	856	852	848	843	839	834	830	825	821	816	812	807	802	797	792	787
710	867	863	859	855	850	846	842	837	833	828	824	819	814	809	804	799	795	790
712	870	866	861	857	853	848	844	839	836	830	826	821	817	812	807	802	797	792
714	872	868	864	859	855	851	846	842	837	833	828	824	819	814	809	804	799	794
716	875	871	866	862	858	853	849	844	840	835	831	826	822	816	812	807	802	797
718	877	873	869	864	860	856	851	847	842	838	833	828	824	819	814	809	804	799
720	880	876	871	867	863	858	854	849	845	840	836	831	826	821	816	812	807	802
722	882	878	874	869	865	861	856	852	847	843	838	833	829	824	819	814	809	804
724	885	880	876	872	867	863	858	854	849	845	840	835	831	826	821	816	811	806
726	887	883	879	874	870	866	861	856	852	847	843	838	833	829	824	818	813	808
728	890	886	881	877	872	868	863	859	854	850	845	840	836	831	826	821	816	811
730	892	888	884	879	875	871	866	861	857	852	847	843	838	833	828	823	818	813
732	895	890	886	882	877	873	868	864	859	854	850	845	840	836	831	825	820	815
734	897	893	889	884	880	875	871	866	862	857	852	847	843	838	833	828	823	818
736	900	895	891	887	882	878	873	869	864	859	855	850	845	840	835	830	825	820
738	902	898	894	889	885	880	876	871	866	862	857	852	848	843	838	833	828	822
740	905	900	896	892	887	883	878	874	869	864	860	855	850	845	840	835	830	825
742	907	903	898	894	890	885	881	876	871	867	862	857	852	847	842	837	832	827
744	910	906	901	897	892	888	883	878	874	869	864	859	855	850	845	840	834	829
746	912	908	903	899	895	890	886	881	876	872	867	862	857	852	847	842	837	832
748	915	910	906	901	897	892	888	883	879	874	869	864	860	854	850	845	839	834
750	917	913	908	904	900	895	890	886	881	876	872	867	862	857	852	847	842	837
752	920	915	911	906	902	897	893	888	883	879	874	869	864	859	854	849	844	839
754	922	918	913	909	904	900	895	891	886	881	876	872	867	862	857	852	846	841
756	925	920	916	911	907	902	898	893	888	883	879	874	869	864	859	854	849	844
758	927	923	918	914	909	905	900	896	891	886	881	876	872	866	861	856	851	846
760	930	925	921	916	912	907	902	898	893	888	883	879	874	869	864	859	854	848
762	932	928	923	919	914	910	905	900	896	891	886	881	876	871	866	861	856	851
764	936	930	926	921	916	912	907	903	898	893	888	884	879	874	869	864	858	853
766	937	933	928	924	919	915	910	905	900	896	891	886	881	876	871	866	861	855
768	940	935	931	926	922	917	912	908	903	898	893	888	883	878	873	868	863	858
770	942	938	933	928	924	919	915	910	905	901	896	891	886	881	876	871	865	860
772	945	940	936	931	926	922	917	912	908	903	898	893	888	883	878	873	868	862
774	947	943	938	933	929	924	920	915	910	905	901	896	891	886	880	875	870	865
776	950	945	941	936	931	927	922	917	912	908	903	898	893	888	883	878	872	867
778	952	948	943	938	934	929	924	920	915	910	905	900	895	890	885	880	875	869
780	955	950	945	941	936	932	927	922	917	912	908	903	898	892	887	882	877	872

Peters, J. P., and Van Slyke, D. D.: *Quantitative Clinical Chemistry.* Vol. II. (*Methods*) Baltimore: The Williams and Wilkins Co., 1932.

Appendix F

BTPS (body temperature, saturated) correction factors

Tabled values are multiplication factors used to correct volumes of gas to volumes occupied at 37°C with the gas saturated with water vapor. These are called BTPS correction factors (Body Temperature, Ambient Pressure, Saturated) and should be used to report all lung volumes and capacities.

BTPS

Exhaled Gas t°C	Factors to Convert Gas Volume to 37°C Saturated P_B mm Hg		
	750	760	770
20	1.102	1.102	1.101
20.5	1.100	1.099	1.099
21	1.097	1.096	1.096
21.5	1.094	1.093	1.093
22	1.091	1.091	1.090
22.5	1.089	1.089	1.088
23	1.086	1.085	1.085
23.5	1.083	1.082	1.082
24	1.080	1.079	1.079
24.5	1.077	1.077	1.076
25	1.074	1.074	1.073
25.5	1.071	1.071	1.070
26	1.069	1.069	1.068
26.5	1.066	1.065	1.065
27	1.063	1.062	1.062
27.5	1.061	1.060	1.060

Glossary

Acetylcholine—a chemical released from certain nerve endings, especially those innervating skeletal muscles.

Actin—one of the contractile protein filaments in muscles.

Action potential—a sudden change in electrical activity across a nerve or muscle membrane, usually due to a rapid flow of sodium ions across the membrane into the cell.

Actomyosin—the interaction of actin and myosin protein filaments in muscle.

Adaptation—a more or less persistent change in structure or function, especially as caused by repeated bouts of physical exercise.

Adenosine diphosphate (ADP)—one of the chemical products of the breakdown of adenosine triphosphate (ATP) for energy during muscle contraction.

Adenosine triphosphate (ATP)—a chemical that serves as the immediate source of chemical energy for most of the energy-consuming reactions of the body, especially for muscle contraction. ATP is split into adenosine diphosphate and phosphate to produce energy.

Adipose tissue—fat tissue.

Adrenaline—a chemical liberated from the adrenal medulla and from sympathetic nerve endings. Important effects include cardiac stimulation and constriction of blood vessels with a consequent rise in blood pressure.

Adrenal cortex—outer portion of the adrenal gland. The cortex produces many hormones, especially cortisol and aldosterone.

Adrenal medulla—inner portion of the adrenal gland. The medulla produces adrenaline and nor-adrenaline in a ratio of about 3:1.

Adrenocorticotrophic hormone (ACTH)—See corticotropin.

Aerobic—utilizing oxygen.

Aerobic endurance—the ability to persist in physical activities that rely heavily upon oxygen for energy production.

Aerobic power—the maximal volume of oxygen consumed per unit of time. Also known as maximal oxygen uptake or maximal oxygen consumption.

Afferent fibers—sensory nerve fibers, i.e., those which conduct impulses toward the central nervous system and especially the brain.

Alactic acid oxygen debt—that part of the oxygen debt which is not accompanied by an increase of lactic acid in the blood.

Aldosterone—a hormone released from the adrenal cortex. Aldosterone causes sodium retention by the kidney.

Alpha motoneuron—nerves that cause skeletal muscle fibers (extrafusal fibers) to contract.

Alveolus—tiny air sacs of the lungs. Plural: alveoli.

Amphetamine—a synthetic drug related to adrenaline. Amphetamines cause stimulation of the central nervous system.

Anabolic—pertaining to the synthesis of complex substances from simpler substances, especially to the synthesis of body proteins from amino acids.

Anaerobic—without oxygen.

Anaerobic endurance—the ability to persist in physical activities of short duration that require high rates of energy expenditure. These high rates of energy expenditure cannot be met solely by aerobic metabolism.

Antidiuretic hormone (ADH, Vasopressin)—a hormone released by the posterior pituitary. Antidiuretic hormone causes water retention by the kidneys.

Arteriovenous oxygen difference—the difference in oxygen content between the arterial blood and the mixed venous blood in the right atrium of the heart.

Atrophy—reduction in size of cells and tissues.

Autoregulation—the regulation of blood flow to an organ or tissue by direct effects of localized changes of chemicals or temperature in the organ or tissue.

Biopsy—the extraction of small pieces of tissue for chemical analysis.

Bradycardia—decreased heart rate, especially at rest.

Calcitonin—a hormone released from the thyroid. Calcitonin decreases levels of blood calcium.

Calorie—a unit of heat energy required to raise the temperature of a kilogram of water 1 degree Celsius under specified conditions. (Also known as a large calorie or kilocalorie.)

Carbohydrate—a chemical compound consisting of carbon, hydrogen and oxygen atoms in specified arrangements. Carbohydrates are major components of foods such as bread, potatoes, and rice.

Cardiac—pertaining to the heart.

Cardiac output—the volume of blood pumped from a ventricle of the heart per unit of time; cardiac output is the product of heart rate and stroke volume.

Cardiorespiratory endurance—See aerobic endurance.

Cardiovascular—pertaining to the heart and blood vessels.

Carotid sinus—a widening of the carotid artery where it divides into internal and external branches.

Catabolism—the degradation of complex substances into simpler structures, for example, the breakdown of fats and carbohydrates for energy production.

Catecholamines—a class of chemicals which includes adrenaline and nor-adrenaline.

Central nervous system—the brain and spinal cord.

Chemoreceptors—sensory nerve endings sensitive to changes in their chemical environment. Such receptors are located in the aortic arch and the carotid sinuses.

Citric acid cycle—Krebs cycle.

Collagen—a fibrous protein that serves as the major component of ligaments and tendons.

Concentric contraction—contraction of a muscle resulting in shortening of the muscle.

Continuous work—work uninterrupted by rest pauses.

Corticotropin—a hormone released by the anterior pituitary. Corticotropin stimulates the growth and secretory activities of the adrenal cortex.

Cortisol—a hormone secreted by the adrenal cortex. Cortisol results in conservation of carbohydrate stores in the body at the expense of fat and protein.

Creatine phosphate (phosphocreatine)—a chemical that can donate its phosphate to adenosine diphosphate to rapidly replenish tissue stores of adenosine triphosphate.

Cross bridges—the linkages between actin and myosin filaments during muscle contraction.

Cyclic adenosine monophosphate (cyclic AMP)—a chemical implicated in the action of many hormones.

Cytochromes—proteins in the electron transport system of the mitochondria.

Depolarization—reduction in the electrical charge across the resting cell membrane.

Diastole—relaxation of the heart.

Diffusion—the net movement of chemicals such as oxygen, carbon dioxide and sodium from an area of high concentration to an area of lower concentration.

Dry bulb thermometer—an ordinary temperature recording instrument.

Eccentric contraction—a muscle contraction incapable of overcoming the resistance imposed; the overall muscle length increases.

Efferent nerve—a motor nerve.

Electrocardiogram (EKG, ECG)—a recording of the transmission of an action potential through the heart.

Energy—the capacity to perform work.

Endurance—the ability to persist in performing some physical activity.

Epinephrine—adrenaline.

Ergometer—a device which can measure work done, e.g., a bicycle ergometer.

Erythropoiesis—the production of red blood cells.

Erythropoietin—a hormone secreted by the kidneys. Erythropoietin stimulates the bone marrow cells to produce red blood cells.

Extracellular fluid—fluid not within the cells, e.g., interstitial fluid, blood plasma.

Fast twitch fibers—skeletal muscle fibers most active in short-duration, intensive exercise, e.g., in sprints and jumps.

Fatigue—the inability to maintain a given level of physical performance.

Fibrinolysis—the breakdown of fibrin strands produced during the clotting of blood.

Flexibility—the range of motion of the body's joints.

Follicle-stimulating hormone (FSH)—See follitropin.

Follitropin—a hormone secreted by the anterior pituitary. Follitropin causes increased growth and hormone-secreting activity of the ovaries and testes.

Foot-pound—the work required to move one pound of resistance one foot in distance.

Frank-Starling effect—the increased contraction of the heart muscle caused by stretching of the muscle fibers upon increased filling of the chambers.

Gamma motor nerve—a nerve that innervates the intrafusal fibers within muscle spindles.

Glucagon—a hormone that is secreted by the pancreas. Glucagon causes more glucose to be released from the liver into the blood.

Glucocorticoids—a class of hormones secreted from the adrenal cortex. Glucocorticoids tend to spare carbohydrate at the expense of protein and fat. Cortisol is the most important glucocorticoid in man.

Gluconeogenesis—the synthesis of glycogen or glucose from amino acids and other substances.

Glucose—blood sugar.

Glycogen—a polymer of glucose. Glycogen is the storage form of carbohydrate in animals.

Glycogenolysis—the breakdown of glycogen to glucose.

Glycolysis—the breakdown of glucose to pyruvic or lactic acid. Also, sometimes used to describe the breakdown of glucose to carbon dioxide and water.

Glycolytic capacity—the capacity to break down glucose to pyruvic or lactic acid.

Growth hormone—See somatotropin.

Hematocrit—the percentage of blood volume that is made up of red blood cells.

Hemoglobin—a protein found in red blood cells. Hemoglobin combines with oxygen.

Homeostasis—the tendency of the body to maintain its internal environment within narrow ranges of temperature, acidity, osmolarity, etc.

Hyperplasia—increased cell number.

Hypertrophy—increased cell size leading to increased tissue size.

Hyperventilation—a rate of ventilation in excess of physiological demand.

Hypoxia—a relative lack of oxygen.

Insulin—a hormone secreted by the pancreas. Insulin lowers blood glucose by increasing the uptake of glucose by the tissues of the body.

Intermittent work—work sessions interrupted by rest sessions.

Intrafusal fibers—muscle fibers located within muscle spindles.

Interstitial fluid—the fluid that lies between cells in the tissue spaces.

Ischemia—a lack of blood flow.

Isokinetic contraction—a muscular contraction through a range of motion at a constant velocity.

Isometric (static) contraction—a muscular contraction in which there is no change in the angle of the involved joint(s) and little or no change in the length of the contracting muscle.

Isotonic contraction—a muscular contraction in which a constant resistance is moved through a range of motion of the involved joint(s).

Kilocalorie (kcal)—the heat required to raise the temperature of 1 kilogram of water 1 degree Celsius under specified conditions.

Kilopond-meter (kpm)—the work done when a mass of one kilogram is lifted one meter against the force of gravity.

Krebs Cycle—a series of enzyme-catalyzed reactions in the mitochondria of cells; involved in the catabolism of fats, carbohydrates, and proteins to carbon dioxide and water.

Lactic acid (lactate)—the end-product of anaerobic glycolysis.

Lactic acid oxygen debt—that portion of the oxygen debt that is associated with a rise in blood lactic acid.

Lean body mass—the body mass that does not include fat tissue.

Ligament—the tough connective tissue that binds bones together at joints.

Lipid—fat, especially triglycerides.

Maximal oxygen uptake (maximal oxygen consumption, maximal oxygen intake, maximal aerobic power)—the greatest volume of oxygen used by the cells of the body per unit of time.

Metabolites—chemical substances generated from the degradation of larger molecules, e.g., carbon dioxide and water are metabolites generated from the breakdown of fats, carbohydrates and proteins.

Mitochondria—the structures located within the cells. Mitochondria contain the enzymes responsible for the generation of adenosine triphosphate by aerobic mechanisms.

Motor neuron—a nerve cell that conducts an impulse from the central nervous system to muscles or glands.

Motor cortex—that portion of the cerebral cortex that generates the nerve impulses leading to voluntary movement.

Motor unit—a motor neuron and all the muscle fibers which it innervates.

Muscle spindle—a sensory organ imbedded in skeletal muscle. The spindle is sensitive to changes in muscle length and especially to stretch.

Myofibril—element of muscle which contains the contractile actin and myosin proteins.

Myoglobin—oxygen-binding protein in skeletal muscle.

Myosin—contractile protein in muscle. Myosin molecules make up the thick filaments in muscle.

Myosin ATPase—the name given to the activity of myosin in catalyzing the breakdown of adenosine triphosphate to adenosine diphosphate and phosphate during muscle contraction.

Neuromuscular junction (motor endplate)—the junction between motor nerve ending and the sarcolemmal membrane of a muscle fiber.

Neuron—a nerve cell, consisting of cell body, axon, and dendrites.

Neurotrophic substance—a chemical transmitted by nerves; causes some growth or development of the structure innervated.

Noradrenaline—a chemical secreted by sympathetic nerve endings and by the adrenal medulla. Noradrenaline increases cardiac output, vasoconstriction, and blood pressure among many activities.

Norepinephrine—noradrenaline.

Obesity—excess body fat.

Osmolarity—a measure of the dissolved particles in a solution that can create osmotic force in the presence of a semipermeable membrane.

Oxidation—the removal of electrons from a chemical.

Oxidative phosphorylation—the production of adenosine triphosphate dependent upon oxidative processes in the electron transport system of the mitochondria.

Oxygen debt—the oxygen uptake during recovery from exercise in excess of the oxygen uptake normally observed during a rest period of similar duration.

Oxygen deficit—the difference between the theoretical oxygen requirement of a physical activity and the oxygen actually used during the activity.

Oxygen uptake—the oxygen used up by the mitochondria of all the body's cells.

Parathyroid hormone—a hormone secreted by the parathyroid glands; increases the level of calcium in the blood.

Partial pressure—in a mixture of gases, the pressure exerted by one of the gases in the mixture. The pressure is due to the heat energy of the gas molecules.

Peripheral nervous system—nerve tissue located outside the brain and spinal cord.

pH—a measure of the acidity of a solution. The possible values of pH range between 0–14, with 7.0 representing a balance between acid and base. Values lower than 7.0 become progressively more acidic, and values above 7.0 become progressively more basic.

Phosphofructokinase—an enzyme involved in the breakdown of glucose to pyruvic acid. The enzyme is especially important in regulation of glycolysis because small changes in its activity can slow or speed the rate of glycolysis.

Phosphorylase—an enzyme involved in the breakdown of glycogen to glucose-6-phosphate. Small changes in the activity of this enzyme help regulate the rate of glycogen breakdown.

Plasma—the fluid portion of the blood.

Power—work performed per unit time.

Renin—an enzyme secreted by the kidney; catalyzes the production of angiotensin I from a plasma protein, angiotensinogen.

Repolarization—the reestablishment of resting membrane potential following depolarization.

Respiratory exchange ratio (R)—the ratio between carbon dioxide produced and oxygen consumed.

Respiratory quotient (RQ)—the ratio between the carbon dioxide produced and oxygen consumed during the metabolism of foodstuffs. Often used as synonym for respiratory exchange ratio (R) even though R may reflect processes other than foodstuff metabolism, e.g., hyperventilation due to acidosis.

Response—a sudden temporary adjustment in physiological function brought on by a single exposure to exercise, e.g., the rise in heart rate associated with an exercise bout.

Sarcolemma—muscle fiber membrane.

Sarcoplasm—the cytoplasm of muscle fibers.

Sarcoplasmic reticulum—a network of channels extending throughout muscle fibers which serves to regulate the availability of calcium to the troponin molecules of the thin filaments.

Sensory fibers—nerve fibers that conduct impulses from the periphery to the central nervous system.

Serum—the fluid exuded from clotted blood.

Sinoatrial node—specialized cells in the right atrium of the heart that serve as the pacemaker of the heart beat because of their rapid rates of depolarization and repolarization.

Slow-twitch fibers—skeletal muscle fibers characterized by relatively slow contraction times and great capacity for the aerobic production of adenosine triphosphate.

Somatotropin—a hormone released from the anterior pituitary; causes growth of many body cells. Also known as growth hormone.

Splanchnic circulation—circulation to the viscera, especially the liver.

Static contraction—a muscular contraction that does not involve changes in the angle of the joint(s) involved.

Steady state—that state of physiological stability wherein the energy demands of the body can be met relatively easily for a prolonged period of time.

Strength—the ability to exert muscular force briefly.

Stroke volume—the amount of blood pumped out of the heart ventricles with each beat.

Submaximal exercise—usually exercise at less than maximal intensity, but may also refer to exercise of less than maximal duration.

Systole—contraction, usually of the heart ventricles.

Testosterone—a hormone secreted by the testes; causes the secondary sex characteristics of the male and is involved in muscle growth.

Thyroxine—the primary hormone secreted by the thyroid gland; increases oxygen uptake by the mitochondria and works with somatotropin to cause cell growth.

Troponin—a protein in the thin filaments of skeletal muscle; inhibits myosin ATPase activity until troponin is inactivated by calcium ions released from the sarcoplasmic reticulum.

Twitch—a single, brief muscle contraction caused by a single stimulus.

Vagus nerve—the tenth cranial nerve.

Vasoconstriction—narrowing of the opening of blood vessels caused by contraction of the smooth muscle cells in the walls of the vessels.

Vasodilatation—widening of the opening of blood vessels caused by a relaxation of the smooth muscle cells in the walls of the vessels.

Index